Thieme

Principles and Practice of Neuropsychopharmacology

A Clinical Reference for Residents, Physicians, and Biomedical Scientists

Vikas Dhikav, MBBS, Postgraduate Training Pharmacology (AIIMS), Post Doctoral Training-Cognitive Neurology (PGIMER Delhi), PhD (Neurology)
Scientist-D (Medical)
ICMR's National Institute of Implementation Research on
Non-Communicable Diseases
Jodhpur, Rajasthan, India

Kuljeet Singh Anand, DM (Neurology)
Professor and Head
Department of Neurology
Atal Bihari Vajpayee Institute of Medical Sciences and
Dr Ram Manohar Lohia Hospital
New Delhi, India

Thieme
Delhi • Stuttgart • New York • Rio de Janeiro

Publishing Director: Ritu Sharma
Development Editor: Dr Gurvinder Kaur
Director-Editorial Services: Rachna Sinha
Project Manager: Shipra Sehgal
Vice President Sales and Marketing: Arun Kumar Majji
Managing Director & CEO: Ajit Kohli

Thieme Medical and Scientific Publishers Private
Limited.
A - 12, Second Floor, Sector - 2, Noida - 201 301,
Uttar Pradesh, India, +911204556600
Email: customerservice@thieme.in
www.thieme.in

Cover design: © Thieme
Cover image source: © Thieme

Typesetting by RECTO Graphics, India

Printed in India

5 4 3 2 1

ISBN: 978-93-90553-07-5
eISBN: 978-93-90553-08-2

Important note: Medicine is an ever-changing science undergoing continual development. Research and clinical experience are continually expanding our knowledge, in particular, our knowledge of proper treatment and drug therapy. Insofar as this book mentions any dosage or application, readers may rest assured that the authors, editors, and publishers have made every effort to ensure that such references are in accordance with the state of knowledge at the time of production of the book.

Nevertheless, this does not involve, imply, or express any guarantee or responsibility on the part of the publishers in respect to any dosage instructions and forms of applications stated in the book. Every user is requested to examine carefully the manufacturers' leaflets accompanying each drug and to check, if necessary, in consultation with a physician or specialist, whether the dosage schedules mentioned therein or the contraindications stated by the manufacturers differ from the statements made in the present book. Such examination is particularly important with drugs that are either rarely used or have been newly released in the market. Every dosage schedule or every form of application used is entirely at the user's own risk and responsibility. The authors and publishers request every user to report to the publishers any discrepancies or inaccuracies noticed. If errors in this work are found after publication, errata will be posted at www.thieme.com on the product description page.

Some of the product names, patents, and registered designs referred to in this book are in fact registered trademarks or proprietary names even though specific reference to this fact is not always made in the text. Therefore, the appearance of a name without designation as proprietary is not to be construed as a representation by the publisher that it is in the public domain.

Thieme addresses people of all gender identities equally. We encourage our authors to use gender-neutral or gender-equal expressions wherever the context allows.

Contents

Contents

Preface

Principles and Practice of Neuropsychopharmacology: A Clinical Reference for Residents, Physicians, and Biomedical Scientists deals with drugs used in the treatment of neurological and psychiatric diseases from both clinical and biomedical perspectives. There is a considerable overlap between these two faculties, and neurologists often use the drugs used in psychiatry and vice versa. Therefore, there was a need to bring out a comprehensive volume to address the merger of topics of mutual interest in a single book of contemporary pharmacology.

The book has 18 chapters with easy-to-understand illustrations, tables, and flowcharts. It also contains details of recommendations from societal and medical bodies from both India and overseas, wherever applicable. Case examples are given to fit the needs of clinicians and details of neurochemical alternatives to suit the basic requirements of neuropsychopharmacologists. Hope the readers like it. For any comments, criticisms, and suggestions, the authors are just a click away!

Vikas Dhikav
Kuljeet Singh Anand

Contributors

Kuljeet Singh Anand, DM (Neurology)
Professor and Head
Department of Neurology
Atal Bihari Vajpayee Institute of Medical Sciences and Dr Ram Manohar Lohia Hospital
New Delhi, India

Rhythm Joshi, MSc (Clinical Research)
Research Scholar
Department of Clinical and Translational Research
Jamia Hamdard University
New Delhi, India

Rupa Mishra, PhD (Psychology)
Research Scholar
Department of Psychology
SGT University
Guruguram, Haryana

Vatsala Sharma, MD (Psychiatry)
Senior Resident
Department of Psychiatry
Institute of Human Behaviour and Allied Sciences
New Delhi, India

Vikas Dhikav, MBBS, Postgraduate Training Pharmacology (AIIMS), Post Doctoral Training-Cognitive Neurology (PGIMER Delhi), PhD (Neurology)
Scientist-D (Medical)
ICMR's National Institute of Implementation Research on Non-Communicable Diseases
Jodhpur, Rajasthan, India

History of Neuropsychopharmacology

Vikas Dhikav

Clinical Case Example

- A 17-year-old girl is hearing voices "coming from the heavens," which forces her to address people and inform them of ways to reach the "heavenly abode." She's been experiencing this for the past 1 year and is unkempt with slurring of speech. The girl yells at everyone and says "she knows God" and wants to be left alone. What is the treatment advised for this condition?

Answer: The girl has a diagnosis of schizophrenia. In the modern world, she would have been offered atypical antipsychotics. But in the bygone era, she may have had to undergo trephination or may have been labeled as a demon and treated accordingly.

What Is Neuropsychopharmacology?[1–5]

Neuropsychopharmacology is a discipline that emerged in the early 20th century.[1] This branch of pharmacology connects the behavioral response to drugs with the interactions of signaling molecules at the cellular level. Thus, neuropsychopharmacology deals with the effects of drugs on the nervous system and studies the effects of drugs on behaviors. This also helps to understand how the components of the central nervous system communicate and coordinate with each other. Neuropsychopharmacology peeps into the basic brain systems' mediating behaviors and figures how these systems may be disrupted in psychiatric and neurological disorders. Drugs of this class belong to heterogenous groups with the following names:

- Generic (chemical): Olanzapine.
- Trade name: Clonotril (Clonazepam).

- Abbreviated chemical name: Tetrahydrocaninabinol (THC).

The historical development of this discipline is very interesting. From the time of Hippocrates (460–377 BC), when superstitions used to rule the roost, the practice of neuropsychopharmacology has come a long way. The main Hippocratic attempt has been to separate the practice of science from religion and superstition.

Western History[6–9]

Ebers Papyrus (Egypt) described more than 700 drugs in detail, and his collection included beer, turpentine, berries, poppy, salt, lead, and crushed precious stones. Those Egyptian remedies were an integral part of the therapeutic armamentarium.

Paracelsus (1493–1541) opposed the idea of using many drugs for a single illness and advocated the other way round, that is, one drug for many illnesses.[7] Polypharmacy[8,9] is common even now, but an effort is being made to curb the same.[8] Polypharmacy not only complicates drug therapy by producing potential drug interactions but also influences compliance.[8]

Indian Ideology

Mood elevating effects of many drugs were known to humans over 5,000 years back.[1] *Rauwolfia serpentina* has been used in India for centuries for the treatment of snake bites and also for the treatment of "insanity."

From a mythological perspective, the use of *Sanjeevni Botti* in the Hindu epic *Ramayana* for treating an unconscious Laxmana, the brother of Lord Rama, is an example of a plant-derived medicinal herb capable of arousing a person from unconsciousness. To many, this would appear to be a fairy tale, as there is no evidence, and unfortunately even now, there is no specific drug that can wake a patient up from an unconscious state.[2]

Dhanvantri, the Indian God of Medicine, helped perfecting many herbal drugs. Sushruta described >700 herbs, and Charaka in his book *Charaka Samhita* mentioned many drugs (about 650) of animal, plant, and mineral origin.

Alcohol has been used since the time of the ancient Greeks and Romans. There are written records of the use of cannabis in India and in Middle East of that era in treating mental illnesses.[3]

Belladona or deadly nightshade was discovered in India during the British period. It was used by tribals to allay their fatigue. Women too used the drug solution to dilate the pupils. It is still used by professional models sometimes and also used by ophthalmologists to dilate pupil for detailed fundus examination. Tobacco and coffee have been popular psychostimulants in human history around the world. Likewise, opium has been used extensively in the treatment of a variety of diseases

in the premodern neuropsychopharmacology era (**Fig. 1.1**).

Kick Start

Opium was used in ancient world.[6] It was the discovery of antihypertensive and antipsychotic drug (Rauwolfia) from India that actually began the revolution in modern neuropsychopharmacology. This galvanized the thoughts of many that the drugs could be used to treat "insane behaviors." The drug was touted to be used in hypertension. However, a sizable number of patients got depressed. Therefore, an inquiry into the mechanism of depression caused by the drug was initiated, and it was found that *Rauwolfia serpentina* (**Fig. 1.2**) has neuron-depleting properties. This formed the basis of the so-called amine theory of depression.

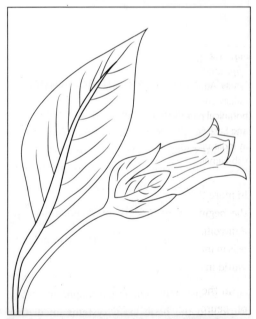

Fig. 1.1 Opium is obtained from the juice of poppy plant. It is a therapeutic drug and also one that can be abused. Opium poppy has been cultivated in India since the 10th century. *Dhanvantari Nighantu,* an ancient Indian medical treatise of the 10th century, lists opium as a remedy for a variety of ailments.

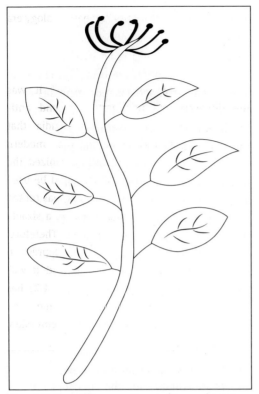

Fig. 1.2 *Rauwolfia serpentina*, Indian snakeroot or *sarpagandha*, is a species of flowering plant in the family Apocynaceae. The plant grows abundantly in Indian conditions and can easily be found in Indian botanical parks. It is native to the Indian Subcontinent and East Asia. It is a perennial undershrub that grows in India up to an elevation of 1,000 m, mainly in the sub-Himalayan region.

In more than one ways, this can be considered as the beginning of modern psychopharmacology. Rauwolfia was used for hypertension and psychosis in India in the 1940s and across the rest of the world in the 1950s.

In the early part of 20th century, the science of neuropsychopharmacology was very rudimentary and even potentially harmful. Even famous psychiatrists such as Kraepelin and Bluler were aware of just basic drugs such as morphine, scopolamine, chloral hydrate, alcohol, barbiturate, and bromides.

Jacques-Joseph Moreau, the French psychiatrist, is credited with the introduction of drugs to study mental disorders in the mid-1950s.[7]

Gaining Momentum

Cocaine and opium were popular central nervous system drugs during the early 1800s. In the 1950s, when methods for the development of modern neuropsychopharmacology started evolving, science reached the desired pace. Laboratories were established around the world. In India, dedicated institutes such as the National Institute of Mental Health and Neurosciences and the Institute of Human Behavior and Allied Sciences for the study of human behaviors were established in the 1960s and 1990s, respectively.

At present, neuropsychopharmacology is a very dynamic science having both basic and clinical aspects. This book deals mainly with the latter, starting from the basics.

The Explosion[10–12]

Delay and Deniker introduced chlorpromazine, the drug that has changed the lives of many schizophrenics in the 1950s. This pleomorphic drug, in terms of mechanism of action, is useful in several diseases. Chlordiazepoxide was introduced by Sternbach, and this initiated an era in which sleep disturbances and general anxiety became amenable to treatment. Before its introduction in modern medicine in 1954, the drug was used as an antiseptic and a dye agent.[4]

Over the decades, the prescription of antidepressant, antianxiety, and antipsychotic drugs became a common practice among psychiatrists.[5] Clinical trials to demonstrate the effectiveness of each class of drugs and drug subcategory are quite common nowadays. Psychiatric research post-1960 has seen many additions to the psychotherapeutic drug range. For example, research has demonstrated the serotonin-dopamine antagonists such as risperidone and clozapine as efficacious against positive and negative symptoms of schizophrenia. Further, advances in Alzheimer's disease, antidepressants, and anticonvulsants have seen the quality of life for many improve. With continued research, assessing the clinical viability of many new and innovative psychotherapeutic medications is on the rise.

Progress

The early 19th century saw the use of drugs as recreational agents and that gave scientists some insights about the site of action of these chemicals, for example, the brain. Simple chemicals, for instance, tea, opium, etc., were being extensively used by Oriental people and this phenomenon essentially became a "living laboratory." Popularity of coffee, tobacco, and alcohol made studying behavioral psychopharmacology easier.

The arrival of morphine and chloral hydrates in patients provided useful information about the use of these drugs and their pharmacological effects. Likewise, chlorpromazine and thioridazine in the 1950s laid the foundation in such a way that it literally led to the birth of "psychopharmacology." Over the next few years, drugs like antidepressants, antianxiety, and antipsychotics were introduced. New drugs such as serotonin, and dopamine antagonists such as risperidone and clozapine, were found to be useful against positive and negative symptoms of schizophrenia and are extensively used at present. The arrival of drugs useful for treatment of Alzheimer's disease and antiepileptic drugs have brought improvement in the lives of many patients.[11] It is surprising that not many workers in the field of psychopharmacology are aware that the term "psychopharmacology" was first used in 1548, more than 400 years before it is thought to have originated.[12]

The Present

At present, the science of neuropsychopharmacology is growing at a rapid pace. It is one of the areas where drugs are being introduced at a regular interval, perhaps more than any other branch. So much so that it has been said that we live in the age of psychopharmacology.[10] Thus, this is posing a challenge to clinicians in terms of using a drug safely and effectively in treating patients, transforming itself into a science as well as art form. The art can be learnt by examining several patients, but the science has to be learnt through books, journals, seminars, conferences, etc. This book is an attempt to provide an overview to both basic and clinical neuroscientists an understanding of the subject with a special emphasis on clinical neuropsychopharmacology.

References

1. Kalmár S. The importance of neuropsychopharmacology in the development of psychiatry. Neuropsychopharmacol Hung 2014;16(3):149–156 Review
2. López-Muñoz F, Alamo C, Cuenca E, Shen WW, Clervoy P, Rubio G. History of the discovery and clinical introduction of chlorpromazine. Ann Clin Psychiatry 2005;17(3):113–135
3. Ban TA. Neuropsychopharmacology and the genetics of schizophrenia: a history of the diagnosis of schizophrenia. Prog Neuropsychopharmacol Biol Psychiatry 2004;28(5):753–762 Review
4. Perez-Caballero L, Torres-Sanchez S, Bravo L, Mico JA, Berrocoso E. Fluoxetine: a case history of its discovery and preclinical development. Expert Opin Drug Discov 2014;9(5):567–578
5. López-Muñoz F, Alamo C. Monoaminergic neurotransmission: the history of the discovery of antidepressants from 1950s until today. Curr Pharm Des 2009;15(14): 1563–1586 Review

6. Central Narcotic Bureau. Available at: http://cbn.nic.in/html/opiumcbn.htm. Accessed August 22, 2016

7. International Network History of Neuropsychopharmacology. Available at: http://inhn.org/archives/ban-collection/1957-the-year-of-neuropsychopharmacology.html. Accessed May 28, 2019

8. Dhikav V, Singh P, Anand KS. Medication adherence survey of drugs useful in prevention of dementia of Alzheimer's type among Indian patients. Int Psychogeriatr 2013;25(9):1409–1413

9. Dhikav V, Sethi M, Singhal AK, Anand KS. Polypharmacy and use of drugs potentially inappropriate medications in patients with dementia and mild cognitive impairment. Asian Journal of Pharmaceutical and Clinical Research 2013;7(2):218–220

10. Braslow JT, Marder SR. History of psychopharmacology. Annu Rev Clin Psychol 2019; 15:25–50

11. History of psychopharmacology. Available at: https://pubmed.ncbi.nlm.nih.gov/30786241. Accessed November 22, 2021

12. Lehmann HE. Special lecture: before they called it psychopharmacology. Available at: https://www.nature.com/articles/npp199369.pdf?origin=ppub. Accessed May 28, 2019

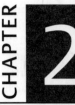
Functional Neuroanatomy in Neuropsychopharmacology

Vikas Dhikav and Rupa Mishra

Clinical Case Example

- An 85-year-old man whose wife passed away 5 years ago and has no children presents with slow onset of memory difficulties. He forgets names and spends hours recalling them but is unable to do so. Gradually, he has noted that he is increasingly becoming unable to care for himself independently due to cognitive decline and experiences two to three episodes of urinary incontinence too. Impaired communication secondary to altered mental status has occurred few times in the past as well. MRI of the brain shows diffuse cortical and temporoparietal atrophy, especially marked in medial temporal lobes.

Answer: This patient has a diagnosis of Alzheimer's disease, where hippocampus and entorhinal cortex are the earliest involved areas. Later, temporal lobes and parietal areas get involved.

Introduction to Functional Neuroanatomy[1]

Early anatomists named most brain structures (in Latin, for the most part) according to their similarity to commonplace objects (**Box 2.1**). This perhaps made remembering the names easier. This trend of using these names continues now to date.

The brain has gray and white matter; the former contains large surface area studded with

Box 2.1: Examples of common parts of names of brain and their counterparts
• Amygdala = almond.
• Hippocampus = sea horse.
• Genu = knee.
• Cortex = bark.
• Pons = bridge.

multiple cells bodies (called neurons), and the latter contains axons in the subcortical area. Therefore, the brain is basically an assembly of functionally interconnected areas (**Fig. 2.1**).

The outer surface of the brain has *gyri* and *sulci* and is divided into lobes, for example, frontal, temporal, parietal, and occipital. The names are divided into various lobes, based upon their proximity to the corresponding areas of the skull.

Macroanatomy of the Central Nervous System[1,2]

The brain is the *organ* of the mind. The mind is composed of multiple distinct, innate faculties. As they are distinct, each faculty must have a separate seat or "organ" in the brain.

A midsagittal section through the brain shows gross structure and its anatomical divisions into

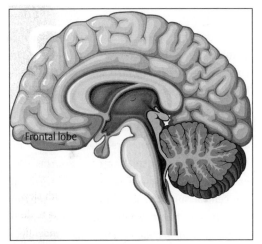

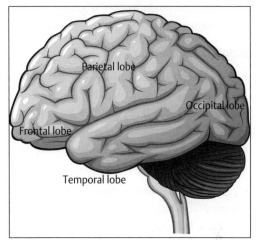

Fig. 2.1 Parts of the brain. The brain is a large organ and is also a soft tissue consisting of neurons. It is the coordination center of sensory, motor, and intellectual activities. It is made up of 100 billion neurons that communicate with the help of trillions of connections between them known as synapses.

Fig. 2.2 The brain is made up of many areas that work together with perfection. The cortex is the outermost layer of the brain cells. Thinking and voluntary movements begin in cortex. The brainstem is between the spinal cord and the rest of the brain. Basic functions like heart rate, breathing, and blood pressure are controlled here. The basal ganglion coordinates messages between multiple areas. The cerebellum is at the base of the brain, toward the hind side, and is responsible for coordination and balance. The lobes of the brain, for example, frontal lobe is important for problem solving, judgment, and motor functions. Parietal lobes are needed for sensory functions, handwriting, and body positions (stereognosis). Likewise, temporal lobes are needed for learning and memory, and visual systems are located in occipital lobes.

the brainstem (medulla, pons, and midbrain), which is linked to diencephalon (hypothalamus, thalamus).

Two cerebral hemispheres are linked by corpus callosum, a large tract that helps the brain to communicate. The brain has four closed spaces that communicate with each other and contain cerebrospinal fluid (CSF) (two lateral ventricles, and the third and fourth ventricle).

The Brain[3]

The brain just constitutes 2% of the body weight but consumes 20% of the energy. Human brain contains 100 billion cells, more than the total stars in the observable universe! There are more neuroglial cells than neurons in the brain, indicating the pace at which the neurons need energy as these play supporting roles. To be able to obtain energy, nerve cells are in close approximation with the capillaries. The brain bathes in CSF, which is formed from the blood and is considered to be ultrafiltrate of plasma.

CSF contains most of the low-molecular weight nutrients and electrolytes but is low in proteins (**Fig. 2.2**).

Cerebrospinal Fluid

CSF is an extracellular fluid of the central nervous system (CNS), which is secreted by ependymal cells of the choroid plexus. CSF circulates to subarachnoid space and ventricles and is reabsorbed by arachnoid villi. The main function is to act as a cushion to the brain and maintain stable interstitial fluid environment. Total volume of CSF at any point of time in the brain is about 150 mL.

Choroid plexus produces CSF (500 mL/d), which is reabsorbed and recycled several times a day.

Blood–Brain Barrier

It is formed by the network of capillaries in the ventricles, which is named choroid plexus. Extracellular space (ECF) and CSF are separated by the blood–brain barrier (BBB), which is formed by tight junctions between endothelial cells (**Fig. 2.3**).

Specific transport sites exist for the transport of glucose and many essential amino acids into the ECF. Thus, BBB plays a structural and functional role in maintaining homeostasis.

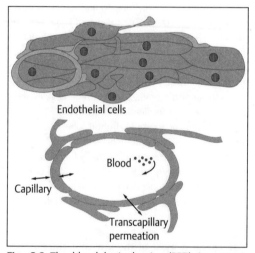

Fig. 2.3 The blood–brain barrier (BBB) is a semipermeable membrane that separates the blood from the cerebrospinal fluid (CSF). This constitutes a barrier to the passage of cells, particles, and large molecules. Brain is the only organ that has such a "security" system wherein drugs have to overcome it to be effective in neurological conditions! Ever since the time of Paul Ehrlich, the barriers present between various tissues have attracted physicians' attention and now in modern neuropsychopharmacology, more so, as methods are being developed to find out ways so that drugs can penetrate this barrier more effectively. Surprisingly, more than 90% of the potential drugs that could become therapeutic blockbusters are unable to enter the BBB. So, this is one challenge in modern neuropsychopharmacology.

Cerebrum[4]

This is the large, convex area of the brain, which is made up of two cerebral hemispheres. This contains depressions called *sulci* and elevations known as *gyri*. Names of the cortices have been derived from the bones that overlay them. Brodman has divided cortex into 50 discrete areas, depending upon cellular structure and function the particular area performs. For example, stimulation of motor area in front of the central sulcus sends commands to muscles of limbs and has, therefore, been named *motor area*. This *primary motor cortex* has been given further names, depending upon which muscles it controls when stimulated.

Likewise, if parts of the brain are stimulated, then sensory experiences are felt in various parts of the body. These areas make up for something called somatosensory areas. These areas help the brain to obtain representation of external environment.

Similar areas for language, vision, and hearing have been identified using probes or accidentally discovered in patients undergoing neurosurgical processes.

Cerebral Cortex

Cerebral cortex is a six-layered structure. It includes most of the two symmetrical cerebral hemispheres. The cerebral hemispheres contain the limbic cortex. The majority of the surface of the cerebral hemispheres is called the neocortex. The majority of cerebral cortex lies exposed, but some part is buried in the frontal lobes (i.e., insula—responsible for taste, sensation, and memory).

The cortex is made up mostly of glia (supporting cells), cell bodies, dendrites, and interconnecting axons of neurons. Neuron cell bodies are grayish brown, which is why the cortex is called gray matter. Beneath the cerebral cortex run millions of axons sheathed in myelin (white matter), which connects the neurons of the cerebral cortex with those located elsewhere.

Cerebral oximetry is an evolving technique that is aimed at measuring blood pressure so that better management of patients with hypertensives can be done. Site of action of several drugs like clonidine, hydralazine, and methyldopa has been demonstrated using the deoxyglucose method.

Cerebellum

Cerebellum is a conspicuous bulbous structure protruding from the posterior brain, which is also sometimes known as "small brain." It has distinctive narrow folds (folia) similar to sulci in neocortex. Cerebellum is involved in the aspects of learning and coordination of skilled or smooth movement. It plays important roles in posture, walking, equilibrium, etc.

Brainstem[5]

The brain can be divided into brainstem (medulla, pons, and midbrain), which is linked to diencephalon that is made up of thalamus and hypothalamus. Two cerebral hemispheres are linked by corpus callosum, which is a large bundle of fibers. These two halves communicate via corpus callosum. Just beneath the cerebral cortex, we have two ventricles that contain CSF. Brainstem consists of all structures from the thalamus to the spinal cord. Regulatory functions include eating, drinking, body temperature, sleep and waking, basic movements, motor learning, etc. (**Fig. 2.4**).

Basal Ganglia

In the coronal section, a large mass of neuronal cell bodies is visible and is called basal ganglia. This is made up of caudate nucleus, putamen, and substantia nigra. Basal ganglia lie beneath the anterior portion of the lateral ventricles. The major parts include caudate nucleus, putamen, and the globus pallidus (**Fig. 2.5**).

Basal ganglia and its structures are involved in the control of movements. The region is concerned with control of movements and is malfunctional in Parkinson's and Huntington's

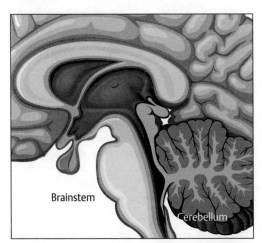

Fig. 2.4 Brainstem is the area of the base of the brain that lies between the deep structures of cerebral hemispheres and cervical part of spinal cord. It is divided into midbrain (metencephalon), pons (metencephalon), and medulla oblongata (myelencephalon). Vital functions are controlled by the brainstem.

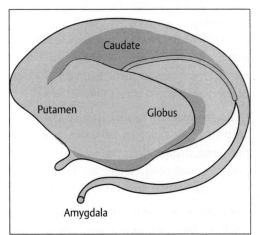

Fig. 2.5 Basal ganglia are a group of structures present near the thalamus and are involved in control of movements. They are involved in some of the common neurological disorders like Huntington's disease and Parkinson's disease.

diseases, both of which are movement disorders. Parkinson's disease results from degeneration of the connections between the midbrain, caudate nucleus, and putamen. Atrophy of basal ganglia occurs in Huntington's disease, where the patients develop movement disorders and neuropsychiatric symptoms along with dementia (**Fig. 2.6**).

Limbic System

One of the most interconnected areas of the brain is known as limbic system (limbic = border). This is made up of hippocampus, which is the seat where short-term memory is processed and sent to cerebral cortex for further storage (**Fig. 2.7**). This is aided by entorhinal cortex, which is considered to be the storage site for maps for navigation. Also, in the dentate gyrus, there are place cells which help us to navigate. The 2014 Nobel Prize was awarded to scientists who discovered place cells in the hippocampus. Fornix and septum also play important role as loops of the limbic system.

Hippocampus and entorhinal cortex have well-defined roles in Alzheimer's disease (AD). This is one of the first regions that undergo atrophies, and overall, in temporal lobe, there is reduction in blood flow, as shown by single photo emission computerized tomography (SPECT). Such changes correlate with cognitive deficits as well. The same can be demonstrated using CT or MRI as well.

Hippocampus is located next to the lateral ventricle in the temporal lobe. This, along with the fornix, mammillary bodies, and cingulate gyrus are involved in learning and memory. Loss of hippocampal gray matter is the hallmark of AD.

Amygdale (almond) is related to rage, fear, and emotions. This is involved in psychotic disorders such as schizophrenia.

Limbic cortex is a three-layer structure covering the periphery of the brainstem on the ventral surface of the lateral ventricles. It is known for

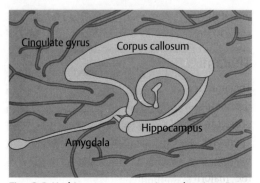

Fig. 2.6 Limbic system; ever since the time Papez described the famous "circuit," it has been at the forefront of memory disorders. Involvement of this system in psychiatric disorders like schizophrenia and neurodegenerative disease such as Alzheimer's disease (AD) is profound. Hippocampal neuron loss in the latter is a major accompaniment responsible for loss of memory.

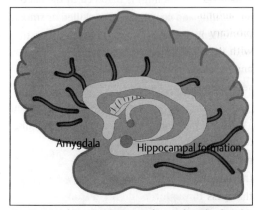

Fig. 2.7 Limbic structures are located on both sides of the thalamus under the cerebrum. It includes hypothalamus, hippocampus (memory center), amygdale, and nearby areas such as parahippocampal and entorhinal area. Limbic structures are not only functionally well-connected, they also have good anatomical connections. Apart from emotions, learning, and memory, limbic system is involved in control of endocrine and autonomic functions.

its role in emotion, learning (emotional), and memory. Limbic system also plays a role in spatial learning and olfaction (memories of odor).

Fornix is a bundle of axons which connects hippocampus with other regions of the brain, including the mammillary bodies (containing some of the hypothalamic nuclei).

Thalamus

Thalamus is a relay center in the brain located near the middle of the cerebral hemispheres. Fibers project to primary sensory areas in the neocortex. There are separate nuclei for vision, touch, and hearing. This is not a "passive" structure because the majority (80%) of its connections are not from sensory neurons, but from the neocortex (including motor areas).

Hypothalamus

Hypothalamus controls all aspects of motivated behavior (pleasure and pain) and several regulatory behaviors such as temperature. It is an autonomic system located superior to the pituitary gland and has reciprocal connections with it. It is considered to be a "master gland" and is closely involved in the regulation and secretion of hormones.

Reticular Formation

Reticular formation has a constellation of several nuclei at the base of the brainstem. It forms the bundles of fibers as well as the projections that pass through the forebrain from the spinal cord. It performs a host of regulatory vegetative functions. Reticular formation has connections with cerebral cortex and thalamus.

White Matter Fibers of the Brain

a) **Projection fibers**
  - Cerebral cortex with lower levels of the brain or spinal cord.

b) **Association fibers**
  - Connect two areas of cerebral cortex on same side of the brain.

c) **Commissural fibers**
  - Connect same cortical regions on two sides of the brain.

d) **Corpus callosum**
  - Primary location of commissural fibers.

Spinal Cord[6]

Spinal cord is a long cylinder of nerve tissue, which is continuous with the brain. It is surrounded by the vertebral column. Spinal nerves are 31 pairs in number. A *dermatome* is a sensory region of skin supplied by a spinal nerve. Dorsal nerves of spinal cord have sensory functions, while the ventral nerves have motor functions (Bell–Megandie law). Spinal nerves are mixed in their functions. White matter forms tracts, which may be ascending or descending (**Figs. 2.8** and **2.9**).

Microanatomy of the Central Nervous System[7]

The Neurons

The neurons are the building blocks of CNS. They are small microscopic structures that have complex neuronal interconnections. Cerebral cortex forms the largest part of the brain and contains approximately 10^{10} neurons, that is about 80% of total brain neurons.

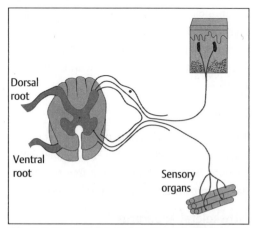

Fig. 2.8 The nerve pathway is involved in reflex actions and is the sensory nerve ending which carries sensations before it is passed onto the motor structure and there is a synapse in between.

11

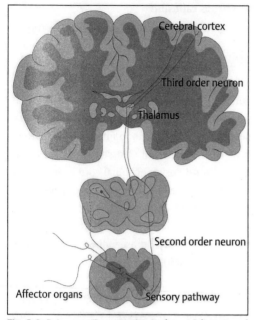

Cerebral cortex

Third order neuron

Thalamus

Second order neuron

Affector organs

Sensory pathway

Fig. 2.9 Pain sensations starting in the periphery travel to the dorsal nerve root ganglion. Thereafter, they are directed, via spinal cord, to the thalamus where they eventually enter the cerebral cortex.

Neurons are surrounded by plasma membranes, which are made up of phospholipid bilayers and contain both intrinsic and extrinsic proteins and cholesterol. Plasma membranes act as a barrier for the cells and do not allow passage of high-molecular weight substances and charged molecules. Plasma membranes are traversed by a number of proteins which may act as voltage-sensitive ion channels and neurotransmitter receptors.

Cytoplasm

This is a fluid-filled compartment that contains enzymes responsible for cellular metabolic reactions. This also contains the free ribosomes that are responsible for local protein synthesis.

Cytoskeletal Apparatus

The shape of neurons is conditioned by neuronal skeleton, which is composed of fibrous proteins. This is of two types:

a) *Internal*: This provides a track to the neurotransmitters and other chemicals to move along the neurons. This moves along the length of axons.

b) *External*: This is cortical cytoskeleton. This helps neurotransmitter receptors and ion channels to the plasma membranes. This also helps in exocytotic processes.

Brain-specific proteins link cytoskeleton internally to microtubules and to the plasma membranes, and neuronal cell adhesion molecules help in such attachments. Such attachments in case of ion channels like sodium is done by another protein known as *ankyrin*. That is why sodium channels concentrate in the region called nodes of Ranvier.

It is of interest that paired helical filaments, which are part of the cytoskeleton, are involved in AD. Microtubule-associated protein *tau* is a part of neurofibrillary tangles that form inside the cells in patients with AD.

Nucleus and Nucleolus

The neurons contain a large number of organelles with specific cellular functions. Together with proteins, deoxyribonucleic acid (DNA) is "the brain" of brain cells like any other cells in the body. Nucleolus lies close to the nucleus and is involved in the ribosomal synthesis and the transfer of messenger ribonucleic acid (mRNA) from nucleus to cytoplasm. Now, it is known that mRNA is involved in synthesis of proteins such as microtubule-associated proteins, which help in structural integrity and differentiation of neurons.

Endoplasmic Reticulum

Smooth endoplasmic reticulum is involved in lipid synthesis and protein glycation process. Rough endoplasmic reticulum contains the ribosomes attached to the endoplasmic reticulum and are the main sites of protein synthesis.

Vesicles

The fact that neurons contain vesicles is a unique feature. These are tiny vesicles (30–100 nm in diameter) and have smooth coatings. Rough-coated vesicles contain a protein called clathrin. Such vesicles are involved in recycling of membrane components once action of neurotransmitter vesicles gets over.

Golgi Apparatus

This is a complex of vesicles and folded membranes found in the neurons of cytoplasm, which is involved in secretion and intracellular support. This is situated near the nucleus and is responsible for the following functions:

- Protein glycation.
- Membrane assembly.
- Protein sorting.

Lysosomes

This is an organelle in the cytoplasm of neurons cells. It contains degradative enzymes which are enclosed in a membrane. The debris, which gets collected inside the cells, is sorted by lysosomes.

The Neuroglial Cells

Not all cells in the brain are neurons! The rest, which are greater in number, are known as glial cells or neuroglial cells (**Box 2.2**).

They are different from neurons and do not have excitable membranes like neurons. Their main role is to provide support to the neurons. These are of two types: *microglia* and *macroglial* cells. Macroglial cells divide into astrocytes, oligodendrocytes, and ependymal cells. Microglial cells act as phagocytes (**Fig. 2.10**).

Astrocytes

Astrocytes are named as such due to their long narrow cellar process that gives them a star-like shape. They transfer nutrients from the blood

Box 2.2: Glial cells of the brain
• Astrocyte—miscellaneous functions.
• Ependymal cells—line cavities.
• Microglia—phagocytes (modified macrophages).
• Oligodendrocytes—form myelin.
• Schwann cells (located in peripheral nervous system [PNS])—form myelin.

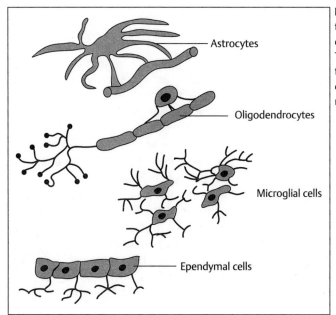

Fig. 2.10 Glial cells found abundantly in the brain surround the neurons and are considered to be the supportive cells. These cells are the most numerous in the brain. They include oligodendrocytes, astrocytes, ependymal, Schwann, microglia, and satellite cells.

Astrocytes

Oligodendrocytes

Microglial cells

Ependymal cells

to the brain. They also have several other roles such as:

- Remove GABA.
- Provide glutamine for GABA synthesis.
- Protect neurons against high potassium.

It seems that they provide metabolic buffers to protect the neurons by buffering potassium ions. Developmentally, they help form neuronal connections and modulate synaptic connectivity. They also help to remove neurotransmitters from the synaptic cleft. Their antioxidant activity protects neurons against toxic substances.

Oligodendrocytes

These occur both in gray and white matter. Insulating myelin sheath around the brain neurons and providing myelin sheath are their main roles. It is notable that these functions are subserved by Schwann cells.

Microglia

These are small cells that are modified macrophages. They protect the CNS from the bacteria or other invaders via phagocytosis. They also conduct antioxidant activity. Brain damage is associated with proliferation of neuroglial cells. This process is known as gliosis. Note that the scar tissue is also associated with gliosis.

Molecular Neuroanatomy[8-10]

Neuroscience landscape is changing fast as new tools and technologies are being generated. New methods of brain gene expression, atlases, and genetically coded proteins for monitoring and manipulating neuronal activities are being developed. This involves the identification of molecular machinery of neurons and neuroglial cells along with their connections and physiological properties. Physical constraints of brain structures can be overcome by technical advances. This budding discipline can integrate various disciplines, leading to specific behaviors in terms of neuronal networks. Techniques for imaging and mapping circuits are proving to be useful.

References

1. Nervous system slides.ppt. Available at: www. gwd50.org/site/handlers/filedownload. ashx?moduleinstanceid=11678. Accessed June 30, 2016

2. The Nervous System: Central Nervous System. Available at: academic.udayton. edu/.../Ch%209%20Central%20Nervous%20 System%20Part%20I. Accessed June 30, 2016

3. Central Nervous System (CNS). Available at: www.austincc.edu/rfofi/BIO2305/2305 LecPPT/2305CNS.ppt. Accessed June 30, 2016

4. Introduction to Neuroanatomy. Available at: www.columbia.edu/itc/hs/medical/ neuralsci/2005/lab/NA_Intro2005_I.ppt. Accessed June 30, 2016

5. The Neuroanatomy of the Brain: Neuroanatomy Learning Module. Available at: http://www.neuroanatomy.ca/module_list. html. Accessed June 30, 2016

6. Neuroanatomy of the Brain Regions. Available at: http://www.onlineveterinaryanatomy. net/content/neuroanatomy-brain-regions-powerpoint-presentation. Accessed June 30, 2016

7. Recent Advances in Cerebral Oximetry. Available at: https://www.ncbi.nlm.nih. gov//29026526. Accessed May 7, 2020

8. Pullock, JD, Wu, DY, Satterlee JS. Molecular Neuroanatomy: Generation of Progress. Available at: https://www.cell.com/trends/ neurosciences/fulltext/S0166-2236(13) 00212-9. Accessed May 8, 2020

9. Neuroanatomy of Synapses and Cell Systems. Available at: https://link.springer.com/ chapter/10.1007/978-3-642-84298-6_8. Accessed May 13, 2020

10. Pollock JD, Wu DY, Satterlee JS. Molecular neuroanatomy: a generation of progress. Trends Neurosci 2014;37(2):106–123

Neurotransmitters

Vikas Dhikav

Introduction

Neurotransmitter is a substance released from the axon terminal of a neuron which binds to the receptor and produces physiological response.[1-5] In the early years of the 20th century, the neural basis of neurotransmission was discovered. During this period, the functions of acetylcholine (ACh) and adrenaline were realized, the oldest known neurotransmitters.[6] **Fig. 3.1** shows a general introduction to the process of neurotransmission. Details of the process are shown in **Fig. 3.2**. Metabolic mechanisms of handling neurotransmitters are illustrated in **Fig. 3.3**.

As per conventional wisdom, neurotransmitters are synthesized in the neuron and become localized in the presynaptic terminal after synthesis.[7-10] They bind to the receptor site on the postsynaptic membrane and are removed from its specific site of action by a specific mechanism. Glutamate and aspartate are abundant neurotransmitters found in cerebral cortex, spinal cord (aspartate), striatum, dentate gyrus (hippocampus), cerebellum, and spinal cord. The neurotransmitter has excitatory influences on basal nuclei.[11]

Glycine is the major inhibitory neurotransmitter of the brain and spinal cord, which is found in interneurons of spinal cord (Renshaw cells) and neurons of subthalamic nuclei projecting to globus pallidus.[11]

Neurotransmitters exhibit their pharmacological effects by acting on the receptors. Receptors are genetically coded proteins embedded in cell membrane, which mediate

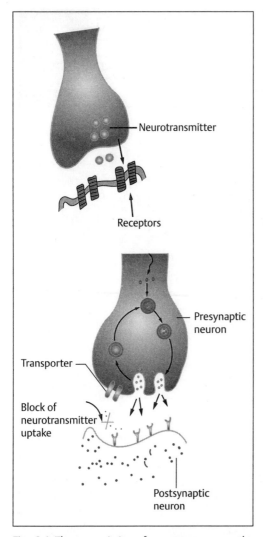

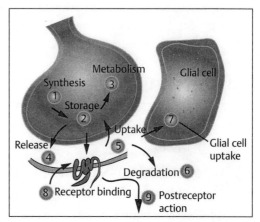

Fig. 3.2 Neurotransmitters released into the synapse cleft do not remain there and are subject to either inactivation or reuptake by presynaptic neurons. Reuptake refers to when the presynaptic neuron takes up most of the neurotransmitter molecules intact and reuses it again for synaptic action. Transporters present presynaptically are special membrane proteins that facilitate reuptake process. For example, serotonin is taken back up into the presynaptic terminals and is stored for future action. Commonly used antidepressants like selective serotonin reuptake inhibitors (SSRIs) block the reuptake process.

Fig. 3.1 The transmission of a message across the synapse occurs by chemical means. Neurotransmitters are chemicals that travel across the synapse and allow communication between neurons via the receptors that are present on the postsynaptic membranes. Neurons in the brain can have thousands of synapses. Both temporal and spatial summation can occur within a neuron. The likelihood of an action potential depends upon the ratio of inhibitor and stimulator potentials at a given moment. Transmission across the synaptic cleft by a neurotransmitter is extremely fast, taking fewer than 10 μs. Most individual neurons release at least two or more different kinds of neurotransmitters (as opposed to Dale's one neuron–one neurotransmitter hypothesis). A neuron may respond to more types of neurotransmitters than it releases.

neuropsychopharmacological effects. They could be ligand-gated or voltage-gated. The effects they produce could be ionotropic or metabotropic. Receptors are located at postsynaptic or presynaptic which may be heteroreceptor or autoreceptors.[10]

It was Sherrington who proposed that cells in the nervous system "talk" to each other, using a group of chemicals (now known as neurotransmitters). He also suggested that there is a gap between cells, and this is known as synapse. The neurotransmitters flow across the synapse and produce the responses.[6]

Precursors, for example, levodopa and noradrenaline, are raw materials that eventually get converted into dopamine and adrenaline, respectively. Making of neurotransmitters is known as biosynthesis, and these are stored in

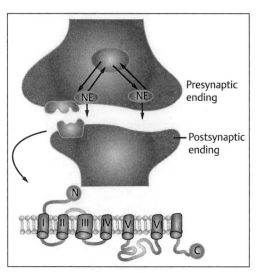

Fig. 3.3 Inactivation and reuptake in presynaptic neurons are the two major events that take place at the synapse. For example, acetylcholine (ACh) is broken down by acetylcholinesterase (AChE) into acetate and choline which are recycled. Serotonin and catecholamine molecules are converted into inactive chemicals. Catechol-o-methyltranferase (COMT) and monoamine oxidase (MAO) are enzymes that convert catecholamine transmitters into inactive chemicals that are eliminated in urine. The major physiologically important fate of a neurotransmitter is postsynaptic action.

Box 3.1: Categories of neurotransmitters

- *Ester*:
  - ◊ ACh.
- *Biogenic amines*:
  - ◊ Catecholamines:
    - □ Dopamine, norepinephrine, and epinephrine.
  - ◊ Indolamines:
    - □ Serotonin (5-hydroxytryptamine [5-HT]).
    - □ Histamine.
- *Amino acids*:
  - ◊ Gamma-aminobutyric acid (GABA).
  - ◊ Glycine.
  - ◊ Aspartate.
  - ◊ Glutamate.
- *Neuropeptides*:
  - ◊ Substance P.
  - ◊ Endorphins and enkephalins.
  - ◊ Somatostatin, gastrin, cholecystokinin, oxytocin, vasopressin.
- *Purines*:
  - ◊ Adenosine.
  - ◊ Adenosine triphosphate (ATP).
- *Small molecules, e.g., gases and lipids*:
  - ◊ Nitric oxide.
  - ◊ Carbon monoxide.
  - ◊ Cannabinoids.

---

vesicles (Golgi bodies). The neurotransmitter, once synthesized, will be transported via neurofilaments and microtubules. Docking of calcium involves influx, leading to vesicle movement and eventual exocytosis. Neurotransmitter reaches into synaptic gap and produces pharmacological action by binding to postsynaptic receptors. Reuptake into presynaptic neurons helps recover the neurotransmitter (Cognitive Neurosciences Society, 2019). **Box 3.1** lists several neurotransmitters found in the brain.

Receptor Types

Ionotropic

Ionotropic receptors work very fast and play an important role in fast neurotransmission. Each ionotropic receptor is made of several subunits, which together form the complete receptor, for example, GABA$_A$ receptors have a pentameric structure. At the center of the receptor is a channel or pore to allow flow of neurotransmitter, leading to generation of physiological effects. At rest, receptor channels are closed, and when neurotransmitter binds to the channel, it immediately opens. When ligand leaves binding site, channel quickly closes.

Metabotropic

Metabotropic receptors work more slowly than ionotropic receptors as their pharmacological effects involve a series of steps to produce combined effects. Although it takes longer for postsynaptic cell to respond, response is somewhat longer-lasting compared to ionotropic receptors. These receptors comprise a single protein subunit, winding back-and-forth through cell membrane seven times (transmembrane domains). They do not possess a channel or pore like ionotropic receptors. Rather, they span the cell membrane like snakes; hence, they are known as serpentine receptors.[10]

Details of both these and other receptor types are described in the chapter on pharmacodynamics.

It is important to differentiate between a few terms here. Neurotransmitters are chemicals synthesized within the axon, travel short distances, and are fast acting.

Neuromodulators, on the other hand, are also synthesized within the cell body of neurons, travel farther distances via diffusion, but are slower acting. Neurohormones are synthesized in endocrine glands, also travel to far distances, and produce pharmacological effects by binding to receptors on the cell or nuclear membrane.

Early Years

In the beginning, it was believed that only ACh and adrenaline were present inside the brain. Later, it was realized that the brain also contains dopamine, serotonin, and several other neurotransmitters. Gaddum and his colleagues showed that 5-HT (also called serotonin) was present in the brain and had neurotransmitter properties. Lysergic acid dimethyl was found to be hallucinogenic during the early 1950s, and this was the period which witnessed the advent of several psychopharmacotherapeutic agents.

Neurochemical Basis of Neurotransmission

After a presynaptic neuron is stimulated, the delay is very short (e.g., 0.3 ms) for the postsynaptic neuron to respond. This is too long for electric transmission, which is lightning fast. If we stimulate the postsynaptic neuron, no response in the presynaptic one occurs. Polarization of communication between neurons occurs only when presynaptic neuron stimulates the postsynaptic neuron. Stimulation of presynaptic neuron may result in postsynaptic inhibition, too, in some neuronal circuits. All the events described here are difficult to explain in terms of direct passage of electrical currents between neurons. All this happens in a series of complicated steps (**Fig. 3.1**). However, to be able to call a putative chemical as a neurotransmitter,

Box 3.2: Criteria for the neurotransmitters
• Must be found in the neurons.
• Must be synthesized there.
• Must be released.
• Must have receptors.
• Degradative mechanisms should exist.
• Should produce some specific physiological/ pharmacological effect.

Table 3.1 Major classes of neurotransmitters

Neurotransmitter	Receptors	Functions
Monoamines (dopamine, norepinephrine, serotonin)	GPCRs	Slow changes in excitability
ACh	GPCRs	Slow changes in excitability
Amino acids (GABA, glycine)	Ion channels	Rapid inhibition
Glutamate (excitatory)	Ion channels	Rapid excitation

Abbreviations: ACh, acetylcholine; GABA, gamma-aminobutyric acid; GPCRs, G-protein–coupled receptors.

certain criteria are needed (**Box 3.2**). Major classes of neurotransmitters are given in **Table 3.1**.

What Is a Neurotransmitter?

This is a chemical substance synthesized, stored, and released by a neuron. However, there are several criteria that need to be fulfilled before a chemical can be called a neurotransmitter. However, these are general guidelines rather than rigid rules as enlisted in **Box 3.2**.

- Following depolarization, the substance is released in the synaptic cleft.
- There are specific receptors for the neuro-transmitter present in the synaptic cleft.
- If the chemical substance is applied by artificial method, say using ionotophoresis, then the result produced should be same as that of natural stimulation.
- Specific antagonists available must be able to block the effect produced by the neurotransmitter.
- A specific mechanism for terminating the action of putative neurotransmitter should be there.
- Specific receptors could be found for some of the receptors in the presynaptic location. These, when stimulated, inhibit the release of neurotransmitter. These are known as "autoreceptors."

Several drugs act on the neurotransmitter systems, and they are used to treat psychiatric and neurological illnesses (**Fig. 3.4**). The entire process of release of a neurotransmitter from presynaptic neuron is explained in **Fig. 3.5**.

Types of Neurotransmitters

Neurotransmitters capable of binding to the receptor on the brain neuron surfaces are of several types[5]:

- Amino acids: This is a class of neurotrans-mitters that are organic molecules con-taining an amino group (NH_2).

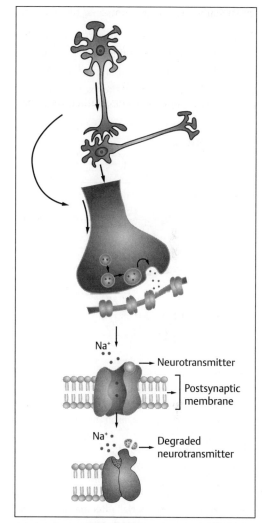

Fig. 3.4 Drugs acting on the synapse work by doing one or more of the following to neurotransmitters, which are secreted in the synapse. They may increase the synthesis, causing vesicles to leak, increasing release (e.g., alpha-2 blockers), decreasing reuptake (SSRIs), blocking the breakdown into inactive chemical (antiacetylcholinesterases [anti-AChE]), or directly blocking postsynaptic receptors (e.g., propranolol or cyproheptadine).

- Peptides: Peptides contain a chain of two or more amino acids, smaller than proteins.
- Proteins: These are long chains of amino acids which contain carbon, hydrogen, oxygen, nitrogen, and, usually, sulfur.

Synapse

Otto Loewi, Dale, and Sherrington worked exhaustively to propagate this concept of synapse and chemical neurotransmission across decades. Synapse is a "gap" between the axon of one nerve

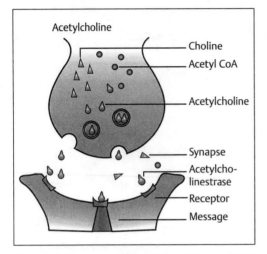

Fig. 3.5 Process of neurotransmitter release. Impulses from action potential generated in cell body open ion channels for Ca^{2+} ions, and this increases Ca^{2+} concentration in the axon terminal which, in turn, initiates the release of the neurotransmitter. Neurotransmitter released from its vesicle after crossing the "gap" or synaptic cleft attaches to a protein receptor on the dendrite. Interaction of neurotransmitter with receptors open postsynaptic membrane ion channel for Na^+. After the action is over, the neurotransmitter is either degraded by an enzyme or taken back into the presynaptic membrane by a transporter or reuptake pump.

and the dendrite of the next one. The average neuron has 1,000 synapses with other neurons. Dendrites receive incoming information from other neurons. Synapses make up most of the surface area of the neuron and the branches of neurons (dendritic), and their spines can number in the thousands.

Mechanism of Action of Neurotransmitters

Broadly, neurotransmitters could have stimulatory or inhibitory effects. Some of the receptors such as GABA are linked to several metabolic steps and hence produce slow effects. Others such as nicotinic receptors are linked to sodium channels. This allows a large amount of sodium ions to enter the cells and hence produce rapid effects.[8]

There are dozens of different neurotransmitters in the neurons. Each neuron generally synthesizes and releases a single type of neurotransmitter (**Table 3.2**).

Acetylcholine

ACh is present in both central nervous system (CNS) and peripheral nervous system (PNS) (**Fig. 3.6**). It is the first neurotransmitter described and is the most abundant of them all. Apart from the brain, it is released at the NMJ and autonomic synapses. It is synthesized

Table 3.2 Major neurotransmitters and their roles

Neurotransmitter	Role
Acetylcholine	Controls muscle tone, movements, and memory
Dopamine	Mediates pleasure and reward system in the brain. It also has inhibitory control
GABA	Major inhibitory neurotransmitter in the brain
Glycine	Major inhibitory neurotransmitter in the spinal cord
Norepinephrine	Acts both as a neurotransmitter and hormone. Mediates flight and flight response
Serotonin	Mediates mood, motivation, has some role in memory and pain pathways
Glutamate	Most abundant excitatory neurotransmitter in the brain

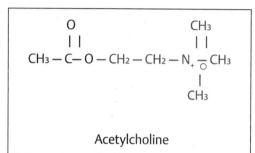

Fig. 3.6 Acetylcholine (ACh) is a quaternary amine synthesized locally in the brain. Peripherally synthesized ACh does not enter the blood–brain barrier (BBB); hence, all functions ascribed to it are the functions of local ACh. Several drugs like donepezil can boost the function of ACh in the brain.

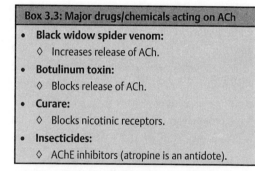

Box 3.3: Major drugs/chemicals acting on ACh

- **Black widow spider venom:**
  ◊ Increases release of ACh.
- **Botulinum toxin:**
  ◊ Blocks release of ACh.
- **Curare:**
  ◊ Blocks nicotinic receptors.
- **Insecticides:**
  ◊ AChE inhibitors (atropine is an antidote).

Box 3.4: Major areas of ACh and its roles

- Dorsolateral pons—rapid eye movement sleep.
- Basal forebrain—perceptual learning.
- Medial septum—formation of memories.
- Basal ganglia—extrapyramidal motor responses.
- Vestibular nucleus—motion sickness.

as a combination of acetyl-coenzyme A (CoA) and choline; the former comes from Krebs cycle in the mitochondria, and the latter is present in the food (eggs, legumes). In the PNS, it is not only responsible for controlling muscle tone but also a major neurotransmitter at NMJ. ACh is synthesized by enzyme choline acetyltransferase and is degraded by the enzyme acetylcholinesterase (AChE). Major drugs/chemicals acting on this system are listed in **Box 3.3**.

ACh is the most abundant neurotransmitter of excitatory type, with a widespread distribution throughout the brain. ACh, present in several areas, perform vital functions with clinical implications (**Box 3.4**). Also, ACh is an attractive therapeutic target in certain disorders like Alzheimer's disease. Inhibition of degradation of ACh is useful in treating this disorder. ACh receptors are described in **Fig. 3.7**.

Clinical Aspects

Cholinergic system undergoes degeneration in Alzheimer's disease, the leading cause of dementia. The degeneration occurs in ACh stores of the brain, for example, nucleus basalis of Meynert.[9]

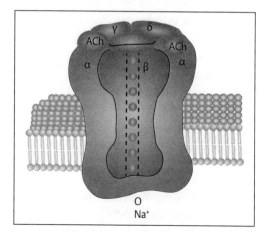

Fig. 3.7 Acetylcholine (ACh) receptors, like many other ligand-activated neurotransmitter receptors, consist of two major subtypes: metabotropic muscarinic receptors and the ionotropic nicotinic receptors. The nicotinic receptors are ligand-gated receptors that allow passage to Na^+ ions.

Monoamines

Monoamine neurotransmitters include dopamine, norepinephrine, epinephrine, and serotonin. These are also called as catecholamines due to the presence of catecholamine nucleus.[3]

These are released both in CNS and PNS and have wide-ranging roles in mood, arousal, emotion, and cognition. The most prominent of their roles in neuropsychopharmacology pertains to mood. Dopamine is important for mood, motivation, memory, and movements (4Ms), and serotonin too has important roles in mood, emotions, and memory. Epinephrine and norepinephrine have roles in arousal and attention. The pathways for synthesis of dopamine and serotonin are given in **Flowcharts 3.1** and **3.2**.

Individual Catecholamines

Dopamine, norepinephrine, epinephrine, and serotonin are catecholamines. Cell bodies producing these are found primarily in the brainstem and branch profusely; hence, they produce widespread areas of physiological effect. They are important in neuropsychopharmacology as biogenic amine theory of depression is based upon monoamines and so is dopaminergic theory of schizophrenia. Dopaminergic system has an involvement in Parkinson's disease. Several features make monoaminergic system special (**Box 3.5**) in brain functioning. Their location in the brain is given in **Table 3.3**.

Dopamine

Dopamine is concentrated in neurons of the ventral tegmental area (VTA) and in the substantia nigra of the basal ganglia. Dopamine is

Box 3.5: Characteristics and functions of monoaminergic system
• *Characteristics*:
◊ Diffuse.
◊ Fine, unmyelinated axons.
◊ Metabotropic synapses.
• *Functions*:
◊ Sleep.
◊ Arousal.
◊ Mood.
◊ Hunger.

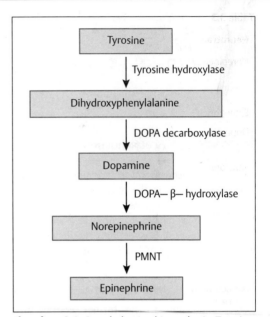

Flowchart 3.1 Catecholamine biosynthesis. Tyrosine, a small amino acid, is transported in the neurons of brain or adrenal medulla where the synthesis takes place. Tyrosine hydroxylase, the key enzyme of biosynthesis, converts phenylalanine into dihydroxyphenylalanine (DOPA). The enzyme DOPA decarboxylase then converts DOPA to dopamine. The enzyme dopamine β-hydroxylase then converts dopamine to norepinephrine. The last step of catecholamine biosynthesis is the conversion of norepinephrine to epinephrine, which involves a methylation reaction, in the presence of phenylethanolamine N-methyltransferase (PMNT).[4]

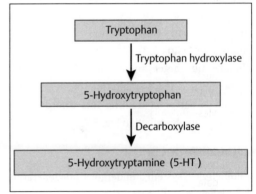

Flowchart 3.2 Serotonin biosynthesis. Serotonin, also known as 5-HT, is a monoamine neurotransmitter. It is derived from tryptophan and is found in the gastrointestinal tract, blood platelets, and CNS.

Table 3.3 Location and projections of catecholamines

Neurotransmitter	Nucleus/cell body	Terminals
Norepinephrine	Locus coeruleus, lateral tegmental area	Widespread effects in cerebral cortex, spinal cord, basal forebrain, thalamus, hypothalamus, brainstem, spinal cord
Epinephrine	Medulla	Thalamus, brainstem, spinal cord
Dopamine	Substantia nigra, ventral tegmental area, arcuate nucleus	Basal ganglia, limbic system, cerebral cortex, cerebellum
Serotonin	Raphe nucleus	Widespread projections in cerebral cortex, cerebellum, brainstem, spinal cord

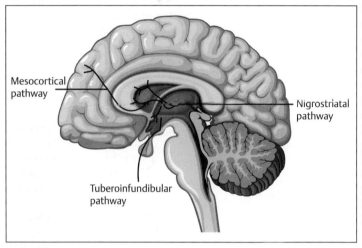

Fig. 3.8 Various dopaminergic tracts in the brain. There are four major dopaminergic pathways, for example, mesolimbic pathway (generates positive symptoms of schizophrenia), mesocortical pathway (produces negative symptoms) when it undergoes hypofunctioning, nigrostriatal pathway (produces side effects like extrapyramidal symptoms and tardive dyskinesia), and tuberoinfundibular pathway, blockade of which can cause hyperprolactinemia.

considered important for motion, mood, reward, etc. It has a major role in schizophrenia. Details of dopaminergic tracts are given in **Fig. 3.8**.

Main dopaminergic systems are as follows:

- Nigrostriatal: The cell bodies located in substantia nigra and project to caudate nucleus and putamen. Blockade of this system leads to extrapyramidal symptoms.
- Mesolimbic system: It is commonly known as the reward system. The cell bodies are located in the VTA and project to nucleus accumbens (prefrontal subcortex), amygdala, and hippocampus. Emotional symptoms of schizophrenia are thought to be generated here.
- Mesocortical system: Mesocortical system is needed for short-term memory,

planning, and strategy preparation. The cell bodies are located in the VTA and project to prefrontal cortex.

Norepinephrine

Norepinephrine was first discovered in the sympathetic branch of the autonomic nervous system. Cell groups containing norepinephrine are found in the locus coeruleus (LC), which projects all over the brain and partakes in the sleep–wake cycle, attention, and vigilance.

Norepinephrine is synthesized from dopamine. The cell bodies of most norepinephrine neurons are located in the regions of pons, medulla, and thalamus. Norepinephrine receptors could be excitatory or inhibitory. LC in the pons is rich in norepinephrine projections. The activation of

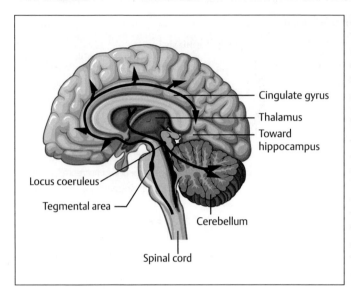

Fig. 3.9 Diffuse adrenergic projections in the brain. The noradrenergic neurons, when activated, exerts diffuse effects on large areas of the brain. The effects are alertness and arousal. Anatomically, the noradrenergic neurons originate both in the locus coeruleus (LC) and the lateral tegmental field. The axons of the neurons in the LC act on adrenergic receptors present in the amygdala, cingulate gyrus, cingulum, hippocampus, hypothalamus, neocortex, striatum, and thalamus. On the other hand, axons of neurons of the lateral tegmental field act on adrenergic receptors in hypothalamus.

neurons in this area leads to increased vigilance. Arousal response leads to sexual behavior. Details of adrenergic projections are given in **Fig. 3.9**.

Epinephrine

Sympathoexcitatory by nature, it is found in the adrenal medulla and in cell groups of the medulla (oblongata). It produces excitatory postsynaptic potentials (EPSPs) and inhibitory postsynaptic potentials (IPSPs), depending on the post-synaptic receptor. Its effects are implicated in movement, attention, learning, and addiction.

Serotonin

Serotonin is also known as 5-HT. The cell bodies are found in raphe nucleus, pons, and medulla (part of the reticular formation). The projections are mainly to the cerebral cortex, hippocampus, and basal ganglia. Serotonin has roles in many behaviors such as mood, control of eating, sleep, arousal, and pain pathways. It also plays important roles in the higher cognition and emotions. Fig. 3.10 describes various receptors related to serotonin.

Serotonin is extensively distributed in the brain. It is derived from the amino acid

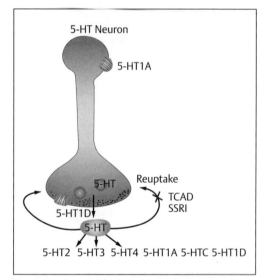

Fig. 3.10 Serotonin is one of the neurotransmitters with maximum number of receptors. At least 15 types and subtypes are known in this case, and they have multiple transduction mechanisms as well. Serotonin receptors have defined roles, for example, 5-HT1A has role in anxiety/depression (buspirone stimulates it), 5-HT1D has a role in migraine (sumatriptan stimulates), 5-HT2 has roles in various central nervous system (CNS) behaviors and in cardiovascular system (CVS) (blocked by atypical antipsychotics), and 5-HT3 has roles in nausea and vomiting, especially due to chemotherapy and radiotherapy (blocked by ondansetron).

tryptophan. Depletion of serotonin in the brain leads to depression (monoamine theory of depression).

Serotonin was first identified as an element found in the blood which aided its clotting and produced vasoconstriction (serum tonic). 5-HT neurons are found mostly in the raphe nuclei that are located in the brainstem and that innervate all major brain areas. It is manipulated by antipsychotic drugs.

Amino Acids

Some amino acids that work as neurotransmitters do not need to be converted into active moieties to have action on synapses. Examples include glutamate (excitatory), GABA, and glycine (inhibitory). They play a major role in synaptic communication and are very effective over short distances due to their rapid action.

Gamma-Aminobutyric Acid Receptors

This is a pentameric structure with two major GABA binding sites per receptor. Benzodiazepines and the newer hypnotic drugs bind to allosteric sites on the receptor to potentiate GABA-mediated channel opening. Barbiturates act at a distinct allosteric site to also potentiate GABA

inhibition (GABA-mimetic action). GABA is synthesized from glutamate (**Fig. 3.11**). Various drugs binding to GABA are described in **Fig. 3.12**.

Benzodiazepines and nonbenzodiazepines act as CNS depressants. Picrotoxin blocks the GABA-gated chloride channels. Loss of GABA-ergic transmission contributes to excessive excitability and can play an important role in the pathogenesis of a serious neurological disorder like epilepsy where the impulses spread uncontrollably.

Bicuculline too is a GABA receptor blocker that inhibits $GABA_A$ receptor function and is a potent convulsant. Both of these drugs are used experimentally to produce seizures in animals. Benzodiazepines and barbiturates increase $GABA_A$ receptor function (potentiate) and are

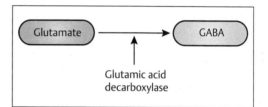

Fig. 3.11 Gamma-aminobutyric acid (GABA) is the major inhibitory neurotransmitter in the central nervous system (CNS). It is synthesized from decarboxylation of glutamate, involved in regulating anxiety, which may be related to eating or sleep disorders.

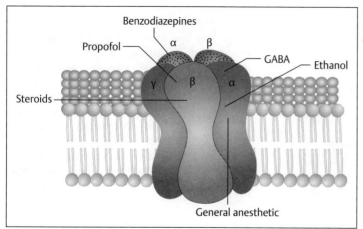

Fig. 3.12 Gamma-aminobutyric acid (GABA) receptors with its various ligands.

anticonvulsants. GABA$_B$ receptors are G–protein-coupled receptors (GPCRs) and largely presynaptic in location where they inhibit transmitter release. Baclofen, an agonist of GABA$_B$, is a muscle relaxant which is used as an antispastic drug.

Glutamate

Glutamate is a fast-acting excitatory neurotransmitter. This is the main excitatory neurotransmitter of the CNS. It is found in almost all CNS structures. Since this is a major neurotransmitter in the brain and spinal cord synapses, it is involved in almost all brain functions. Glutamate is synthesized within the brain from glucose (via KREBS cycle/α-ketoglutarate pathway in the body) and via glutamine (from glial cells in the brain). The actions of glutamate are terminated by uptake through excitatory amino acid transporters in the neurons and astrocytes. All agonists of glutamate stimulate receptors and increase excitation in the neuronal pathways. Behavioral effects vary depending on neural integration and the nature of the neurons activated. In high doses, all agonists induce seizures. Agonists and antagonists are listed in **Box 3.6**. Various glutamate receptors are given in **Fig. 3.13**.

Glycine

Glycine has a major role in the spinal cord, where it mediates inhibition of synaptic transmission. Glycine receptor is an ionotropic chloride channel analogous to the GABA$_A$ receptor. Strychnine, a competitive antagonist of glycine, removes spinal inhibition to skeletal muscle and induces a violent motor response. Glycine seems to be secreted by neurons in the lower brain stem at the same time as GABA.

Peptides

Endogenous opioids are peptides with analgesic properties which mediate "stress analgesia." The examples include endorphins, enkephalins, dynorphins, etc. Apart from mediating stress analgesia, they are involved in regulation of pain for different brain areas.[4] Also, the enhancement of flight or flight response is mediated via them. Some evidence suggests their linkage with memory via hippocampus and amygdale. Details are given in **Table 3.4**.

Neuromodulators and Neurohormones

Neuromodulators are fatlike substances which are water insoluble. Examples include cannabis or tetrahydrocannabinol (THC) and *anandamide*

Box 3.6: Glutamate agonists and antagonists
• Glutamate agonists:
◊ AMPA.
◊ NMDA.
◊ Kainate.
• Glutamate antagonists:
◊ PCP.
◊ Ecstasy.
◊ Can lead to memory loss, inebriation, and apathy.

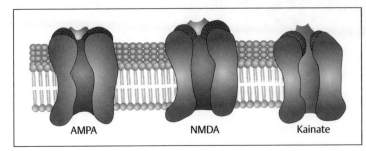

AMPA   NMDA   Kainate

Fig. 3.13 Subtypes of glutamate receptors, each of which bind to glutamate but are activated by different agonists. AMPA, amino-3-hydroxy-5-methyl-4-isoxazolepropionic acid; NMDA, N-methyl-o-aspartate.

Table 3.4 Major peptides and their functions

Neurotransmitter	Functions
Substance P	First peptide neurotransmitter discovered; role in pain
Gut hormones (gastrins)	Angiotensin, neuropeptide Y, cholecystokinin
Releasing factors	Thyrotropin, somatostatin, corticotrophin
Opiates	Encephalins, endorphins; pain pathways
Tachykinins	Substance K, substance P
Insulins	Insulin, insulinlike growth factors I and II

(after Sanskrit word = *anandum*). Another example is adenosine which is a nucleoside; sugar molecule bound with one of the two amino acids (purine or pyrimidine). This is involved in dilation of blood vessels, especially during sleep. Caffeine acts as an adenosine antagonist, which can cause headaches, drowsiness, and difficulty in concentrating. Caffeine can neutralize these effects.[4]

Neurohormones are not produced in the brain and work in various organ systems. Cholecystokinin, neuropeptide Y, substance P, thyroid hormone-releasing hormone, etc., are examples of the same. These are used in brain areas that control these organs.[4]

References

1. Amino acid derivatives: synthesis of neurotransmitters, nitric oxide, and additional derivatives. Available at: http://themedical biochemistrypage.org/aminoacidderivatives.php. Last accessed April 3, 2021
2. Burnstock G. Autonomic neurotransmission: 60 years since Sir Henry Dale. Annu Rev Pharmacol Toxicol 2009;49:1–30
3. Stjärne L. Catecholaminergic neurotransmission: flagship of all neurobiology. Acta Physiol Scand 1999;166(4):251–259
4. Bennett MR. Non-adrenergic noncholinergic (NANC) transmission to smooth muscle: 35 years on. Prog Neurobiol 1997; 52(3):159–195
5. Karczmar AG. The Otto Loewi lecture. Loewi's discovery and the XXI century. Prog Brain Res 1996;109:1–27, xvii
6. Eccles JC. Developing concepts of the synapses. J Neurosci 1990;10(12): 3769–3781
8. Bertrand D. Neurocircuitry of the nicotinic cholinergic system. Dialogues Clin Neurosci 2010;12(4):463–470
9. Van der Zee EA, Keijser JN. Localization of pre- and postsynaptic cholinergic markers in rodent forebrain: a brief history and comparison of rat and mouse. Behav Brain Res 2011;221(2):356–366
10. Cognitive Neurosciences Society. Available at: www.cogsci.ucsd.edu. Last accessed April 3, 2021
11. Kansas University Medical Centre. Available at: www.classes.kumc.edu/sah/resource. Last accessed April 3, 2021

Pharmacokinetic Principles in Neuropsychopharmacology

CHAPTER 4

Vikas Dhikav

Introduction

Pharmacokinetics deals with the movements of drugs inside the body.[1-3] For example, if someone took tablet fluoxetine for depression, then it will go to mouth, esophagus, stomach, intestines, and finally be exposed to liver. Metabolites of several drugs not only prolong their action but also mediate their pharmacological response (**Flowchart 4.1**).

Routes of Drug Administration

The drugs in neuropsychopharmacology can be administered by a variety of routes:

- **Enteral (through alimentary tract):**
    - ◊ Oral.
    - ◊ Sublingual or buccal.
    - ◊ Rectal.
- **Parenteral (through injection):**
    - ◊ Intravenous (IV).
    - ◊ Intramuscular (IM).
    - ◊ Subcutaneous (SC).
    - ◊ Intradermal.
    - ◊ Intraperitoneal.
    - ◊ Intrapleural.
    - ◊ Intracardiac.
    - ◊ Intra-arterial.
    - ◊ Intrathecal.

Oral Route

This is the most convenient and oldest route of drug administration. Most of the drugs can be given by this route. Buccal cavity offers very little in terms of absorption until small intestine. Nausea, vomiting, and diarrhea can occur. Moreover, this is a slow route and unreliable in emergencies. Oral absorption, in general,

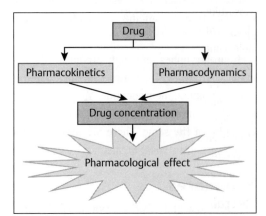

Flowchart 4.1 Pharmacological effects of drugs (pharmacodynamics). Drugs in neuropsychopharmacology have good penetration in the blood–brain barrier (BBB) and remain in continued flux in cerebrospinal fluid (CSF). While it is freely permeable to lipid-soluble drugs, it is impermeable to most of the water-soluble drugs. Also, the penetration of biological fluids like saliva can occur. The drugs can hence be measured in saliva or CSF apart from blood. However, the blood remains most common fluid used for monitoring. In addition, drugs of this class (e.g., antidepressants and antiepileptics) can change electrolyte levels, for example, sodium; hence, monitoring is required.

depends upon passive diffusion which, in turn, depends upon ionization and lipid solubility. Some drugs like levodopa have carrier-mediated transport, and food in the gut interferes with its absorption. Some disorders that affect GI motility may affect absorption of orally administered drugs. Splanchnic blood flow, drug particle size/ formulations like capsules/coated tablets, or timed-release formulations can affect the absorption of drugs. One should be aware of drug interactions which are possible in the gut.

Sublingual

Sublingual (Latin) route means "under the tongue" and refers to the pharmacological route of administration by which drugs diffuse into the blood through tissues under the tongue isosorbide dinitrate, prochlorperazine, etc. The drugs with high first-pass metabolism are suitable candidates for the sublingual absorption. Drugs like buprenorphine, which is a mu agonist and used in opioid detoxification, are used via this route. Since this route is not subjected to first-pass metabolism, drugs given via this route do not enter the liver portal system (so no first-pass effect). Glyceryl trinitrate reliving angina is a famous example of this route in cardiac medicine.

Rectal

This is not a popular route as the drug absorption is not reliable. However, it can be used for local action. Also, this is useful for patients who are vomiting or those who are unable to take by mouth (infants). It is used for febrile seizures (rectal diazepam).

Cutaneous (Transdermal Patches)

This route is often used in general medicine for the local effect on skin. However, if the drug is sufficiently lipophilic, then absorption occurs and systemic effects are produced. Estrogen patches and nicotinic patches are examples from general

medicine. In neuropsychopharmacology, drugs like rivastigmine patches are given to patients with dementias. Likewise, rotigotine patches have been used in the treatment of Parkinson's disease. Allergic reactions to the patches can occur.

Nasal Sprays

Absorption of the drug occurs via mucosa overlaying the lymphoid tissue in the nasal cavity. This route may be important for the drugs that are inactive in the gastrointestinal tract (GIT). Peptide hormone analogs such as antidiuretic hormone (ADH) and calcitonin are examples. In neuropsychopharmacology, zolmitriptan sprays for the treatment of acute migraine are popular.

Subcutaneous and Intramuscular

These are commonly used parenteral routes. These are faster than oral routes, and the rate of absorption depends on site of administration, local blood flow, and the volume of drug injected. Adding another agent, for example, lidocaine with adrenaline can prolong the duration of action of lidocaine. Insulin is often given as SC injection, and lorazepam is IM administered. SC injection of sumatriptan is given in acute attack of migraine.

Intrathecal

This is a special route where the drug is injected directly into the subarachnoid space via lumbar puncture. This is suitable for regional anesthetics, cancer chemotherapeutics, and antibiotics for central nervous system (CNS) infections (e.g., meningitis). Patients must be guarded against the risk of infections.

Intravenous

IV route is the fastest and most certain route of drug administration as the bioavailability is 100%. Bolus injections of the drug expose organs to high concentrations of the drugs. Peak concentration depends on rate of injection. This is used commonly for antiepileptics. This route has most uncomplicated distribution and pharmacokinetics in general.

After biotransformation, the drug will form an active metabolite, which will mediate the pharmacological effects of this drug.

Generally, the drugs of general classes are metabolized in liver and eliminated by urine. Drugs of neuropsychopharmacology class too have same pathway, but may have absorption, entry into the blood–brain barrier (BBB), high volume of distribution (Vd), and interindividual differences in rates of metabolism. For example, drugs of antidepressant classes (selective serotonin reuptake inhibitors [SSRIs], tricyclic antidepressants [TCADs]) may have poor metabolism in about 10% cases, and such patients need lower than usual doses. Similar mechanisms have been described in case of antipsychotics for Asian patients who are poor metabolizers and have developed toxicity after being exposed to high doses.

CNS Pharmacokinetics[1]

Mostly, the principles of pharmacokinetics in case of drugs remain identical, but pharmacokinetics of neuropsychopharmacological agents is unique in many ways:

- Most drugs are lipid soluble.
- Extensively metabolized and form active metabolites (e.g., norfluoxetine).
- Concentrated in the brain and cause CNS-related side effects.
- Highly protein bound (e.g., benzodiazepines),
- Large Vd; hence, hemodialysis is not effective in overdose.

Drugs can enter into the brain directly if they are small nonpolar molecules such as ethanol. Drugs of large molecular weight may need transporters to enter BBB in case they have high molecular weight. Exploitation of BBB transport pathway is a useful strategy to make the entry of drugs in the brain easier, and this has been under development for last decade or so. Under this scheme, transporters or ligands are targeted so that they are able to carry the drugs in larger amounts. Their chemical properties have also been experimentally modified. Lipidization is another approach where the lipid solubility of the drugs has been modified to enhance transcellular passage of drugs to the brain.

A student of neuropsychopharmacology will have to take these properties into account to be able to understand these principles successfully. However, for better understanding and clarity, the author will go through the general principles of pharmacology first.

Before proceeding further, let us know what pharmacokinetics is. Pharmacokinetics deals with absorption, distribution, metabolism, and elimination.

Absorption

It is the process by which the drugs get absorbed in the systemic circulation. Both rate and extent of absorption are important. The drugs of CNS class are lipid soluble and hence have good oral absorption. Some drugs are given by routes other than oral route as well. More lipid soluble and less water soluble, that is, it has high lipid-water partition coefficient and will be absorbed rapidly (**Figs. 4.1** and **4.2**).

Distribution of drugs in the body is dependent upon its route of administration and target area. Every drug has to be absorbed, by diffusion, through a variety of bodily tissue. The permeability of a drug into the tissues depends on the ratio of its water-to-lipid solubility. Within the body, drugs may exist as a mixture of two interchangeable forms, either water (ionized-charged) or lipid (nonionized) soluble. The concentration of two forms depends on characteristics of the drug molecule (pKa, pH at which 50% of the drug is ionized) and the pH of fluid in which it is dissolved.

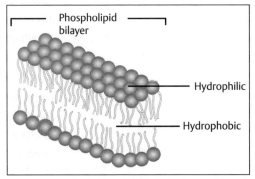

Fig. 4.1 Lipid-soluble (hydrophobic), uncharged, unionized drugs will cross the membrane rapidly than lipid insoluble (hydrophilic or water soluble), charged, and ionized drugs.

Bioavailability is the amount of drug that reaches into systematic circulation without metabolism. Bioavailability is useful to compare two different drugs or different dosage forms of same drug. Rate of absorption depends, in part, on rate of dissolution of drugs (which, in turn, is dependent on chemical structure, pH, partition coefficient, surface area of absorbing region, etc.). Also, first-pass metabolism is a determining factor in bioavailability.

Several factors can affect drug absorption of psychoactive drugs:

- Site: Majority of the drugs are absorbed from the upper part of small intestine. Some acidic drugs like aspirin have good oral absorption from stomach as well. Phenobarbitone too may have considerable absorption from stomach. However, since the surface area of intestine is large, the drugs are absorbed mostly from intestine (**Fig. 4.3**).

- Food: Some drugs can be given with or without meals, for example, donepezil. Likewise, absorption of some drugs such as levodopa gets reduced by protein meals.

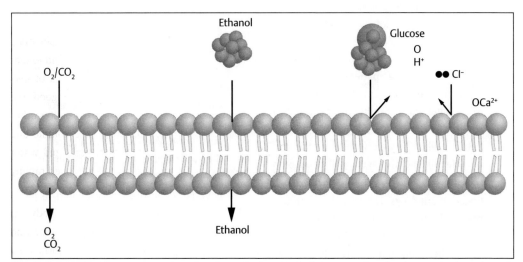

Fig. 4.2 Molecules like oxygen, carbon dioxide, and ethanol, which have small molecular weight, pass through easily via the cell membranes of intestines; however, amino acids and glucose need special transporters.

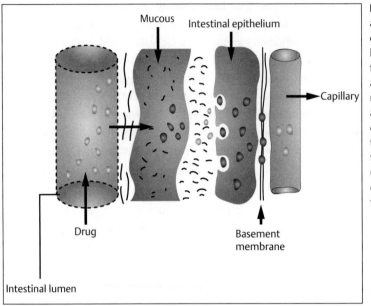

Mucous Intestinal epithelium

Capillary

Drug

Basement membrane

Intestinal lumen

Fig. 4.3 Most drugs are absorbed from the upper art of intestine. Some agents like phenobarbitone are sufficiently acidic so that they are absorbed via stomach too. Too much increase in peristaltic activity, as in diarrhea, reduces drug absorption by increasing the transit of the drug across the gastrointestinal tract (GIT). Also, enhanced gastric emptying time may ensure that absorption will be more.

Interaction of monoamine oxidase (MAO) inhibitors with foods such as cheese, beer, wine, and meat is a famous one.

- First-pass metabolism: Drugs such as levodopa are extensively metabolized in the wall of the gut and are therefore given with carbidopa. Carbidopa, an inhibitor of dopa decarboxylase, blocks intestinal metabolism of levodopa and is able to increase its absorption by double. Likewise, drugs such as TCADs are metabolized to the tune of 50%; hence, blood levels are reduced. In some patients, toxicity of TCADs is likely to occur due to difference in the metabolism. Studies involving debrisoquine metabolism have shown that patients who show a difference in the rate of metabolism to this agent will also have a difference in metabolism to TCADs.

- Concomitant drugs: Drugs such as trihexyphenidyl, used in treatment of Parkinson's disease, have high-anticholinergic activity and hence can potentially slow down absorption of other drugs.

- Sustained release formulation: Generally, as a rule, long-acting formulations of the drugs with a long half-life are not made. However, donepezil is an exception to the general rule, it seems. The drug is available as a sustained-release formulation despite having a half-life of 80 hours! This is because the immediate release formulation could be toxic.

- Dosage form: Drugs given in aqueous solutions are more rapidly soluble than when given in oily solution, suspension, or solid form. Dosage form (tablets and capsules), rate of disintegration, and dissolution are the limiting factors in their absorption. After dissolution, the smaller the particle size, the more efficient will be absorption. That is why aspirin granules have faster absorption compared to paracetamol in migraine.

- Blood flow: The blood flow to the area decides how much and how fast the drug can get absorbed in the circulation.

- pH: Most drugs are either weak acids or weak bases. Majority of drugs are weak electrolytics; hence, their ionization can generate ions that diffuse into cells depending upon pH around or inside the cells.

Drugs like atropine, phenobarbitone, and sulfadiazine, and most other drugs, are examples of weak electrolytes. Nonelectrolytes are substances that do not ionize in water at all and therefore do not conduct an electric current in solution. Examples of nonelectrolytes include sucrose and glycerol, etc.

Weak acids become less ionized in an acidic medium and weak bases become less ionized in an alkaline medium. The opposite happens in basic medium. Unionized drug is lipid soluble and hence diffusible.

Rate, extent of absorption, bioavailability, and concomitantly administered drugs play an important role in determining the final pharmacological outcome of psychopharmaceutical drugs (**Fig. 4.4**).

Distribution[4,5]

Distribution means spread of the drug. Drugs will take whatever volume of body fluids that is available to them for distribution. It is mathematically calculated as Vd.

Vd is an abstract concept that provides information on how and where is the drug distributed in the body. Clinically, it is used to calculate loading dose and half-life of the drug. Drugs acting in the brain have a very large Vd, for example, cocaine (140 L), clonazepam (200 L), and amitriptyline (1,000 L).

It is difficult for the drug to stay in the organ it is supposed to act upon. Often, the drugs that achieve high concentrations in the perfused organs leave that and distribute widely. This is important in case of drugs like thiopentone. Distribution of drugs depends upon lipid solubility and protein binding. Low-protein binding and high-lipid solubility generally means high Vd. Drugs of CNS class are lipid soluble and hence have an extensive distribution into tissues.

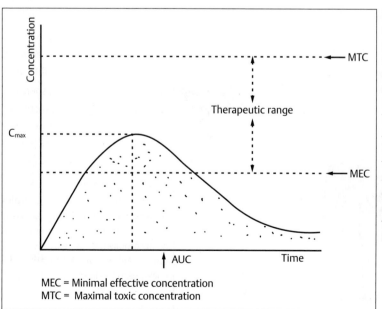

MEC = Minimal effective concentration
MTC = Maximal toxic concentration

Fig. 4.4 Absorption of the administered dose is proportional to the amount of drug in intestines. Bioavailability is proportional to the area under the curve (AUC) in a concentration curve. Thus, we have k = dose/AUC. Because oral administration is full of barriers, the fraction, F, that is available by entering the general circulation may not be significant. Thus, fraction (f) = k(AUC) or k = FD/AUC.

Therefore, hemodialysis is not effective in case of overdose.

Many drugs such as thiopentone, which is an inducing agent, undergo redistribution, which make it short-acting drugs. Likewise, midazolam, used as an inducing agent, in the treatment of seizures, and short-duration sedation, undergoes quick redistribution.

It is generally assumed that the body is a series of interconnected well-stirred compartments within which the drug remains fairly constant. But the movement of drugs between compartments is important in determining when and for how long a drug will be present in body. Fat constitutes a large, nonpolar compartment of the body but has a low blood supply (less than 2% of cardiac output). So, drugs are delivered relatively slowly and stay there for longer.

Although redistribution can potentially occur in case of lipid-soluble drugs having ability to enter BBB, it is more often the case of CNS-active agent (**Fig. 4.5**).

Vd is a theoretical volume which determines the loading dose. Clearance is a constant and determines the maintenance dose.

Mathematically, clearance (CL) = kVd, where CL and Vd are independent variables and k is a dependent variable.

Volume of distribution is the apparent volume into which the drug appears to be distributed to provide the same concentration as it currently is in blood plasma. It is calculated by:

Amount of the drug in the body/plasma concentration. Volume of distribution is useful in calculating half-life of the drug and gives an idea about duration of action of drug.

Vd is an important pharmacokinetic parameter that informs us about the duration of action of drugs and can also help in calculation of half-lives of drugs. The larger the Vd, the greater is duration of action of drugs. Vd is also helpful in case of deciding about the use of dialysis in case of drug overdose.

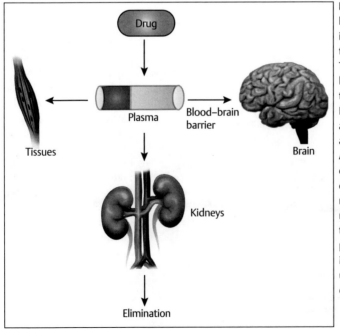

Fig. 4.5 Equilibrium of drug in brain and tissues. Drug molecules interact with target sites to affect the central nervous system (CNS). The drug must be absorbed into the bloodstream and then carried to the target site(s), for example, brain. Pharmacokinetics is the study of drug absorption, distribution within body, and drug elimination over time. Absorption depends on the route of administration. Drug distribution depends on how soluble the drug molecule is in fat (to pass through membranes) and on the extent to which the drug binds to blood proteins (albumin). Drug elimination is accomplished by excretion into urine and/or by inactivation by enzymes in the liver.

Most drugs, which are lipid soluble, distribute freely, while the ones that are water soluble may be bound to plasma proteins. Protein-bound drugs become longer acting, and proteins act as depots for the drugs. Benzodiazepines are examples of highly protein-bound drugs. Roughly, the partition coefficient can determine the distribution fate of the drugs. For example, drugs with high partition coefficient (>1) are likely to go to different tissues (likely to be lipid soluble), while drugs with low partition coefficient (<1) are likely to stay there in plasma (water soluble). Drugs with molecular weight more than 200 Dalton are unlikely to penetrate widely and have a large Vd.

Metabolism

Metabolism means inactivation of the drugs. Some drugs, on the contrary, are activated by metabolism and are known as prodrugs, for example, levodopa, fluoxetine, morphine, oxcarbazepine, eslicarbazepine, and pethidine. It is noteworthy that there are considerable interindividual variations in the way the drugs of this class are metabolized. Drugs like phenobarbitone can induce metabolism of drugs such as warfarin, leading to failure. Induction by phenobarbitone is dose-dependent and takes 2 to 3 weeks to develop.

Metabolism is brought about in two phases (phase I and II reactions). The purpose of metabolism is to convert a lipid-soluble molecule to a more water-soluble molecule in order to excrete in kidney. The main function of phase I reactions is to prepare chemicals for phase II metabolism and subsequent excretion, while the phase II reaction is the true "detoxification" step in the metabolism process (**Fig. 4.6**).

Possibility of active metabolites with identical or different properties as parent molecule exists with several drugs of CNS classes. Biliary excretion involves active transport, and drugs of high-molecular weight are secreted like this.

Prodrugs may produce a short- or a long-acting metabolite; the latter will make them stay in the body and have residual effects for long periods. Drugs like fluoxetine form a long-acting metabolite, making it a very long-acting drug. Mostly, liver enzymes inactivate the drug molecules into metabolites.

Microsomal enzymes belong to cytochrome P450 (CYP) monooxygenase family of enzymes, which oxidize most of the clinically administered drugs. They act on structurally unrelated drugs. Most of the enzymes metabolizing the drugs belong to P450 class, the activity of which is genetically determined. However, some people lack such activity, and this can lead to higher drug plasma levels (adverse actions). Some persons have high levels, and this may lead to lower

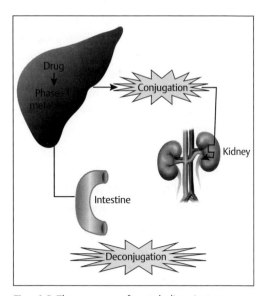

Fig. 4.6 The purpose of metabolism is to convert a lipid-soluble drug into a water-soluble drug. This way it is easy for the drug to be excreted from the body. Metabolite hence formed should bind to the endogenous product, and this process is known as conjugation. If the product is excreted in the intestine instead of the urine, the reabsorption can occur, and this is known as enterohepatic circulation. This can make a drug longer acting. Phenytoin has some degree of enterohepatic circulation.

35

plasma levels (and reduced drug action). This is the basis of interindividual variations. Several drugs are metabolized by P450 enzyme systems, and they can either induce activity (apparent tolerance) or inactivate an enzyme system, and this can significantly change the plasma levels of drugs.

Drug metabolizing enzymes are found, apart from the liver, in the small intestine, lungs, kidneys, placenta, etc. They consist of >50 isoforms, and it has been estimated that 90% or more of human drug oxidation can be attributed to 6 main enzymes, for example, CYP3A4, CYP2D6, CYP1A2, CYP2C9, CYP2E1, and CYP2C19. In different people and different populations, the activity of cytochromal oxidases differs.

A number of drug metabolizing enzymes play a role in disposing off the drugs of CNS class. Mainly, cytochromal enzymes are involved; however, CYP3A4 is the main enzyme isoform responsible for metabolism of clinically administered drugs. In case of CNS active drugs, CYP2D6 is responsible. This enzyme is pleomorphic and is involved in several clinically important drug interactions.

A number of drugs can induce or inhibit their metabolism, leading to severe drug interactions. It is not unusual for a patient with a psychiatric or neurological disease to have several drugs. Some of the inducers and inhibitors are given below:

- **Inducers:**
  ◇ Cigarettes.
  ◇ Alcohol.
  ◇ Rifampin.
  ◇ Glucocorticoids.
  ◇ Antiepileptic drugs.
  ◇ Spironolactone/sulfonamides.
- **Inhibitors:**
  ◇ Flagyl (metronidazole).

◇ Amiodarone.
◇ Ciprofloxacin.
◇ Erythromycin.
◇ Dextropropoxyphene.
◇ Isoniazid/imipramine/imatinib.
◇ Pills (oral contraceptive pills).

It may be worthwhile discussing some of the commonly occurring drug interactions:

- Although we discussed that all antiepileptic drugs have enzyme-inducing activity, sodium valproate is an exception. This drug can boost the levels of concomitantly administered drugs. One example is lamotrigine. This is a new antiepileptic drug, effective in generalized and partial seizures. However, when the drug is given with valproate, it may have increase in its plasma levels. This may cause toxicity of lamotrigine. Therefore, the dose of lamotrigine has to be reduced when used with sodium valproate.

- Likewise, clonazepam and valproate combination can cause thalamic synchronization, leading to increase in the risk of a status absence like situation. Therefore, this combination may prudently be avoided.

- Some drugs, like carbamazepine, can act as their own inducer (autoinducer).

- Phenobarbitone can induce metabolism of warfarin, making control of international normalized ratio difficult.

- Fluvoxamine is a potent inhibitor of microsomal enzymes, leading to elevation of blood levels of many concomitantly administered drugs.

- Benzodiazepines can potentiate the effect of many drugs like opioids and TCADs.

Elimination

Kidneys are the most common organ of elimination, and the process is majorly passive mostly. Some drugs may have a high-molecular weight and some carriers via renal tubules may be required to expel them from the renal tract. However, kidneys are not alone in elimination (**Figs. 4.7** and **4.8**).

Some drugs that have high-molecular weight (e.g., bromocriptine) are eliminated via bile. Similarly, drugs such as lithium are eliminated by saliva, and there is a method of detecting the drug in saliva as well.

Some unconventional routes such as breast milk and sweat also play some role in eliminating the drugs. Drugs eliminated by breast milk are

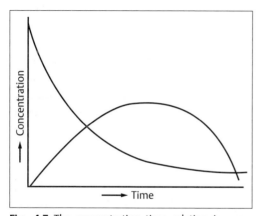

Fig. 4.7 The concentration–time relation in cases of drugs reflect the bioavailability; also, calculated as area under curve (AUC). The area depends upon the rate of elimination from the body and the dose administered. The total amount eliminated may be assessed by adding up or integrating the amount of drugs eliminated in each time interval from zero to infinite time. This amount corresponds to the fraction of dose administered which reaches into systemic circulation in an unchanged manner. In clinical trials in neuropsychopharmacology, this curve is very important, and the drug concentration time profile can be drawn graphically by measuring the time concentration several times after giving the drug. This can predict the pharmacokinetic behavior of the drug. Renal system acts as the site where potential drug interactions can occur. For example, the renal elimination of drugs such as lithium may be blunted by nonsteroidal anti-inflammatory drugs (NSAIDs), leading to increase in its plasma levels.

predictably avoided during breastfeeding. Such drugs include lithium, antiepileptics, etc. Drugs with high-sedation potential, for example, benzodiazepines are also avoided as this may lead to the problem.

Clearance of drugs represents the capacity for drug removal by various organs and is defined as the volume of blood from which all the drug is removed per minute and is usually expressed as mL/minute. Both clearance and distribution volume are model-independent parameters. Thus, plasma drug concentrations are determined by the rate at which drug is administered, its clearance (Cl), and volume of distribution (Vd). Likewise, the rate of elimination can be determined from clearance (Cl) and Vd.

CL can be calculated by:

Rate of elimination/plasma concentration

CL is the ability of organs of elimination (e.g., kidney, liver) to "clear" drug from the bloodstream. It is the volume of fluid which is completely cleared of drug per unit time. Units are in L/h or L/h/kg. It is a pharmacokinetic term used in determination of maintenance doses.

CL is the volume of blood in a defined region of the body which is cleared of a drug in a unit time. CL is a more useful concept in reality than $t_{1/2}$ or k_{el} since it takes into account blood flow rate. CL varies with body weight. It also varies with degree of protein binding.

Half-life is the time taken for the drug concentration to fall to half its original value. The elimination rate constant (k) is the fraction of drug in the body, which is removed per unit time.

Half-life denotes how quickly a drug is removed from the plasma by metabolism or excretion. Since drug requires a minimum concentration in the plasma to produce pharmacological action, a drug which is eliminated quickly requires more frequent dosing than a

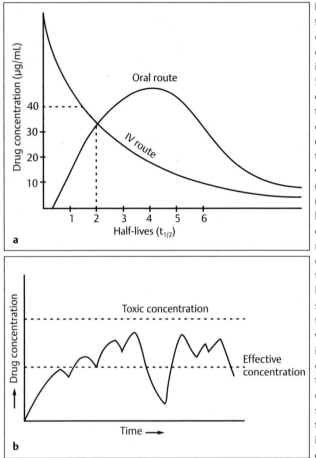

Fig. 4.8 (a) Half-life is the time required for the concentration of drug in the plasma to decrease to one-half of its initial value. For example, if the initial concentration of drug is 100 mg and if the half-life is 1 hour, only 50 mg will remain in the plasma at the end of 1 hour; a drug achieves steady state in 4 to 5 half-lives, and after that if no further doses are given, then it is eliminated out. Some drugs like buspirone may take a week or 2 to achieve steady state, while drugs like tricyclic antidepressants (TCADs) take longer to achieve the same. **(b)** Steady state occurs after a drug has been given for approximately five elimination half-lives. At steady state, the rate of drug administration equals the rate of elimination and plasma concentration–time curves found after each dose should be approximately superimposable. At the steady state, the rate of drug in is equal to the rate of the drug out. It is important when interpreting drug concentrations in time-dependent manner or assessing clinical response. This is important as these drugs become clinically effective only after achieving steady state. There are several factors that come in the way when the drugs achieve the steady state, and it is clear that it is not half-life alone that explains the same.

drug with a long half-life. Half-life, thus, not only indicates the duration of action of drug but also determines the frequency of administration of dose of the drug for therapeutic effectiveness. Half-life, however, cannot determine dose of the drug.

Drugs can be eliminated in the following two main ways (**Table 4.1**):

- **Zero order:**

    These drugs have a limited capacity for elimination, and hence, this mode of elimination is considered to be saturable. Therefore, fixed dose of drugs is not recommended. This is because a fixed dose can lead to disproportionately high blood levels. Since drugs following zero order are very few in number and have the chance of producing toxicity in high concentrations, their plasma level monitoring is routinely recommended. Drugs such as phenytoin follow zero order. However, phenytoin is a special case as it follows zero order in high dose. Therefore, starting the patient with a fixed dose of 300 mg at night, which many neurologists use, may produce side effects in a sizable number of cases. Giving the drug in a 100-mg tablet three times daily is a better way of prescribing the same.

- **First order:**

    Most commonly, drugs are metabolized by first-order kinetics. In this form

Table 4.1 Comparison of zero-order and first-order kinetics

Zero order	First order
• The concentration of drug decreases linearly with time • Rate of elimination is constant regardless of the dose given • No true half-life ($t_{1/2}$), as it becomes a function of the dose	• The drug concentration decreases exponentially with time • The rate of elimination of drug is proportional to the concentration; higher the concentration, greater is the elimination • Half-life of the drug ($t_{1/2}$) is constant regardless of the dose given
• Not a common mechanism of elimination, except in case of drugs like phenytoin	• This is the most common way in which drugs are eliminated

of stretchable kinetics, the drugs are eliminated, depending upon the plasma concentrations, unlike zero order, where the rate of elimination is constant, regardless of the dose given. Since the rate of elimination can increase proportionately, drugs handled by this type of elimination do not develop toxicity easily unlike zero-order drugs.

Drug Dosages

Loading Dose

Loading dose of the drug is an initial large dose used to achieve plasma steady state concentration quickly. This will ensure a quick therapeutic response. It is usually given for a short period before therapy continues with a lower maintenance dose, which needs to be done later on. The use of loading doses of drugs can be complex and error prone. Loading doses are not without adverse reactions and hence need to be carefully calculated and used. For example, phenytoin is given as a loading dose for quick control of seizures. It is calculated as a function of volume of distribution and target concentration:

Loading dose = Vd × target concentration. Loading dose of phenytoin is commonly used to control seizures.

Maintenance Dose

Maintenance dose = CL × target concentration. Once the patient is loaded, then maintenance dose of phenytoin is given.

Therapeutic Drug Monitoring

This involves evaluation of serum/plasma/salivary/cerebrospinal fluid (CSF) concentration of the drug to predict the therapeutic response. Mostly, serum is used for estimation of plasma concentrations. Some drugs such as TCADs have large interindividual variations and hence are not amenable to plasma monitoring. The guidelines are given below.

In general, the therapeutic drug monitoring is useful when the drug in question:
- Has narrow therapeutic range.
- Has a direct relationship between the drug or drug metabolite levels in plasma and the pharmacological or toxic effects.
- Therapeutic effect cannot be easily accessed by the clinical observations.
- Large individual variability in steady-state plasma concentration exists at any given dose.
- Appropriate techniques are available to determine the drug and metabolite levels in body fluids.

Several drugs used in nervous system diseases are the candidates for therapeutic drug monitoring:

- Antidepressants and mood stabilizers:
    ◇ Lithium.
    ◇ TCADs.
- Antiepileptic drugs:
    ◇ Phenytoin.
    ◇ Phenobarbitone.
    ◇ Carbamazepine.
    ◇ Valproic acid.
    ◇ Ethosuximide.

While doing therapeutic drug monitoring, both the parent drugs and their metabolites should be taken into account. Some drugs such as lithium, however, have been monitored with great therapeutic successes. Both the therapeutic and toxic concentration of the drugs have been identified in patients with unipolar and bipolar disorders.

Therapeutic Window[6–8]

Some drugs have a useful range of concentration over which a drug is therapeutically beneficial. Therapeutic window may vary from one patient to another. Drugs with narrow therapeutic windows require smaller and more frequent doses or a different method of administration (e.g., amitriptyline). Drugs with slow elimination rates may rapidly accumulate to toxic levels and hence one can choose to give one large initial dose, following only with small doses later on.

Drug Interactions

CNS drugs are commonly involved in drug interactions, especially in elderly and those with liver disease or history of alcoholism. Therefore, it is important to know the potential for drug interactions. In a nation like India, where an elderly receives several drugs at the same time (polypharmacy), it is even more important to

consider the potential for drug interactions that have the potential to harm the patient. Drug–drug interactions are common.

Fluoxetine increases plasma concentrations of amitriptyline by inhibiting its metabolism. This is a pharmacokinetic drug interaction. If fluoxetine is given with tramadol, then serotonin syndrome can result. This is a pharmacodynamic drug interaction.

Polypharmacy in Elderly

Polypharmacy and the use of potentially inappropriate medications (PIMs) is a common clinical problem among the elderly worldwide. A reported definition of polypharmacy is the intake of five or more drugs. Alternatively, it has also been defined as the introduction of at least one unnecessary medication over and above the required ones. An elderly reporting to the Department of Neurology receives eight drugs on an average. This may be because of concomitant hypertension, diabetes, and dyslipidemia, which may actually make the count of drugs as five.

If there is any other illness such as dementia and Parkinson's disease, then this value will go further and become eight or well over eight. There are several ways to avoid the same.

Pharmacokinetics in Elderly

The body changes considerably in old age. The muscle mass becomes less, and the body fat increases. This ensures that the lipid-soluble drugs become longer acting. The baroreceptor sensitivity becomes less in old age. Hence, the antipsychotics that have the potential to cause postural hypotension are likely to result in considerable morbidity in old age. The lean muscle mass of the elderly with high body fat ensures that the Vd of hydrophilic drugs decreases and that of the fat-soluble drugs like diazepam and haloperidol increases. This implies that there is an increase in half-life and the drug takes longer time. Decrease in oxidative dephosphorylation and renal capacity too contribute to increase in half-lives of drugs in old age. Polypharmacy and drug interactions take a toll as well. Since there is lesser amount of plasma protein, drugs like aspirin develop higher plasma concentrations (**Fig. 4.9**).

Absorption of drugs become slow in old age, and the drugs spend considerable time in the intestine. "Dose dumping" is hence likely. Metabolism too becomes slowed down due to deficiency in the oxidative degradation of drugs. This would mean the drugs become longer acting. Glomerular filtration becomes less with the passage of time; hence, drugs accumulate in old age. "Start low and go slow" is a useful general rule in old age.

Pharmacokinetics in Children

Children have higher capacity of drug metabolism compared to adults due to greater liver mass relative to their body weight. Therefore, children may need higher per kg doses of the drugs compared to adults.

This may explain higher frequency of rashes to lamotrigine in older children and hepatotoxicity to sodium valproate in younger children due to greater amounts of toxic metabolites. Neonates may differ from older children with regard to Vd of many drugs like phenobarbitone and phenytoin and hence may need larger doses. So, the dictum "children are not smaller adults" applies here and should be kept in mind while calculating the drug doses.

By 1 year, the glomerular filtration rate (GFR) may reach at the same level as that of the adults. Since the fluid intake in children is higher, the drugs may have a more rapid renal clearance compared to adults.

Pharmacokinetics in Pregnancy

Pregnancy poses a special challenge in drug treatment of neuropsychiatric diseases. This is because there is nausea and vomiting, and this

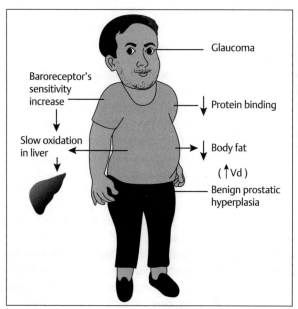

Fig. 4.9 Reduction in renal and hepatic clearance occurs with an increase in volume of distribution (Vd) due to greater amount of fat. Prolongation of elimination half-life occurs henceforth. There is an increase in baroreceptors sensitivity and receptors; so, even small doses produce a greater response, leading to increase sensitivity to psychotropic drugs. Likewise, sensitivity to anticoagulants and cardiovascular drugs is increased as well.

Glaucoma

Baroreceptor's sensitivity increase

↓ Protein binding

Slow oxidation in liver

↓ Body fat

(↑Vd)

Benign prostatic hyperplasia

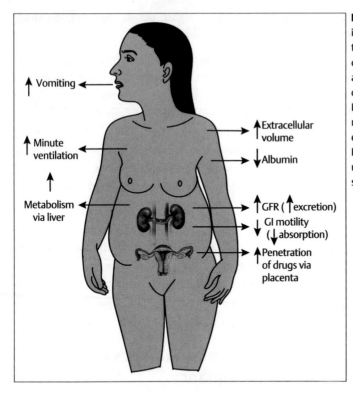

↑ Vomiting

↑ Minute ventilation

↑

Metabolism via liver

↑ Extracellular volume

↓ Albumin

↑ GFR (↑ excretion)

↓ GI motility (↓ absorption)

↑ Penetration of drugs via placenta

Fig. 4.10 Ventilatory changes occur in pregnancy and this may influence the pulmonary absorption of inhaled drugs. This is important in drug abusers which commonly inhale cocaine or in smoking addiction. Likewise, as the glomerular filtration rate (GFR) increases, the renal drug elimination may be enhanced. Influence on drug metabolism is unpredictable, and it may remain same or increase or decrease.

can lead to hemoconcentration. Notably, lithium levels go up if this happens. Likewise, some drugs may have higher Vd like aminoglycosides as there is increase in the extracellular fluid volume. There is increase in free drug levels of nonsteroidal anti-inflammatory drugs (NSAIDs) due to decreased albumin. One of the important concerns is that the drugs that are given to pregnant women have the potential to affect the developing baby (e.g., phenytoin, valproate, lithium); hence, when treating a woman of child-bearing potential, possibility of pregnancy should be kept in mind to avoid teratogencity (**Fig. 4.10**).

References

1. Suthakaran C, Adithan C. Therapeutic drug monitoring—concepts, methodology, clinical applications and limitations. Available at: http://medind.nic.in/haa/t06/i1/haat07i1p22.pdf. Last accessed March 31, 2021

2. Oie S. Drug distribution and binding. J Clin Pharmacol 1986;26(8):583–586

3. Crooks J, O'Malley K, Stevenson IH. Pharmacokinetics in the elderly. Clin Pharmacokinet 1976;1(4):280–296

4. Kristensen MB. Drug interactions and clinical pharmacokinetics. Clin Pharmacokinet 1976;1(5):351–372

5. Palleria C, Di Paolo A, Giofrè C, et al. Pharmacokinetic drug-drug interaction and their implication in clinical management. J Res Med Sci 2013;18(7):601–610

6. Suzuki E. Drugs interactions and pharmacokinetics of psychotropic drugs. Seishin Shinkeigaku Zasshi 2015;117(1):49–55

7. Kubo Y. Carrier-mediated transport of cationic drugs across the blood-tissue barrier. Yakugaku Zasshi 2015;135(10):1135–1140

8. Rico-Villademoros F, Slim M, Calandre EP. Amitriptyline for the treatment of fibromyalgia: a comprehensive review. Expert Rev Neurother 2015;15(10):1123–1150

Pharmacodynamics of Neuropsychopharmacological Agents

Vikas Dhikav

Introduction

The term "pharmacodynamics" means mechanism of drug actions. Knowledge of how a drug works increases the therapist's confidence that the drug is being used appropriately. Usually, a drug produces pharmacological response by binding to the proteins called receptors, but there exist several other mechanisms as well (**Box 5.1**). Pharmacodynamics deals with the action of a drug on the body, including drug–receptor interactions, dose-response phenomena, and mechanisms of therapeutic and toxic action. Many drugs inhibit enzymes, and enzymes control a number of metabolic processes. This is a very common mode of action of many drugs. For example, angiotensin-converting enzyme (ACE) inhibitors block angiotensin convertase enzyme. However, most drugs act on the receptors. Some drugs modulate the activity of ion channels (like antiepileptic drugs), and carriers are blocked by others (e.g., tiagabine). A drug binding to the receptors produces a pharmacological response, leading to clinical change in the patient, for example, euthymia in a depressed patient or seizure control in a patient with epilepsy. **Fig. 5.1** gives details of what happens when a drug binds to the receptor.

Box 5.1: Major sites of drug action
Drugs act on the following:
• Receptors.
• Enzymes.
• Ion channels.
• Carriers.

Some drugs antagonize, block, or inhibit endogenous receptors, while the others stimulate receptors. Detailed examples are given in **Box 5.2**.

A drug can act by one of the following general principles:

- Stimulation (amphetamines stimulate the brain).
- Depression (benzodiazepines [BZDs] depress the central nervous system [CNS]).

Drugs could act as full agonists, partial agonists, or antagonists, depending upon if they have 50%

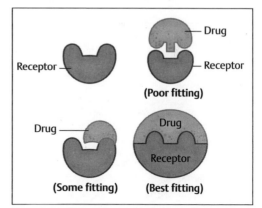

Fig. 5.1 Illustration depicting drug–receptor interaction. Most drugs act or bind on the *receptors*, which are mostly the protein molecules present in or on the cells. Receptors form the tight bonds with the *ligand*. This interaction depends upon exacting requirements (size, shape, stereospecificity, etc.). The binding drugs can be *agonists* (salbutamol) or *antagonists* (propranolol). Receptors have *signal transduction* mechanisms to convert binding into clinically meaningful pharmacological response. Drugs may augment or disrupt the signal transduction mechanisms associated with the drugs and their receptors.

intrinsic activity, 100% intrinsic activity, or no activity at all (**Fig. 5.2**). Drugs given together may support each other (like BZDs and opioids) or be synergistic. Likewise, they may have antagonistic combinations too (like tricyclic antidepressants [TCADs] can block action of donepezil, which is cholinergic drug). Drugs may not have any interactions with each other too, like analgesics given to a manic patient.

Box 5.2: Pharmacological classes with examples
• Antagonists of cell-surface receptors (beta blockers).
• Antagonists of nuclear receptors (e.g., corticosteroids).
• Enzyme inhibitors (monoamine oxidase [MAO] inhibitors).
• Ion channel blockers (calcium channel blockers [CCBs]).
• Transport Inhibitors (selective serotonin reuptake inhibitors [SSRIs]).

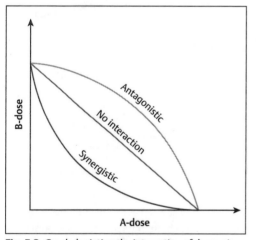

Fig. 5.2 Graph depicting the interaction of drugs given together. Two drugs given together can have agonistic or antagonistic interactions. For example, selective serotonin reuptake inhibitors (SSRIs) and tricyclic antidepressants (TCADs) given together may have risk of serotonin syndrome due to agonistic or synergistic interaction of blocking the reuptake of serotonin. Similarly, cyproheptadine, an antiserotonergic drug, can block the excessive effect of serotonin causing sexual dysfunctions. This effect can be therapeutic.

Receptors[2,3]

Drugs of psychopharmacological class, like any other, act on receptors. A receptor is a macro-molecular component of the organism which binds the drug and initiates its effect. G-proteins are the most common type of receptors and involve a lot of intermediate steps when the drug binds to them and produces pharmacological response (**Fig. 5.3**). This is followed by ion channel receptors called ionotropic receptors (**Fig. 5.4**).

Drugs, when they bind to receptors, often behave as "keys" that "unlock" the receptors so that the pharmacological responses get generated (**Fig. 5.5**).

Most receptors are proteins that have under-gone various posttranslational modifications

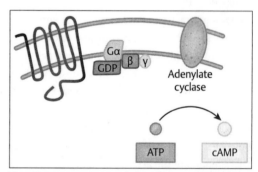

Fig. 5.3 G-protein–coupled receptors (GPCRs) are seven transmembrane receptors (7-TM), which have seven helical structures like a snake and are therefore known to belong to a serpentine family of receptors. These sense the drugs outside the cells and activate a signal cascade inside the cells. There are two main pathways that they operate with: cAMP pathway and phosphatidylinositol pathway (PIP2). When a drug binds to GPCRs, then it causes a conformational change in the receptor, which can activate an associated G-protein, leading to exchanging of GDP for GTP. Alpha subunit of G protein (Gα) together with GTP can dissociate it from other subunits (β and γ), and this can activate or inhibit the activity of adenylate cyclase, which is capable of modulating activity of protein kinases that are able to produce multiple cellular effects, depending upon the type of G-proteins involved.

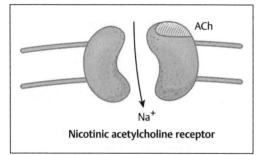

Nicotinic acetylcholine receptor

Fig. 5.4 A nicotinic receptor is a typical example of an ion channel that is fast conducting. This is an integral membrane protein that can be blocked by tubocurarine or hexamethonium, both of which act as muscle relaxants. Several toxins such as snake toxins and shellfish can paralyze the body by blocking these receptors.

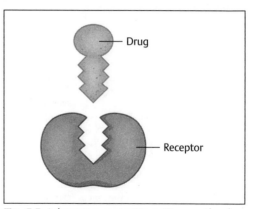

Fig. 5.5 A hormone, neurotransmitter, or the drug (the key, commonly called as ligand) binds to the receptors on the target cells (the lock) and produces the desired action.

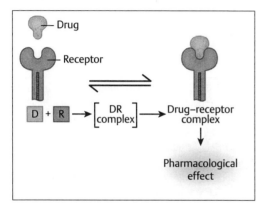

Fig. 5.6 Receptors are involved in the chemical signaling after the drug binds to their surface. Activated receptors directly or indirectly regulate several biochemical processes like ion conductance, protein phosphorylation, enzymatic activity, DNA transcription, etc. However, it starts with the drug binding to the receptors, producing some conformational changes. This changes the drug–receptor interaction to drug–receptor complex, which is a prerequisite to pharmacological response.

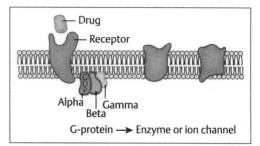

Fig. 5.7 Binding of receptors to the drugs can bring about changes that are typically seen with 7-transmembrane receptors. However, apart from producing routine changes like modifying enzyme activity, G-protein–coupled receptors (GPCRs) have a "cross-talk" with ion channels and can modify their activity. This is a classic example where one receptor type can influence the other receptor type.

such as covalent attachments of carbohydrate, lipid, and phosphate. A drug binds to them and produces pharmacological response. A chemical signal is the most common way in which response is produced and is often a chain of events, except ion channels where it is a direct action (**Fig 5.6**). A series of events take place where

one group of receptors can influence the activity of others (cross-talk), which is common with G-proteins and ion channels (**Fig. 5.7**). Receptors are not just important pharmacologically, but antibodies developed against the receptors can also produce diseases, for example, myasthenia gravis (**Fig. 5.8**). Drugs could behave both as competitive and irreversible antagonists of receptors (**Fig. 5.9**).

Drugs can oppose actions of other drugs and chemicals by receptor antagonism, which

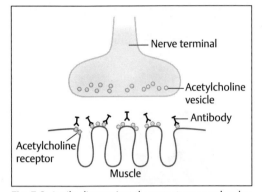

Fig. 5.8 Antibodies against the receptors may develop and can contribute to diseases like myasthenia gravis. This antibody test is used to help diagnose the disease (acetylcholine receptor antibody test). Chronic fatigue and muscle weakness are the symptoms associated with this disease. Development of antibodies against NMDA receptors can cause anti-NMDA encephalitis, a potentially fatal disease.

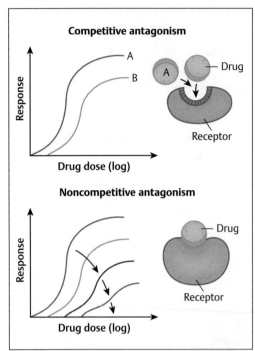

Fig. 5.9 Drugs can act as competitive antagonists (e.g., propranolol blocks action of beta-adrenergic receptors in the treatment of akathisia and tremors induced by valproate in the treatment of epilepsy). In this type of inhibition, the endogenous substrate (adrenaline, noradrenaline) cannot bind to the receptor, and the drug occupies and blocks it. In this case, the block is surmountable in case the stress occurs; the dose of propranolol can change social phobia. In the noncompetitive type of drug block, the bond between the drug and the receptors is of irreversible type, for example, phenoxybenzamine which is used to treat hypertension in pheochromocytoma.

is a receptor protein or any other micro- or macromolecule. Receptor antagonists are of two types—reversible and irreversible. Vmax is reduced by reversible antagonists, while it is unaffected by irreversible antagonists.

Drugs binding to the receptors via covalent bond bind strongly, and the drug receptor complex will have to be separated (**Fig. 5.10**).

Suppose acetylcholine (ACh) produces bradycardia, atropine can produce tachycardia by blocking muscarinic receptors on the heart. Similarly, blood pressure elevation in pheochromocytoma is extreme. A long-acting antagonist phenoxybenzamine is the drug of choice. This is an example of irreversible antagonism. One can guess that irreversible antagonism will make the drug longer acting.

Neuropsychopharmacological Agents[3,4]

A drug used in neurology or psychiatric practice is little different from many others used in general.

Such a drug mimics the action of neurotransmitter at the same site, or binds to nearby site and facilitates neurotransmitter binding. Several targets exist for CNS drugs to exploit and produce pharmacological response (**Fig. 5.11**).

The drug may also block actions of neurotransmitter at same site (antagonist). The drug acts on several different types of receptors (**Box 5.3**). Several drugs of varied classes can work in the CNS (**Table 5.1**).

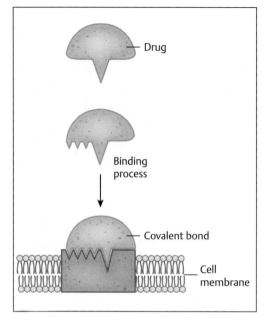

Fig. 5.10 Illustration depicting covalent bonding. A covalent bond is a powerful bond between the drug and the receptor. A traditional example is aspirin binding to the enzyme cyclooxygenase, which is used extensively in the secondary prevention of thrombotic stroke. It should be noted that, conventionally, the drug–receptor interaction is considered to be reversible but covalent bond is irreversible. Potency of agonist does not get affected in the presence of this type of antagonist, unlike in case of reversible antagonists. Duration of action of drugs of this type is long.

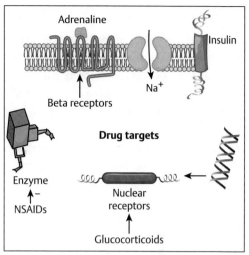

Fig. 5.11 Several drug targets in neuropsychopharmacology.

Box 5.3: Receptors are of several types

- G-protein-coupled receptors (GPCRs) (adrenaline, ACh).
- Ion-gated channels (nicotinic, gamma-aminobutyric acid [GABA] A).
- Intracellular receptors (corticosteroids, sex hormones, T3, T4, vitamin A, and vitamin D).
- Growth factor receptors (also called tyrosine kinase receptors, growth factor receptors act upon them).
- Cytokine receptors (Janus kinase [JAK] receptors use JAK signal transducer and activator of transcription [STAT] pathway).

Table 5.1 Neurotransmitters, receptors, and the drugs

Neurotransmitters	Receptors	Drugs
Glutamate	NMDA	Riluzole
GABA	GABA$_A$, GABA$_B$	Benzodiazepine, baclofen
Glycine	Glycine receptors	Strychnine
Acetylcholine	Nicotinic, muscarinic	Donepezil
Serotonin	5-HT$_{1A}$	Buspirone
Noradrenaline	Alpha receptors	Phenoxybenzamine
Dopamine	D2 receptors	Haloperidol

Abbreviations: GABA, gamma-aminobutyric acid; NMDA, N-methyl-D-aspartate; 5-HT, 5-hydroxytryptamine; D2 receptor, dopamine receptor.

Receptor Agonists

Cell-surface receptors transmit chemical signals from the outside to the inside of the cell. Some drugs bind to cell surface receptors but do not activate the receptors to trigger a response. When cell surface receptors bind to the molecule, the endogenous chemical cannot bind to the receptor and cannot trigger a response. The compound is said to "antagonize" or "block" the receptor and is referred to as a receptor antagonist. Several drugs like buspirone, sumatriptan, and buprenorphine are agonists (partial) of various receptors.

Receptor Antagonists

Most antagonists attach to binding site on receptor for endogenous agonist and sterically prevent endogenous agonist from binding. If binding is reversible, it is called as competitive antagonist, and if the binding is irreversible, then it is called as noncompetitive antagonist. However, antagonists may bind to remote site on receptor and cause allosteric effects that displace endogenous agonist or prevent endogenous agonist from activating receptor (noncompetitive antagonists).

Drug Receptor Selectivity

Alterations to a drug's chemical structure may influence potency and its binding ability. Examples include amphetamine and methamphetamine, where the potency has changed after modification of chemical structure. Many drugs have multiple sites of action and many such actions are responsible for side effects. Examples include TCAD-induced side effects such as sedation, dry mouth, blurred vision, etc.

Drug Action in Central Nervous System

Drugs in CNS work on all possible mechanisms or processes that are physiologically needed. For example, in the axons, they may act upon axons to slow or block axonal electrical conduction (antiepileptics, anesthetics, etc.). The synapse is the most common site of drug action as most drugs act here. Drugs may affect the synthesis, storage, release, or reuptake of the neurotransmitters. The best example of this class will be antidepressants. Receptors, on the other hand, can be activated or blocked, for example, by BZDs ($GABA_A$) and antipsychotics (haloperidol), respectively.

Receptors may undergo sensitization or upregulation or desensitization or downregulation.

Prolonged or continuous use of receptor blockers like beta blockers can upregulate the beta-adrenergic receptors. This is important in case of depression. Likewise, inhibition of synthesis or release of hormone/neurotransmitter can cause desensitization of neurotransmitters. This may happen after prolonged/continuous use of agonist or inhibition of degradation of neurotransmitters or the neuronal uptake of an agonist can result in desensitization.

Synergism is a Greek word that means working together. It is of two types:

- Addition (1 + 1 = 2).
- Potentiation (1 + 0 = 2).

Addition: Two drugs are combined for their beneficial effects; toxic effects do not add up. Each of these drugs can be used independently also. Nitrous oxide and ether are used together because of this. Nitrous oxide is a good analgesic but poor muscle relaxant. Ether is an excellent muscle relaxant. Both of them are used together.

Potentiation: One drug is active (1), and another drug is inactive (0). L-dopa is an active drug and carbidopa is an inactive drug. Both of them are used together. Carbidopa potentiates L-dopa.

Dose Response Curve

This is a mathematical relationship between the drug dose and the response one gets. It is of two types: Graded and quantal (**Fig. 5.12**). In graded dose response curve (DRC), a gradually increasing dose is used until a satisfactory response is obtained. Potency can be determined by this curve and is expressed in terms of median effective dose (ED_{50}), which is a dose that produces 50% of clinical response. In quantal DRC, a definite number of patients exhibit all or no response. Ratio between lethal dose (LD_{50})/ED_{50} is known as therapeutic index. It is an indicator of safety of drug (**Fig 5.13**). Drugs may have narrow or wider therapeutic index. Barbiturates are examples of narrow therapeutic index, while BZDs have wider therapeutic index.

Few definitions are considered before discussing DRC properly:

- *Dose* is the amount of drug and is denoted by potency. So, potency is the amount of drug. It is indicated by X axis of DRC.

- Efficacy is the clinical usefulness; no matter how potent the drug is, it should have clinical usefulness. It is indicated by Y axis on DRC. Effectiveness is a clinical concept and is different from efficacy, which is measured in clinical trials (**Fig. 5.13**).

- Affinity means attraction for the receptors. A drug with high affinity for receptors works in low dose. Similarly, drug that has high selectivity is safer. Paul Ehrlich, father of microbiology, said 100 years back, "if a drug is selective, it is safer." So, selectivity means safety. For example, prazosin is a selective alpha-1 receptor antagonist. It produces postural hypotension as side effect. Tamsulosin is even more selective (selective alpha-1A antagonist). Risk of postural hypotension with this is barely minimum.

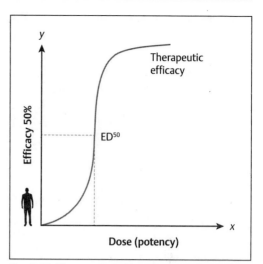

Fig. 5.12 Therapeutic index is the ratio of toxic dose/effective dose. This is a measure of a drug's safety. A large number of therapeutic index means the drug has a wide margin of safety. However, if there is a small number, then it means the drug has a small margin of safety.

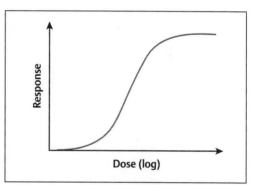

Fig. 5.13 Dose response curve (DRC) is the mathematical relationship between the dose and the response. Traditionally, it is taken as log values of the dose and the percentage of therapeutic response. On X axis, traditionally, the dose is plotted, and on the Y axis, the response is given. Normal shape of DRC is sigmoid, and it cannot be a straight line as the drug response is not easily predictable and is subjected to several factors (e.g., interindividual variations, diseases, etc.). The middle part is a relatively straight line and informs us about the safety of the drug. Parallel and right shift of DRC is produced by competitive antagonists, but noncompetitive antagonists produce flattening of DRC.

- Agonist is a drug that stimulates the receptors. It has full affinity and intrinsic activity. It is of three types: Full, partial, and inverse. Full agonist has intrinsic activity and affinity. Partial agonists have 50% intrinsic activity. Inverse agonist has efficacy but in opposite direction. **Fig. 5.14** explains the concept diagrammatically.

- Antagonist has no intrinsic activity of its own. That means unless there is an agonist along with it, an antagonist cannot act. Propranolol is a reversible antagonist of beta receptors. Parallel and rightward shift of DRC indicates competitive antagonism. Responses of various receptors could be different (**Fig. 5.15**), and it has a correlation with structure and function (**Fig. 5.16**). Cross-talk between receptors can occur (**Fig. 5.17**) and chemicals which mediate their effects are known as secondary messengers (**Fig. 5.18**).

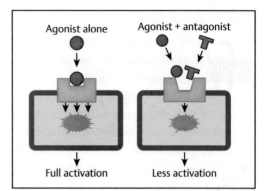

Fig. 5.14 Most of the drugs binding to the receptors resemble their natural agonists. Agonists have intrinsic activity or efficacy or affinity of binding ability or affinity. Partial agonists have half-maximal intrinsic activity and hence produce less activation of the receptors. Examples of such drugs are buprenorphine, buspirone, and sumatriptan. Some tissues like the heart may have large number of spare receptors that increase sensitivity of tissues (e.g., beta-adrenergic receptors). This creates vast amount of reserves and hence even small doses can produce large effects. Some such spare receptors have been identified in the brain also (cerebral cortex, olfactory bulb, etc.).

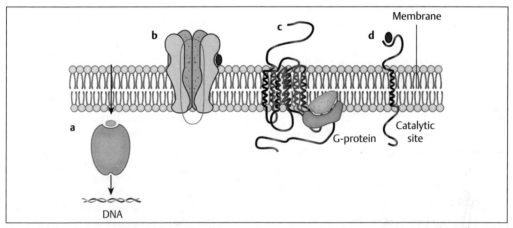

Fig. 5.15 Receptors are of several varieties; for example, some receptors are present within the cells and in the nucleus. Drugs binding to such receptors include steroids, sex hormones, and thyroid hormones **(a)**. Inflow of the currents of sodium or other ion alters electrical potential, and this is important in case of receptors like acetylcholine (ACh), NMDA, and nicotinic receptors also. Ligands of gamma-aminobutyric acid (GABA$_A$) receptors are extensively used in neurological and psychiatric diseases. The responses are produced fast due to rapid conduction **(b)**. G-protein–coupled receptors (GPCRs) are the largest class of receptors, and G-protein is a GTP binding protein with three subunits (α, β, and γ). Endocytosis of such receptors can also occur **(c)**. Certain ligand-bound receptors include receptors for insulin and epidermal growth factor receptors (EGFRs) which get phosphorylated once the ligand binds to them. Inhibition of tyrosine kinase receptors is important in case of neoplastic diseases **(d)**.

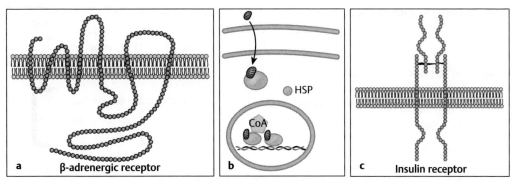

Fig. 5.16 (a) Drugs show a high degree of correlation between the structure of the receptors and their own to produce pharmacological response. **(b)** Slight change in the structure of receptors can change the drug action remarkably. **(c)** Quantitative relation between the drug and the response is determined by receptors. CoA, coenzyme A; HSP, heat-shock proteins.

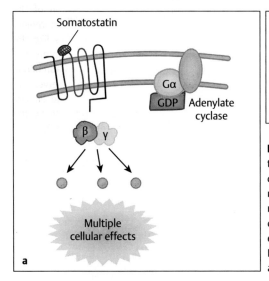

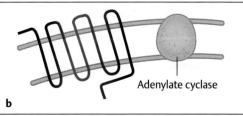

Fig. 5.17 (a,b) Receptors for many biogenic amines that are extensively employed in neuropsychopharmacology for understanding actions of drugs of central nervous system (CNS) class are G-protein–coupled receptors (GPCRs) (histamine, acetylcholine [ACh], dopamine [DA], adrenaline, etc.). G-protein–regulated enzymes include adenyl cyclase and phospholipase C. Importantly, they may have cross-talk with ion channels also, as described earlier.

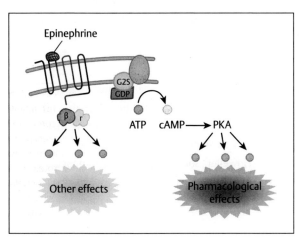

Fig. 5.18 Secondary messengers are small molecules or ions that are found within the cells and mediate pharmacological responses of drugs. cAMP, cGMP, and calcium phospho-inositide are the best-studied secondary messengers.

51

Sites of Drug Action in CNS

A drug can act at various levels in the CNS as opposed to the gut where a single process is likely to be affected rather than multiple ones. For example, in the CNS, entire activity done by the neuron may be the target of drug therapy and includes the following:

- Conduction.
- Synthesis and storage.
- Release and reuptake.
- Degradation.

Likewise, several additional factors should be considered when considering drug action in the brain. For example, in the gut, bones, or vessels, receptors are generally postsynaptic. In the CNS, the action can occur at both pre- and postsynaptic levels. Additionally, ion channels and second messengers can be the drug targets.

Most neurotransmitters can activate multiple receptor subtypes and receptor classes. Selectivity is achieved by targeting the receptors or their subtypes. The drugs have actions on allosteric sites on receptors as well as presynaptic and postsynaptic actions. The drugs may have partial/inverse agonist (activity-dependent) action. The drug may change neuronal plasticity, and neurons may experience adaptive changes as well. Drug metabolism too may play a role.

Interindividual Variations of Drug Responses in Neuropyschopharmacology

Doses of the drugs used vary among individuals widely; so, the prescribers should have idea about this important concept of interindividual variations. The sources of variations can be summarized as follows:

- Pharmacokinetic: Gender and races where differences in rates of metabolism can occur. Additionally, renal impairment can cause differences in the drug responses by

changing plasma levels of drugs. Hepatic diseases of gross nature have certain effect of drug levels. Drug–drug interactions are common in CNS drugs, and one should be cautious of using too many drugs. Finally, drug polymorphisms are beginning to be understood in developing nations and can pose a special challenge when dosages of the drugs described in Western literature are given to Indian patients.

- Pharmacodynamic: Pharmacological responses of certain drugs may be affected by the gender and race as is the case with pharmacokinetic variations. Also, diseases can affect drug responses. Receptor abnormalities or mutations can change drug behavior in vivo. Also, tolerance to the drugs is an important issue in BZD therapy.

Tolerance

Tolerance and dependence are big issues in CNS drugs' administration. Tolerance means the reduced effect of drug, while dependence means that a new physiological milieu has been achieved and discontinuation is difficult or else withdrawal may occur. Tolerance may be metabolic (pharmacokinetic, like metabolism tolerance due to enzyme induction). The same can also be cellular, where adaptive (pharmacodynamic) changes can occur. The behavioral conditioning too can lead to tolerance, where the patient believes that the drug is no longer being effective.

Dependence

Dependence could be serious as stopping the drug could produce full-fledged abstinence syndrome. It is important to know that not all addictive drugs produce physical dependence. However, some nonaddictive therapeutic drugs (e.g., SSRIs) can produce physical dependence. Withdrawal will, however, be mild though.

General Rules of Treating Psychiatric and Neurological Disorders

- Establish a diagnosis and identify the target symptoms that will be used to monitor therapy response. This makes the task simpler. For example, in cerebral palsy, identifying and treating seizures may be an important therapeutic goal.

- Treat any other comorbid conditions when you are selecting an agent to treat—often one can get two birds with one stone! For example, depression with fibromyalgia with duloxetine.

- Choice of agent and dosage: One will have to select an agent with an acceptable side effect profile and use the lowest effective dose. Remember the delayed response for many psych meds and drug–drug interactions.

- Select the agent based on patient's history, current symptom profile, and the side effect profile of the medication—there is no one correct answer in most cases.

- The patient should understand the benefits and risks of the medications, and gross major side effects should be told to the patient. In fertile women, make sure to document teratogenicity discussion, especially with lithium and sodium valproate.

- Have a treatment monitoring program to track and document compliance, side effects, target symptom response, blood levels, and blood tests, as and when appropriate.

- Adverse effects of the CNS agents can be considerable. Hence, it is important that prescribers have experience in prescribing and handling them. Once someone becomes experienced, it is easy to handle them like any other drug class.

Clinical Research in Neuropsychopharmacology

Randomized Clinical Trials

Clinical neuropsychopharmacology keeps growing and changing. Clinical trials provide new evidence of this change. Randomized trials are considered to be the highest form of evidence accepted in modern times for the safety and efficacy of drug treatment using human subjects. Understanding trials will enable us to be aware of foundations of evidence-based methods in a detailed manner. Clinical trial uses placebo or the active drug as a comparator and either confirm or refute the claim that the said drug is more effective than the standard drug.

Blinding

This is a form of experiment in which participants are deliberately kept in darkness about whether the patient is taking placebo or the active drug. Do the patients know what they are taking? It will be difficult for them to exhibit true pharmacological response. It is always going to be mixed with psychological response. Knowing that a patient is getting the placebo can change the way a patient behaves in an experiment. This is known as the Hawthorne effect. To avoid this effect, blinding is used. A person who is not directly connected with the trial (say a nurse or a pharmacist) will be given the task of assigning random numbers to patients and assign them into two groups, for example, containing placebo or active comparator, as per the protocol.

Blinding, therefore, ensures that the psychological bias is removed. Other forms of biases that get eliminated include observer bias.

For example, if the physicians are aware that they have some patients who are "favorites," they willingly or unknowingly may assign them active "drug." External validity of such a trial is limited.

53

So, it is clear that until and unless there is a comparator, that is, placebo or the active drug, it is hard to say that the said effect in a clinical trial is due to the presence of the drug itself and not due to other factors.

Different Types of Clinical Trials

There are many types of clinical trials, but there are four main phases of these trials. These include the following:

Phase I: This is known as pharmacokinetic trial. Normally, 20 to 50 subjects are recruited and an attempt is carried out to determine maximally tolerated dose in this form. Safety data get generated by this type of trial. Nowadays, there is a trend of using pharmacokinetic/pharmacodynamic (pk/pd) data and make more sense about the way a drug works. Comparator or placebo will not be needed here as we are not trying to test the efficacy.

Phase II: This is known as efficacy trial. Around 50 to 300 patients are recruited. Healthy volunteers are generally not taken nowadays as this is increasingly becoming a "mini-phase-III" study. The aim is to further confirm findings of the phase-I trial and to know what happens when the same results are repeated in a large number of cases.

Phase III: These are called as double-blind placebo controlled randomized trials. Normally 300 to 1,000 patients are recruited. Since there are a large number of patients in randomized trials, this has to be a highly organized process. Randomization is the cornerstone. Failing of proper randomization will limit the generalizability of trial. It has placebo or active control, and the evidence of refuting null hypothesis is searched. The alternative hypothesis is accepted if evidence is so found.

Phase IV: This is a pharmacovigilance study and a common type of pragmatic trial. In this form, one will try to observe a drug for possible side effects associated with the drug. Since some side effects are always going to be missed if we take a small sample size, the aim is always to take a large sample. Usually, it is done in a sample size > 1,000. Since it is done after the drug has gotten the final approval for marketing, it is also known as phase IV trial or postmarketing surveillance. It is often termed as "adverse drug reaction monitoring" trial. This is one of the most potent tools to ensure good drug safety. Case reports by clinicians could be the beginning of some thorough clinical studies that could be initiated once we get some hint that the drug is associated with side effect/s. This process is known as signal generation.

A decision to continue with the drug or to withdraw could be taken, based upon the results of phase IV studies. They could also be initiated if we get hints that already-marketed drug is associated with a particular side effect. This happened with zimeldine, a drug of SSRI class, which was withdrawn later. True signals, however, need to be differentiated from false signals. This process is known as "signal-to-noise" ratio.

Trial Designs

There are several ways to classify the trial designs:

- Parallel group design: Patients are randomized either to the treatment arm or to the placebo arm or to the (test) and (control) arm using standard comparators. They are followed-up prospectively to know the efficacy difference as and when they emerge. There could be several variants of these:
  ◊ Sequential crossover: A single patient given placebo who continues taking it and later on gets the drug.
  ◊ Group sequential trials: At certain stages that are defined in the protocol,

one could get an idea about efficacy of clinical trials. They could be evaluated and stopped when desired results are obtained.

◊ Adapted designs: A trial is stopped midway and some changes in design and protocol could be done.

- Factorial design: Normally, patients are assigned one treatment-comparison group and are followed up. In such a trial, a single patient may be randomized in two or more groups.

- Cluster randomized trial: This is parallel group design; the only difference is that rather than the individuals being randomized, a cluster of patients, for example, hospitals and clinics, or groups of patients are randomized.

Trial Centers

Trials could conveniently be done at a single center. However, nowadays, they are preferably done at multiple centers. Multicentric studies are done for the following reasons:

- Sufficient number of cases could be found if more than one center is inducted at the same time.

- To improve generalizability.

Exploratory versus Confirmatory Trial

If we are the first ones to conduct a clinical trial, then it is known as exploratory trial. Others will have to confirm the results; hence, it will be termed as confirmatory trial.

Biases

A clinical trial may or may not show the true difference and hence may be subjected to lot of biases. So, it may have false positive and false negative results. Both biases and contamination can result. There is a possibility of random error also.

There are two main kinds of errors noted in clinical trials:

- Systematic error.
- Random error.

Systematic Error

This can result from the trial design and hence will affect interpretation of results. Mostly, it is related to selection of subjects and outcome measurements. For example, if the investigators know what is being given to which group, they may have a psychological bias and may favor treatment.

Likewise, exclusion of missing subjects due to lack of proper data or compliance may also affect the analysis and interfere with trial results. This may overestimate the benefit offered by the trial. Advanced trial designs seek to eliminate these biases from clinical trials.

Confounding

This is a special form of distorted relationship that may come about due to an extraneous variable, and we may false attribute it to some other variable. For example, if we wish to know the relationship between physical inactivity and brain disease, then a number of potential confounders will emerge. These include smoking, alcohol, weight, sex, age, hyperlipidemia, diabetes, etc.

The most effective method to deal with confounders is to randomize the subjects so that they are distributed equally among both groups. Both known and unknown confounders could be distributed like this.

Random Error

Even in the best of trial designs, errors due to measurements, individual variations, and sampling can occur. Proper recording of data, therefore, may be of value. Most studies will be studying only a part of the sample; therefore, one should keep in mind the possibility of sampling error. This may be reduced by selecting a large number of participants or using special techniques for analysis, for example, meta-analysis. These are termed as "studies of studies."

Interim Monitoring

Safety of the patients in clinical trials is paramount; hence, during interim analysis, an attempt is made to monitor safety of drugs in a periodic manner. Safety monitoring board, ethics committees, and the Drug Controller General of India will ensure that the drug safety data are properly generated. Likewise, if there is major evidence that the desired results have been obtained, then one could stop the trial (stop trial for efficacy).

Final Data Analysis

If there are lots of missing values and also issues about compliance, it may be advisable to conduct intention-to-treat analysis.

Intention-to-Treat Analysis

Intention-to-treat analysis deals with outcomes of the patients who were randomized but subsequently discontinued or changed treatment. This is a pragmatic realization of trial, and it is taken "as if the patients, who were enrolled and randomized, finished trial" as well.

Doing intention-to-treat analysis and using two-sided p value is a good fallback option for clinical trials. Moreover, results could be stratified to reduce random error. Time to event end points could be demonstrated by Kaplan–Meier plots. Size of treatment effect could be calculated from hazard ratios derived from proportional hazard model. Cox regression model could be used to adjust hazard ratio for other factors that might affect prognosis. Subgroup analysis could be done using test for heterogeneity to assess for possible interaction effect between treatment and baseline

variables. Statistical analysis is prespecified in protocol, and one should preferably stick to the same.

Consolidated Standards of Reporting Trials (CONSORT) Guidelines

A trial is published in accordance with the statement and guidelines of reporting.

Trial Profile

A trial profile is provided in the clinical trial to describe the flow of participants through each stage of the randomized controlled trial, that is, enrollment, randomization, treatment allocation, follow-up, etc. Analysis of a clinical trial should be specified, and it should also be mentioned if midterm analysis will be done, and if so, then at what stage. The baseline characteristics of patient, for example, demographic information, history of intercurrent illnesses like brain diseases/risk factors, medical history, treatment history, etc., are noted. Randomized patients should be comparable in order to reduce systematic error.

Case Series

A case series is effectively a register of interesting cases prepared by clinicians. Usually, it is a coherent and consecutive set of cases of a disease (or similar problem), which is derived from a general practice or a defined health care setting, for example, a hospital. The reports are sent to a medical journal. The aim is to analyze cases together to learn about the disease collectively. A case series is the key to sound case control and cohort studies and trials. That means, they can serve as the starting point where the hypothesis or a theory gets generated. Case series are very helpful to learn about symptoms and signs, create case definitions, and receive clinical education, audit and research.

Cross-Sectional Studies

Cross-sectional studies are the "snap shot" of the population and are also known as prevalence studies. This is because the sample size calculations are easy and are not very time-consuming. Few of the strengths include the following: It is done in quick time, does not take long time to complete, one can study several diseases at the same time, and it is very useful to determine the population burden of disease. It is also a good tool to carry out health planning and prioritize health problems. In a population studied at a specific time and place (a cross-section), the primary output is prevalence data, although association between risk factors and disease can be generated. In this regard, the cross-sectional studies resemble case-control studies. However, it should be noted that they are not hypothesis testing studies.

These studies are good for calculating the point prevalence. The period prevalence is the number of cases during the study period divided by the population. If the population is unclear, then this must be specified. Cross-sectional studies are good tools to calculate the point prevalence, as stated earlier; this must, however, be differentiated from lifetime prevalence. Such studies can show the association between two factors, but case-control studies or cohort studies are the best in terms of showing the associations. One should bear in mind the following criteria proposed by Bradford Hill:

- Findings should be consistent.
- There should be a temporal relationship between the stimuli and the occurrence of phenomena.
- Biological gradient should favor the same. For example, in an area with high prevalence of malaria, a new onset fever should be taken as malaria until proved otherwise due to high gradient.
- Plausible mechanism should be given to explain the occurrence.
- Coherence between the occurrence and laboratory values will increase concordance.
- Similar factors could be accounted for.
- Strength of association should be good.

Case-Control Studies

Case-control studies are a popular way of studying the "cause and effect relationship." It can be considered to be the "poor man's" substitute for experimental design, wherein one wants to prove or disprove a given hypothesis. However, this design will give the association and not the "proof" that a given factor is causally related. They are less expensive compared to several other study designs and not too time-consuming. One of the best features of this type of study design is that it allows the investigator to study the noncommunicable or rare diseases. However, if the exposure is rare, then it may not be a good study design. Several biases such as selection bias and recall bias can affect the results.

The cross-sectional study can be repeated, and if the same sample is studied for a second time and followed up, the original cross-sectional study now becomes a cohort study. If during a cohort study, possibly in a subgroup, the investigator imposes an intervention, a trial begins. In the cohort study, case-control studies can be conducted as well using incident cases. This is called as nested case-control study.

Sometimes, the cases are compared with some special controls known as reference groups. For example, if we are studying the hippocampal volume of a group of elderly with or without diabetes, we should have normative data as well who will serve as the "controls" or "internal controls." In such a design, where there is a requirement of normative data, it is not possible to validate data unless the normative data is not there. Therefore, selection of control is an important feature of case-control studies.

Cohort Studies

This is a grand design and can be prospective and retrospective. An example of the prospective design may be infants who are born in heavily polluted areas with lead and following them up for next 5 years for incidence of foot drop. Likewise, all the men and women born in the year 1980 and their frequency of heart disease will be an example of a retrospective cohort. One of the best features of this design is that several outcomes can be studied at the same time, and it is very good to study the incident cases. However, this is time-consuming and at times may not be feasible at all. Relative risk can be calculated as opposed to case-control studies, where the odds of having the disease in the cases are compared with that of the controls.

Open Label Trials

These types of trials are very commonly done in psychiatry and neurology. These clinical trials are done without control groups and are known as uncontrolled trials. Since there is a lack of comparison group, they convey less information. In early stages of clinical research, they may play an important role. They, however, could be succeeded by the large-scale clinical trials to confirm the same. They are often done for finding pharmacokinetic details and also determine the

maximal dose of the drugs. Comparison groups are not included in open label trials, and both doctor and patients know who is getting what. Usefulness of open labeled trials is given in **Table 5.2**.

Uncontrolled trials have an important role in clinical research and provide a ground for evaluating new and untested treatments. They often serve to generate sufficient evidence for further exploration of trials. If it is unethical to include a control group, for example, in surgical trials, uncontrolled trials with before and after evaluation could be the best method of evaluation.

Pharmacovigilance[1-6]

Pharmakon is a Greek word that means "medicinal substances" and vigilare is a Latin word which means "to keep watch"; therefore, pharmacovigilance is keeping a "watch on the medicinal substances" for their safety. The main goal of this activity is to improve the safe and rational use of medicines, thereby improving patient care and public health. This is a very important concept in clinical neuro-psychopharmacology as adverse drug reactions (ADRs) of CNS drugs often top the list.

Adverse drug reactions are long-term effects of the drug interactions, which become probable when several drugs are used at the same time.

Postmarketing surveillance (phase 4) is the most important process to detect such

Table 5.2 Strengths of uncontrolled trials

Strengths	Weakness
• Generate hypothesis	• Investigator bias may occur as investigators may believe in their own treatments
• Provide ground for large-scale treatment	• Interpretation could be difficult and may not be as informative as the controlled trials
• If it is unethical to include a control group, then one can go ahead	• Concurrent control group provides best chance of interpreting the results as immediate comparison is available

drug-related problems that were not identified during the premarketing phases.

The World Health Organization (WHO) defines pharmacovigilance as "the science and activities relating to the detection, assessment, understanding and prevention of adverse effects or any other drug-related problem." Pharmacovigilance covers various areas as mentioned in **Table 5.3**.

Adverse Drug Reaction

An ADR can be defined as any untoward, unintended, noxious, and unpleasant response of a drug, which occurs at doses normally used for the prophylaxis, diagnosis, or therapy of a disease, or for the modification of physiological functions. Types (alphabetical categorization) of ADRs are given below:

- Type A (augmented).
- Type B (bizarre).
- Type C (continuous drug usage).
- Type D (delayed).

Type A (Augmented)

These are related to the principal action of the drug and can occur in anyone during the course of drug treatment. These are mostly dose related and predictable. They usually represent pharmacodynamic effects and are the most common type of drug reactions. Skilled management (e.g., dose reduction) can reduce their incidence.

Type B (Bizarre)

These types of ADRs are not related to the principal action of the drug and are hence not common and only occur in some people. Their occurrence is not part of the pharmacology of the drug and hence they are not dose related. Mostly, they are unpredictable and hence called *idiosyncratic*. Unfortunately, they account for most drug fatalities.

Type C (Continuous Drug Usage)

These types of ADRs are due to long-term use of the drug and include tardive dyskinesia, which can even be permanent. In many countries, written consent from the patient is needed before starting antipsychotic drugs.

Type D (Delayed)

Effects like teratogenicity and carcinogenicity are the examples of this type of ADR. They are not common, but drugs like phenytoin, carbamazepine, and valproate have teratogenicity. Similarly, lithium is a teratogenic drug.

Medication Errors

Medication errors are common in neurology and psychiatric practice as is the case with rest of the practice in medicine. In neuropsychiatry practice,

Table 5.3 Definitions of terms related to pharmacovigilance

Term	Definition	Example
ADR	Harm caused by the use of a drug at normal doses	Sedation by BZD
ADE	Harm caused by the use of a drug	Falls during antipsychotic treatment
Medication error	Preventable event that may cause inappropriate use of a drug or patient harm	High dose of haloperidol for a patient of dementia with aggression
Potential ADE	Situations that could result in harm by the use of a drug but did not harm the patient	Diabetes during antipsychotic treatment

Abbreviations: ADE, adverse drug event; ADR, adverse drug reaction; BZD, benzodiazepine.

since multiple drugs with narrow therapeutic index are used, the chances are significant.

The National Coordinating Council for Medication Error Reporting and Prevention defines medication error as "any preventable event that may cause or may lead to inappropriate medication use or patient harm while the medication is in the control of the health care professional, patient, or consumer." Errors can be harmless or detrimental to the patient.

Such events may be related to professional practice, for example, using high dose or drug combinations that are inappropriate for health care products, procedures, and systems, defective prescribing or wrong order communication; product labeling mistakes, packaging errors, and nomenclature difficulties; compounding problems; wrong dispensing/distribution/administration and defects in patient education, monitoring and use of drugs.

There could be many causes of medication errors, but the major ones include the following three factors:

- *Human factors*:
  - ◇ Heavy staff workload and fatigue due to prolonged hospital duties.
  - ◇ Inexperience, lack of training, poor handwriting, and oral orders.
  - ◇ Professional negligence.
- *Workplace factors*:
  - ◇ Poor lighting, noise, and interruptions in the outpatient departments.
- *Pharmaceutical factors*:
  - ◇ Excessive prescribing.
  - ◇ Confusing nomenclature of drugs, especially drug names resembling each other, for example, chlorpromazine, chlorzoxazone, chlordiazepoxide, etc., or packaging or labeling.

- ◇ Frequency and complexity of calculations needed to prescribe drugs, for example, dosage calculation in loading and maintenance dose in critical care neurological illness.

Adverse Drug Event[1-4]

These are drug-related injuries, with at least a reasonable possibility of it being caused by a number of reasons. The direct pharmacological mechanism of a drug may be related to an individual's particular vulnerability to a drug. Drug interactions may be responsible in some cases. Unexpected therapeutic ineffectiveness (e.g., product quality problems or antimicrobial resistance) could account for adverse drug event (ADE). Medication errors are an important category.

Pharmacovigilance in India[1,2]

The Pharmacovigilance Program of India was started with the objective to safeguard the health of people of India. ADRs are reported from all over the country to the National Coordinating Centre, which also works in association with the global ADR monitoring center in order to contribute to the global ADR database. It monitors the ADRs occurring among the Indian population and helps authorities in taking decision for the safe use of medicines. The main idea of the pharmacovigilance program involves improving patient safety and welfare among the Indian population by monitoring drug safety, thereby reducing the risk associated with use of medicines.

References

1. Medications errors. Available at: http://www.nccmerp.org/aboutMedErrors.html. Accessed on August 9, 2016
2. Pharmacovigilance & Drug safety. Available at: http://www.who.int/medicines/areas/

quality_safety/safety_efficacy/pharmvigi/
en. Accessed on August 9, 2016

3. WHO statement on drug safety. Available at:
http://www.who-umc.org/graphics/28550.
pdf. Accessed on August 9, 2016

4. Center for drug control. Available at: http://
www.cdsco.nic.in. Accessed on August 9,
2016

5. Drug safety. Available at: http://ipc.nic.in/
writereaddata/linkimages/pvpi-2611733
527.pdf. Accessed on August 9, 2016

6. Iturriaga-Vásquez P, Alzate-Morales J,
Bermudez I, Varas R, Reyes-Parada M.
Multiple binding sites in the nicotinic
acetylcholine receptors: an opportunity for
polypharmacology. Pharmacol Res 2015;
101:9–17

Drug Treatment of Headaches

Vikas Dhikav

Clinical Case Example

- A 32-year-old housewife, slightly overweight, presented with a 4-year old history of right-sided hemicrania and depressive features. She has a sharp pain during attack, visible aura, occasional nausea, and vomiting with irritability. She is hypersensitive to sounds and has a desire to rest in a dark, noise-free room. What drugs will be appropriate for this patient?

Answer: Treatment may involve sumatriptan as per need basis and amitriptyline 25 mg at bedtime. Since the patient has depressive features, this is the most likely choice. Initiate the chosen drug at a low dose and titrate up (usually every 2–4 weeks) until benefits occur or side effects prevent any further increase in dose. Initial sedation occurs until tolerance develops. Patient should be encouraged to maintain a headache diary. A 2 to 3 months' trial is needed before decision is made to withdraw. After a year, the drug should be withdrawn even if it has been effective. It should be noted that prophylaxis is best done with monotherapy and multiple agents have not shown any significant benefit.

Introduction[1-4]

Headache disorders are among the most common of central nervous system (CNS) disorders. It has been seen that almost half of the world's population may have experienced headache, at least, once a year. Headache is described as a functional pain in the head as in most patients with headache, there is no sign of tissue damage. Injuring the brain itself does not cause pain but causes altered brain functions. The membrane and blood vessels of the brain are, however, very pain sensitive. Headache may be primary or secondary. Migraine, cluster, and tension type of headaches are common primary headaches. Secondary headaches are caused by intracranial lesions, head injury, cervical spondylitis, dental

or ocular diseases, and temporomandibular joint dysfunction. Sinusitis and depression can also account for headache. Very high blood pressure can be a cause of headache. A significant number of patients with brain tumors can present with a headache.

Several pain-sensitive structures are there in the brain, for example, scalp, aponeurosis, arteries, dura mater, sinuses, falx cerebri, pial surfaces, etc. Inflammation, traction, compression, and malignant infiltration are common neurological causes of headache. Several functional headaches exist where there is no clear-cut mechanism that can be delineated. Tension headache, migraine, trigeminal neuralgia, cluster headache, poststroke headache, and tumor- or trauma-induced headaches are common in practice (**Box 6.1**).

Box 6.1: Types of headaches

- Primary:
  ◊ Migraine headache.
  ◊ Tension-type headache.
  ◊ Cluster headache.
  ◊ Paroxysmal hemicrania.
  ◊ Short-lasting unilateral neuralgia with conjunctival injection (SUNCT).
  ◊ Trigeminal neuralgia.
  ◊ Chronic daily headache.
- Secondary:
  ◊ Medication overuse (rebound).
  ◊ Trauma.
  ◊ Vascular disorders, for example, subarachnoid hemorrhage (SAH), arteriovenous malformation (AVM), vasculitis, etc.
  ◊ Changes in intracranial pressure (ICP).
  ◊ Brain tumors.
  ◊ Infections.

Box 6.2: Trouble indicators in headache

- First or worst headache ("thunderclap headache").
- Progressive or new daily persistent headache.
- Old patient or child.
- Headache associated with fever, rash, stiff neck, etc.
- Headache associated with abnormal mental status or abnormal neurological findings.

Box 6.3: Rules of treating headaches

- Rule out potentially dangerous (secondary) headache:
  ◊ Neoplasm, infection, hemorrhage, etc.
- Thorough history and physical examination of the patient.
- Diagnose headache type.
- Implement treatment.
- Monitor outcome.

Most of the headaches are primary, and secondary headaches are not common and account for < 2% of the headaches. Also, headaches are benign diseases but can be indicative of serious illnesses if any of the warning signs, as listed in **Box 6.2**, are noted.

Although the headache treatment is individualized, there are certain general rules of handling headaches (**Box 6.3**).

Migraine

Migraine is a painful headache syndrome that is preceded or accompanied by sensory symptoms such as light flashes, blind spots, tingling, numbness, nausea or vomiting, and photophobia or phonophobia. It is the most common type of headache. This is also the most common cause of "pulsatile headache," which is typically unilateral.

Migraine is a complex disorder of the brain, characterized by "hemicrania" which is periodic in nature. This is a disorder of brain neuron excitability and is not just a "vascular headache"

that "throbs." It is very common and yet under-recognized clinically. Key to handling migraine is to diagnose by appropriate history-taking and clinical examination. This does not underscore the use of appropriate medications as and when needed. Headache without aura is common.

History[5,6]

Migraine has been known to the mankind for the last 5,000 to 7,000 years, making it perhaps the oldest of all headaches. Galen introduced the term *megrim* (after hemicranias). Egyptians were perhaps first to think of this as a clinical entity and introduced some herbal magical remedies. Later on in the 10th century, Arabians introduced some brutal treatments like iron rod penetration of the scalp for migraine. Similarly, the treatments in 1600s started by Western doctors were no less cruel and included bloodletting, leech therapy, etc. The decade of 1870s saw the arrival of some sensible treatments like cold sponges. In the 1970s, ergot alkaloids were introduced, and ergotamine tartrate came into being in 1925;

in the next decade or so, it became the drug of choice.

Blood flow in the brain theory became popular in the 1970s and it is still the leading one. Wolf delineated pathology of migraine by introducing the concept of "cortical spreading depression." He was able to track his own scotoma by the use of perimetry.

Epidemiology

Migraine is a very common disorder and up to 1 in 4 women and 1 in 10 men may have migraine. As much as 5% of women have headache more than 15 days per month. It is a heavy burden on society in terms of direct and indirect costs; worse is that the majority of patients with migraine have not received an appropriate diagnosis or are not receiving appropriate therapy.

Pathophysiology

Migraine is a neurovascular disorder with altered central neuronal processing, where activation of brain stem nuclei, cortical hyperexcitability, occurs with cortical spreading depression. There is an involvement of trigeminovascular system, liberating neuropeptide release, which causes inflammation in cranial vessels and dura, leading to headache (**Fig. 6.1**).

In a typical migraine attack, headache starts with premonition in migraine, followed by aura and headache, which is accompanied by nausea and vomiting. Patients usually get tired after migraine attack.

Neurovascular dysfunction related to vasodilation of blood vessels is the main cause of headache, which is mediated by the fifth cranial nerve. Neuropeptides are released by parasympathetic nerve fibers. Complex polygenic inheritance may be found. Familial hemiplegic migraine cases have autosomal dominant pattern, while in rest of the migraine cases, polygenic inheritance is

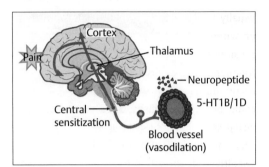

Fig. 6.1 Pathophysiology of migraine. The severe headache phase correlates with the vasodilation produced as a result of several processes. The hallmark of migraine is the involvement of trigeminovascular system triggering neuropeptide release, which causes painful involvement of cranial vessels and dura mater. Neuronal sensitization due to which neurons become highly sensitive to nociceptive stimuli plays an important role in pathophysiology of migraine.

found. This type may have lateralized weakness with aura. Mutation in vascular genes has been found.

Phases of Migraine

There are four phases of migraine: Prodrome, aura, pain, and postdrome.

- **Prodrome:** This is a phase that may begin days before migraine starts. Patients become irritated and behavioral changes may also occur.
- **Aura:** Neurological phenomena like visual symptoms often occur during this phase.
- **Pain phase:** One-sided headache with nausea and vomiting often starts. Photophobia and phonophobia may occur.
- **Postdrome:** This is a period after the headache is over and patients tend to feel very weak or fatigued after this.

Clinical Features[6–9]

Migraine is a hemicrania, and pain is usually moderate to severe. The symptoms are localized usually to one side, and there is an "aura" with or without nausea or vomiting. There is high sensitivity to light (photophobia) or sound (phonophobia); osmophobia (fear of foul smells) occurs during the migraine attack and patients could be irritated easily. Aura usually involves visual symptoms and may involve field defects such as flashes of lights (photopsias), etc. Cognitive impairment and blurring of vision can occur as well. Symptoms gradually build and may last for hours. Focal distances may occur due to constriction of internal carotid arties. Aphasia, numbness, and clumsiness can also occur. Onset of migraine often occurs in teenagers or young adults but can occur at any age. Ophthalmoplegic migraine may lead to pain around the eye and also involve nausea, vomiting, and diplopia. In basllar artery migraine, dysarthria, disequilibrium, tinnitus, and vertigo can occur with visual symptoms. This is two to three times more common in women than in men. Loud noise, flashes of lights, stress, lack of sleep, hunger, menstrual cycle, and oral contraceptive pills are common precipitants.

Pharmacotherapy[10-12]

Avoiding triggers is important. Management of migraine depends in acute phase on nonsteroidal anti-inflammatory drugs (NSAIDs) and several drugs that act on serotonin receptors. It will be worthwhile to review serotonin receptors briefly here before discussing details of pharmacotherapy.

Serotonin and Its Receptors

Serotonin is synthesized from l-tryptophan by hydroxylation and decarboxylation. Serotonin is present in major amount in enterochromaffin cells of the intestine (gastrointestinal [GI] tract). Platelets acquire serotonin as they pass through the circulation. Serotonin is metabolized to 5-hydroxyindole acetic acid.

Serotonin has a rich array of receptors through which it exhibits its pharmacological responses:

- 5-HT1A (5-HT1A to 5-HT1F): These are the major classes of serotonin receptors present in presynaptic neurons. 5-HT1 receptors are coupled to inhibition of cAMP generation. 5-HT1B class of receptors is present in coronary and cerebral circulation, and their stimulation can cause vasoconstriction.
- 5-HT2 (5-HT2A, 5-HT2B, 5-HT2C): Stimulation of receptors of this class leads to constriction of vessels and stimulates smooth muscles of intestines. Platelet aggregation is also stimulated.
- 5-HT3: These receptors are coupled to ligand-gated channels; stimulation can cause nausea and vomiting. These receptors are also important in pain occurrence at the periphery.

Management of migraine starts from elimination of triggers, stressors, and use of mild analgesics (like paracetamol) or NSAIDs (ibuprofen, naproxen) for mild headaches. Certain drugs (**Box 6.4**) tend to worsen migraine and should be dealt with accordingly.

Acute Treatment of Migraine[7-9]

For routine cases, NSAIDs like ibuprofen and paracetamol are good choices. Naproxen is favored due to its rapid absorption and high bioavailability, and peak plasma levels are reached within 2 hours. The drug is available in combination with domperidone and is given at doses of 250 to 500 mg. Prochlorperazine 5 to 10 mg could also

Box 6.4: Drugs worsening migraine
• Oral contraceptives.
• Selective serotonin reuptake inhibitors (SSRIs).
• Nasal decongestants.
• Corticosteroids.

be given. In case they fail, addition of caffeine may help. Naproxen is useful in such cases as well. Sumatriptan is tried in cases that fail on NSAIDs (**Table 6.1**). Analgesics should not be continued for long and may be given for a period of a month. Combination of analgesics should not be used for more than 10 to 15 days a month. Such cases may need to be reviewed for possible prophylaxis. The tablets should be taken at the onset of headache for best results. Intravenous (IV) propofol could be given in intractable cases in subanesthetic cases.

Treatment of Severe Attack of Migraine[10]

For severe headache, triptans or dihydroergotamine with or without antiemetics is indicated. A reassuring advice would be the following: "Migraine cannot be cured but can be controlled." Use of frequent analgesics, however, should be discouraged as it may lead to "medication overuse headache (MOH)" also. Sometimes, antiemetic alone may be able to relieve the headache.

Triptans are the drugs of choice for severe attacks. They are quite effective for acute phase of headache but are not without side effects.[9] These are selective agonists of serotonin receptors (5-HT1B/1D) and are not the analgesics per se. They especially block the release of vasoactive neuropeptides that trigger migraine pain. They are most effective when taken at the onset of pain. They are available in a variety of formulations like oral, basal, and subcutaneous (SC) forms. It should be noted that overuse can cause "MOH."

Dehydration from vomiting should be treated by IV fluids (1–2 L of normal saline). Metoclopramide 10 mg IV or prochlorperazine 5 to 10 mg IV helps to abort severe persistent attacks. Prochlorperazine is also available as rectal suppository (10–25 mg) for those patients who fail to tolerate oral formulations. Dihydroergotamine can be subcutaneously administered or used as an intranasal spray.

It should be noted that both ergotamines and triptans can worsen coronary artery disease (CAD) and are contraindicated. These should also be used with caution in elderly patients or those with known vascular risk factors, for example, hypertension or heart disease.

Opioids such as pethidine or pentazocine are last options for severe headaches.

Ergotamine

Ergotamine is structurally similar to amines, serotonin, norepinephrine, and dopamine and hence interacts with multiple receptors. The

Table 6.1 Doses of commonly used antimigraine drugs in acute attack

Drug	Dosage
Ergotamine tartrate	Available as caffergot (ergotamine tartrate = 1 mg and caffeine = 100 mg)
Dihydroergotamine	60–120 mg
Aspirin	300–900 mg every 4–6 h
Ibuprofen	400–800 mg every 6 h
Naproxen	250–500 mg every 12
Paracetamol	500–650 mg every 6–8 h
Sumatriptan	50–200 mg in 24 h
Rizatriptan	5–30 mg in 24 h
Almotriptan	6.25–12 mg given as a single dose; maximum dose is 25 mg
Zolmitriptan	1.25–5 mg given as single dose; not to exceed 10 mg in 24 h

main pharmacological effect responsible for therapeutic effect is constriction of the blood vessels of the brain. Side effect is constriction of coronary arteries, leading to worsening of CAD. Safety margin is small in overdose. They should be avoided in pregnancy and heart disease. A combination of ergotamine tartrate (1 mg) + caffeine (100 mg) could be given at the onset of symptoms or headache and can be repeated every 30 minutes up to 6 tablets per attack.

Triptans

Classically, triptans have been serotonin receptors (5-HT1B/1D) agonists that cause constriction of the cerebral vessels and bring about pain relief in the headache phase. For these drugs to be effective, they should be taken as early as possible (as headache starts). Apart from constricting cerebral vessels, triptans reduce neuro-inflammation around the brain vessels and also block release of calcitonin-related gene peptide (CGRP).

Therapeutic Potential of Triptans

Triptans, in contrast to ergot alkaloids that possess widespread pharmacological effects, have their pharmacodynamic effect limited to 5-HT1B/1D receptors. Thus, they are more selective than ergots. They are inactive at α_1, α_2, β adrenergic, dopaminergic, or muscarinic receptors. Triptans can rapidly abort the attack. Sumatriptan is given orally in 50 to 100 mg daily or 4 to 12 mg as SC injections. Triptans should not be used in familial hemiplegic migraine and basilar artery migraine. Also, they are avoided in patients with risk factors for stroke, for example, uncontrolled hypertension, diabetes, and obesity. They are tolerated very poorly by those with peripheral artery diseases and cardiovascular diseases. Combination of naproxen with triptans is well tolerated.

They act specifically via receptors present in the CNS and its vascular system. They suppress the excitability of cells in the trigeminal nuclei of serotonergic receptors (5-HT1B/1D) within the brain stem. Triptans produce vasoconstriction of meningeal, dural, and cerebral vessels via stimulation of vascular 5-HT1B receptors. **Fig. 6.2** gives their mechanism of action. Commonly used triptans that are helpful in the treatment of migraine are as follows:

- Zolmitriptan.
- Sumatriptan.
- Naratriptans.
- Rizatriptan.
- Almotriptan.

Sumatriptan

This has been a popular option for migraine and was the first approved drug for acute treatment of migraine. The drug is structurally similar to amines such as serotonin, dopamine, and noradrenaline. The drug is a selective agonist at 5-HT1B/1D receptors and a selective cerebral vasoconstrictor. Since vasodilatation is the cause of migraine, sumatriptan acts by stimulation of 5-HT1B and produces vasoconstriction. Apart from producing cerebral vasoconstriction, the drug may also cause cardiac vasoconstriction

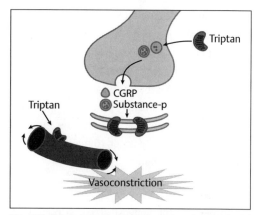

Fig. 6.2 Triptans have agonistic actions in the cranial vessels upon 5-HT1B/1D receptors, leading to their vasoconstriction. This leads to inhibition of proinflammatory neuropeptides. CGRP, calcitonin gene-related peptide.

and hence can cause chest discomfort in many patients. Because of this, it is avoided in patients with known ischemic heart disease.

Pharmacokinetically, it can be administered orally or by injection, nasal spray, or rectal suppository. Administered orally, it undergoes extensive first-pass hepatic metabolism and has poor oral bioavailability. When administered subcutaneously, its absorption is rapid, and the peak plasma concentration is reached within minutes with good bioavailability. It has a shorter duration of action with a half-life of 2 hours. It is used for acute attacks of migraine of moderate-to-severe nature. It can also be used to treat cluster headaches. Myocardial infarction has occurred as a result of coronary vasospasms.

Side Effects

Pain and burning at injection site can occur, with rise of blood pressure. Angina pain can occur due to vasospasm of the coronary vessels.

Zolmitriptan

Zolmitriptan is a second-generation triptan that rapidly relieves migraine attacks. It is available in the form of oral tablets, oral disintegrating tablets, and fast-acting nasal spray. It has oral bioavailability of 40%, with peak plasma concentration reached in about 2 hours. Zolmitriptan is metabolized in the liver to active metabolites, and the drug is poorly protein bound. A 5-mg nasal spray is available for rapid symptomatic relief and may provide symptomatic relief within 1 hour. The drug can be repeated after 2 hours. A total dose of 10 mg is maximum over a period of 24 hours.

Naratriptan

Naratriptan is the longest acting triptan with good bioavailability and a half-life of 6 hours. It has the best oral bioavailability among triptans. It gains peak plasma concentration in 2 to 3 hours

when given orally. It is contraindicated in severe renal and hepatic impairment or peripheral vascular syndrome. A total of 1 to 5 mg of the drug is given over 24 hours.

Rizatriptan

Rizatriptan has oral bioavailability of 40% and has a half-life of 2.5 hours. The drug has the fastest time of onset. A dose of 5 to 30 mg is given over 24 hours.

Almotriptan

The drug is used at dose of 6.25 to 25 mg over 25 hours.

Prevention[10–15]

Preventive treatment is needed for patients in whom migraine interferes with the activity of daily living despite acute treatment. Botulinum toxin type-A is being used increasingly nowadays. Botulinum toxin A compared with placebo was associated with beneficial effects in chronic daily headaches and chronic migraines but was not associated with fewer episodic migraine or chronic tension-type headaches per month.[5,10]

For patients who have migraine with insomnia, a small bedtime dose of amitriptyline at a dose of 10 to 25 mg could be helpful. For patients who are young, stressful, and have CAD, β-blockers are good options. Carbonic anhydrase inhibitor, topiramate, is a therapeutic option for those who are overweight or who are refractory to other drugs (25–100 mg/d). Divalproex could be used for patients with mania and coexisting migraine. A recent meta-analysis demonstrated topiramate in a 100 mg/day dosage as an effective therapy in reducing headache frequency, and it was reasonably well tolerated in adult patients with episodic migraine.[4] Anticonvulsants appear to be both effective in reducing migraine frequency and reasonably well tolerated. The best evidence is for sodium valproate and topiramate.[6]

Prophylaxis

Prophylaxis is used to reduce the number of attacks in circumstances when acute therapy, used appropriately, gives inadequate symptom control. One would have to define the severity of attack.

Types of migraine according to the severity and frequency of attacks are as follows:

- Mild headache: Once a month, normal daily activities are not disturbed.
- Moderate headache: More than once a month; normal daily activities may or may not be disturbed.
- Severe headache: More than three attacks per month; normal activities are difficult to continue; patients need to be treated with both acute and prophylactic medicines.

Prophylaxis is indicated when the headache occurs two to three times a month or there is significant migraine-related disability.

Prophylactic treatment is indicated in the following conditions:

- When there are two or more attacks per month.
- When acute symptomatic treatment is required for more than two to three times per week.
- Drugs used in acute attack are ineffective, intolerable, or contraindicated.
- Headache is severe and associated with neurological symptoms.
- Drugs used need several weeks for the onset of action.
- Treatment continues for 6 months and can be repeated.

While treating migraine, one should avoid opiates or combination analgesics with barbiturates, caffeine, etc., due to potential for abuse. Also, one should restrict the use to no more than 2 days/dose/week. NSAIDs have the lowest potential for medication overuse.

Beta-Blockers

Beta-blockers are most commonly used for prophylaxis against migraine attacks. Propranolol and timolol are often given. The former is given at doses of 8 to 240 mg daily. The patient needs to be observed for bradycardia. They act mainly through blocking β-induced vasodilating effect on intra- or extracranial blood vessels. Propranolol is most often used, but atenolol and metoprolol are other beta-blockers utilized for this indication (**Table 6.2**). Side effects of beta-blockers include fatigue, drowsiness, dizziness, depression, etc. Impotence and bradycardia are contraindications. Other contraindications include old age, asthma, atrioventricular (AV) nodal block, and congestive heart failure.

Beta-blockers undergo extensive first-pass metabolism. Hence, the bioavailability, of drug varies and so does the dosage range. Beta-blockers have actions on serotonin receptors apart from beta-adrenergic receptors. Propranolol has been found to be a good therapeutic option with children with migraine. They could also be potentially good options for patients with heart disease, hypertension, or those who are anxious or have phobic disorders. They could also be suited for young, stressful individuals who have migraine. Nadolol (20–160 mg) is given when depression and other CNS side effects of beta-blockers are a cause for concern due to its hydrophilic nature. Atenolol is another water-soluble beta-blocker, which can be used alternatively. Atenolol (50–200 mg) is a cardioselective beta-blocker; hence, it is safe in asthma, diabetes, and peripheral vascular disease patients.

Amitriptyline

Amitriptyline (10–150 mg) is a tricyclic anti-depressant (TCAD) that prevents the release of plasma peritoneal fluid serotonin from brain mast cells. Hence, amitriptyline prevents vaso-constriction which triggers first phase like all prophylactic drugs do. However, it has a delayed onset of action, about 6 to 8 weeks before the onset of clinical effect. Side effects include dry mouth, blurred vision, and constipation. This is the only antidepressant effective for prophylaxis of migraine. Nortriptyline and doxepin have been tried in patients who cannot tolerate the side effects of amitriptyline (**Fig. 6.3**).

Calcium Channel Blockers

Verapamil, nifedipine, diltiazem, nimodipine, and flunarizine are commonly used calcium channel

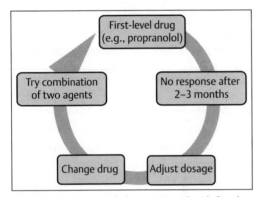

Fig. 6.3 Migraine prophylaxis is started with first-line drugs such as propranolol, valproate, topiramate, or amitriptyline. The drugs are given for 8 to 12 weeks in sufficient dosages and decrease in frequency and severity is noted. However, if there is no relief, then the dose is increased. Finally, if there is no response with the single agent, then combination of two drugs could be used for prophylaxis.

blockers for migraine prophylaxis. They decrease the severity and frequency of migraine through inhibition of Ca^{++} influx into the neurons. Side effects include constipation, ankle edema, and brady or tachycardia.

Dihydroergotamine

This ergot alkaloid is used in the prophylaxis of migraine. It binds to noradrenaline and dopamine receptors and stimulates alpha and serotonin receptors.

Antihypertensives

Lisinopril, ramipril, and candesartan (8–32 mg) have been tried with variable success. These could be good options in patients with hypertension.

Topiramate

This drug is used in refractory migraine, and those with obesity and epilepsy having migraine. The drug is used at doses of 25 to 100 mg daily. Side effects include paresthesia and renal stones.

Divalproex Sodium

This is another antiseptic drug used in migraine prophylaxis at doses of 500 to 1,000 mg daily. GI upset, tremors, and weight gain can occur. Platelet levels may be reduced. Pancreatitis and alopecia can occur.

Table 6.2 Drugs used for prophylaxis of migraine

Drug	Dose	Side effects
Propranolol	80–240 mg daily in three to four divided doses	Fatigue, exercise intolerance, sexual side effects in men. Look for bradycardia, if heart rate becomes less than 60, then avoid. Avoid in asthma
Timolol	10–15 mg twice daily	Similar side effect profile as that of propranolol
Divalproex	250–500 mg twice daily (maximum dose – 1,000 mg/d)	Gastrointestinal upset, alopecia, pancreatitis, polycystic ovary disease, tremors, increase chance of liver side effects, and teratogenicity in pregnancy
Amitriptyline	10–150 mg daily	Sedation, dry mouth, and weight gain

Botulinum Toxin

Botulinum toxin (type-A) has been approved for migraine prevention. The drug is injected around the temporalis muscle for relaxation effect.

Migraine Prevention in Pregnancy

Risks versus benefit ratio should be considered for migraine treatment in pregnancy. Category C drugs that have acceptable risks in pregnancy like amitriptyline could be considered. Labetalol 150 mg/day could be a good option if the patient has concomitant pregnancy-induced hypertension. Valproate and its derivatives should be avoided. Angiotensin-converting enzyme (ACE) inhibitors and angiotensin-receptor blockers (ARBs) too are contraindicated.

Canadian Headache Society Guidelines for Migraine Prophylaxis (2012)

The Canadian Headache Society Guidelines assert that the prophylactic drug of choice for migraine should be based on evidence for efficacy, side effect profile, migraine clinical features, and coexisting disorders. Topiramate, propranolol, nadolol, metoprolol, amitriptyline, gabapentin, candesartan, butterbur, riboflavin, coenzyme Q10, and magnesium citrate) are favored, but divalproex sodium, flunarizine, pizotifen, venlafaxine, verapamil, and lisinopril are weakly favored. First-time treatment options for patients who have not had prophylaxis before could be a beta-blocker and a TCAD, for example, amitriptyline.

Handling a Case of Migraine

One should advise the patient to avoid all the triggers and prevent attacks. Pain medicines should be taken properly. NSAIDs are the drugs taken at the time of starting of headache. Ergots and triptans are given if the case is moderate to severe. Prophylaxis is needed if the attacks become three to four times in a month. A regular

monitoring of the patient with maintenance of headache diary may be needed.

Other Common Headaches[13-15]

Tension Headache

Tension-type headache is a chronic headache that often occurs daily. Tension headache is the most common primary headache disorder. The pain is of mild-to-moderate intensity, and there is a feeling of "pressure or tightness." Duration of headache is 30 minutes to 7 days. The location is on both sides of head and neck. There is no light/sound sensitivity or aura. Mostly, these patients like to get head massage or try to compress their heads by hands when headache occurs.

Patients could be seen wrapping their handkerchief or any other cloths around their head to get relief.

Tension headache often presents as a mild-to-moderate pain described as feeling like a tight band around the head (holocranial). Pericranial tenderness may be found. These patients may have poor concentrations and other nonspecific features. Constant daily headaches can also occur, but headache is not pulsatile like migraine and has no aura. Emotional stress, fatigue, or noise often exacerbates it. Patients need to be reassured about the beginning nature of this type of headache. Treatment involves use of analgesics, either alone or in combination. Such patients respond well to amitriptyline on long term. Some studies have found usefulness of venlafaxine and mirtazapine. Triptans have no role in management. Treatment of comorbid conditions like generalized anxiety and depression is needed. Biofeedback is useful.

Medication Overuse Headache

This is a type of headache made worse by pain killers (mostly NSAIDs). MOH only occurs in people who already had headache and were using the drugs on regular basis. It is mainly due to codeine-containing drugs or opioids like morphine, etc. One needs to stop responsible drugs. Gradual withdrawal of the overdose medications as soon as possible is the treatment of choice. Patients need to be educated about the detrimental effects of long-term analgesic therapy. About half of the chronic daily headaches may have medication overuse. If the cause is migraine, then early prevention should be done as it may have "analgesic sparing effect."

Cluster Headache

This is a severe and excruciating headache that comes in clusters like (every time each year or season), and then pain-free period follows. Pain is penetrating or continuous, nonthrobbing type. Usually, the affected patients are middle-aged men. Activation of cells in ipsilateral hypothalamus can trigger trigeminal autonomic system. Family history of migraine or other headaches may be found.

This is not an uncommon type of headache, predominantly found in men, and is usually mild to moderate in intensity. This has recurring character and come in clusters.

Pain may occur for 15 minutes to 3 hours and may have same clock time each day and several episodes may occur during the day. Pain may occur for several weeks, occurs on the same side, and comes with watering eyes or nasal stuffiness, runny nose, red eye, swollen eyelids, sweating, etc. Agitation and restlessness may occur. Episode often occurs at night and spontaneous remission may occur. Chronic clutter headache with no remission may occur. Alcohol triggers the attacks.

Sumatriptan is effective and subcutaneous injection works better than oral therapy. Inhalation of 100% oxygen can abort an acute attack (12 L/min) for 15 to 30 minutes in one setting. Zolmitriptan nasal spray 5 to 10 mg is useful. Ergotamine with lidocaine has been tried. Lithium is the best-known prophylactic agent, followed by verapamil. Topiramate and valproate have been tried. Ergotamine and prednisolone can also be used. Civamide has also been tried as a prophylactic agent. The drug is a vanilloid receptor agonist and neuronal calcium channel blocker that inhibits the neuronal release of excitatory neurotransmitters (e.g., CGRP and substance P [SP]) and depletes the neurons of the trigeminal plexus of their neurotransmitter content.[3] Refractory cases may respond to suboccipital corticosteroid injections. Occipital nerve stimulation has shown some success.[11]

Hemicranias Continua

This is a separate type of primary headache disorder with continuous hemicranial pain and without remission, which resolves with indomethacin. Horner syndrome transiently may occur.

Headaches Associated with Sexual Activity

Primary headache with sexual activity is known by several other names, for example, benign coital headache, coital cephalgia, benign orgasmic cephalgia, sex-related headache, etc. Headache associated with sexual activity (HSA) is an acute explosive headache that is time-related to sexual intercourse. A special form of headache, characterized by headache induced by watching pornography, has been reported.[8] Even though in ancient times, Hippocrates described a headache resulting from "sexual activity," it was not until the 1970s that attention was drawn to a benign form of headache occurring during sexual activity. HSA is often confused with more serious neurological conditions, such as SAH due to ruptured intracranial aneurysm, etc. Therefore, for patients in whom HSA occurs for the first time, appropriate radiological investigations should be done to exclude intracranial hemorrhage. Counselling and reassurance plays an important role in management, apart from pharmacological prevention, if and when needed.

Indomethacin (25–50 mg/d) or propranolol (40–200 mg/d) are useful preventive treatments. However, treatment is required for cases with regular and frequent episodes. Ergotamine (1–2 mg/d) or calcium channel blocker, diltiazem (60 m, three times daily), have also been found to be helpful. Prophylaxis can be advised for a period of 3 months, and then the patient should be checked for spontaneous remission. For those with mild headaches, reassurance and advice about ceasing sexual activity is sufficient.[7]

Recent Advances in Headaches

A number of extended-release formulations are under development. Traditionally, opioids have been kept away from pharmacotherapy of headaches. Now, long-acting formulation of opioids are underway.[12] Monoclonal antibodies targeting CGRP and its receptors are in development now.[13] In the treatment of migraine, compounds acting on the serotonin 5-HT1F receptors, nitric oxide synthase, and acid-sensing ion channel blockers are under development.[14]

References

1. NNN-Charles.ppt - Headache Research and Treatment Program - UCLA. Available at: hartp.neurology.ucla.edu/IMAGES/NNN-Charles.ppt. Accessed June 8,2016)
2. Pringsheim T, Davenport W, Mackie G, et al; Canadian Headache Society Prophylactic Guidelines Development Group. Canadian Headache Society guideline for migraine prophylaxis. Can J Neurol Sci 2012; 39(2, Suppl 2):S1–S59
3. Diamond S, Freitag F, Phillips SB, Bernstein JE, Saper JR. Intranasal civamide for the acute treatment of migraine headache. Cephalalgia 2000;20(6):597–602
4. Linde M, Mulleners WM, Chronicle EP, McCrory DC. Topiramate for the prophylaxis of episodic migraine in adults. Cochrane Database Syst Rev 2013; (6):CD010610
5. Jackson JL, Kuriyama A, Hayashino Y. Botulinum toxin A for prophylactic treatment of migraine and tension headaches in adults: a meta-analysis. JAMA 2012; 307(16):1736–1745
6. Chronicle E, Mulleners W. Anticonvulsant drugs for migraine prophylaxis. Cochrane Database Syst Rev 2016; (5):CD003226
7. Anand KS, Dhikav V. Primary headache associated with sexual activity. Singapore Med J 2009;50(5):e176–e177
8. Anand KS, Dhikav V. Headaches induced by pornography use. Arch Sex Behav 2012; 41(5):1077
9. Thorlund K, Toor K, Wu P, et al. Comparative tolerability of treatments for acute migraine: A network meta-analysis. Cephalalgia 2016; 37(10):965–978
10. Anand KS, Prasad A, Singh MM, Sharma S, Bala K. Botulinum toxin type A in prophylactic treatment of migraine. Am J Ther 2006;13(3):183–187
11. Proietti Cecchini A, Grazzi L. Emerging therapies for chronic migraine. Curr Pain Headache Rep 2014;18(4):408
12. Jones MR, Carney MJ, Kaye RJ, Prabhakar A, Kaye AD. Drug formulation advances in extended-release medications for pain control. Curr Pain Headache Rep 2016; 20(6):36 Review
13. Schuster NM, Vollbracht S, Rapoport AM. Emerging treatments for the primary headache disorders. Neurol Sci 2015; 36(Suppl 1):109–113
14. Antonaci F, Ghiotto N, Wu S, Pucci E, Costa A. Recent advances in migraine therapy. Springerplus 2016;5:637
15. Recent advances in migraine therapy. Available at: https://www.ncbi.nlm.nih.gov/pmc/articles/PMC4870579/. Accessed September 20, 2020

Antidepressants

Vikas Dhikav

Clinical Case Example

- A 24-year-old girl has a nonpsychotic unipolar depression with no history of hypomania or mania. She has depressed mood, hyperphagia, psychomotor retardation, and hypersomnolence. What agent would be used for her?

Answer: The diagnosis is that of a major depressive disorder. Target symptoms that could be treated are: depression, hyperphagia, psychomotor retardation, and hypersomnolence. For a treatment naive patient, one can start with a selective serotonin reuptake inhibitor (SSRI). Using the side effect profile as a guide, one could select an SSRI that is less sedating. Good choices would be citalopram, fluoxetine, or sertraline. Bupropion would also be a reasonable choice given her hypersomnolence, psychomotor retardation, and hyperphagia condition. Less desirable choices include paroxetine and mirtazapine because of sedation and weight gain in a young female. She may not need reuptake inhibitors because she is treatment naive and may not need a "big gun drug." One should not use a tricyclic antidepressant (TCAD) because of side effects.

Depressive Disorders[1-3]

Depression is a common clinical disorder characterized by low mood, low self-esteem, loss of interest in pleasurable activities, and negative perceptions. Dictionary meaning of the word depression is "low mood or spirits." The term "major depressive disorder" was coined in 1980 and was included in the *Diagnostic and Statistical Manual, version III (DSM-III)*. Most often, onset occurs in middle age and the disorder is reported twice as often in women than men. Lifetime prevalence in men is around 10%, while in women it is 20%. It has been estimated by the World Health Organization that by next 20 years, depression will be second only to ischemic heart disease in terms of disability or disease burden. It should be kept in mind that although depression responds very favorably to treatment, 20% of the patients may have treatment refractory depression. Although there are many evidence-based psychotherapies and drugs available to treat depression, antidepressant medications remain the mainstay of treatment of depression. Antidepressants bring about a lot of changes in the brain and behavior.

Antidepressants elevate the mood, increase physical activity, and can cause mental alertness, increase in appetite, and sexual desires. They improve sleep and reduce premorbid thoughts.

Drugs like doxepin and amitriptyline have been used as popular sedatives in the past. Nowadays, due to availability of better agents such as zolpidem, antidepressants are not used as sedatives–hypnotics anymore.

The World Health Organization has put bipolar disorders among 10 leading medical conditions affecting humans worldwide. Lifetime prevalence of depressive disorders has been estimated to be 10 to 15% by the World Health Organization. Greatest risk of depression is the high risk of suicide. Overall, 120 million people worldwide have depression.

What Causes Depression?[1-5]

First, depression should be differentiated from normal day-to-day sadness. The word "depression" used here means clinical depression. *Monoamine hypothesis of depression* states that there is a deficiency of monoamines such as norepinephrine, serotonin, and dopamine in predisposed patients. Antidepressants can boost the activity of these monoamines in brain. It should be noted that almost all clinically significant antidepressants work either by affecting the action of transporters or by inhibiting enzymes that metabolize catecholamines. Traditionally, depression has been treated with a single drug (monotherapy). Off late, several studies have shown that combination treatment may be more effective in reducing the rate of relapse than single drug used alone. Recently, disturbances of hypothalamic pituitary axis have been linked with suicidal behavior. The disease has several vegetative features (**Box 7.1**).

Drugs for Depression

Drugs used against mental depression are of two types: Older and newer.

- **Older:**
  - ◇ **Monoamine oxidase (MAO) inhibitors:**
    - □ **MAO-A inhibitors:**
      - – Phenelzine.
      - – Moclobemide.
      - – Tranylcypromine.
      - – Isocarboxazid.
    - □ **MAO-B inhibitors:**
      - – Selegiline.
  - ◇ **Tricyclics:**
    - □ Imipramine.
    - □ Doxepin.
    - □ Amitriptyline.
    - □ Trimipramine.
  - ◇ **Tetracyclics:**
    - □ Clomipramine.
    - □ Desipramine.
    - □ Nortriptyline.
    - □ Dothiepin.
- **Newer:**
  - ◇ SSRIs:
    - □ Fluoxetine.
    - □ Fluvoxamine.
    - □ Sertraline.
    - □ Reboxetine.
    - □ Citalopram.
    - □ Escitalopram.

Box 7.1: Diagnostic and Statistical Manual IV criteria for major depression
In the last 2 weeks, a person should have five or more of the following symptoms: • Depressed mood, most days. • Loss of interest/decreased pleasure every day. • Marked loss or weight gain. • Excessive sleep or not enough sleep. • Agitated or retarded motor activity. • Worthlessness/inappropriate guilt. • Fatigue. • Indecisiveness. • Suicidal attempt/or plans for it.

◊ Serotonin–dopamine reuptake inhibitor (SDRI):

  □ Bupropion.

◊ SSRI/selective norepinephrine reuptake inhibitor (SNRI):

  □ Duloxetine.

◊ SNRI:

  □ Venlafaxine.

◊ Selective serotonin reuptake enhancer (SSRE):

  □ Amineptine.

  □ Tianeptine.

◊ Miscellaneous:

  □ Nefazodone.

  □ Trazodone.

  □ Mirtazapine.

  □ Mianserin.

  □ Maprotiline.

  □ Milnacipran.

History of Depression Treatment

Antidepressant drugs were introduced 40 years ago, and apart from depression, they are also used for treatment of other disorders including anxiety disorders, dysthymia, chronic pain, and behavioral problems. Antidepressants were discovered accidentally while investigating antipsychotic efficacy of modifications of phenothiazines. Imipramine was the first antidepressant discovered. Around the same time, monoamine oxidase inhibitors (MAOIs) were identified. Second-generation antidepressants were identified to address problems with first-generation antidepressants. In late 1980s, SSRIs were developed which revolutionized the treatment of depression.[1]

Mechanism of Action[1-7]

Antidepressants inhibit reuptake of monoamines. Some antidepressants are selective inhibitors of serotonin. These are 1,000 to 3,000 times more selective for serotonin compared to norepinephrine. Desipramine and nortriptyline inhibit reuptake of norepinephrine. Therefore, these drugs have brain-activating properties. Importantly, both of them are used in patients with depression having hypersomnia (**Fig. 7.1**).

Most clinically used antidepressants exert important actions on the metabolism of neurotransmitters (e.g., serotonin and noradrenaline) and their receptors. The pharmacologic effects of any of the antidepressant drugs on neurotransmission occur immediately, whereas the time course for a therapeutic response occurs over several weeks.

Antidepressants have a long latency of clinical effect. That means, they start acting only after 3 to 4 weeks. It is not entirely clear as to what is the major cause of this delay. Leading theory

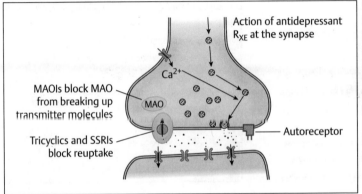

Fig. 7.1 Antidepressants block reuptake-I and this can lead to increase in synapse concentrations of monoamines. SSRIs block reuptake of serotonin, while tianeptine and amineptine enhance their reuptake. MAO, monoamine oxidase; MAOI, monoamine oxidase inhibitors; SSRIs, selective serotonin reuptake inhibitors.

suggests that increased levels of norepinephrine and serotonin lead to downregulation of some inhibitory receptors leading to enhancement of their release into synaptic cleft or greater postsynaptic response. Alternatively, the chronic activation of monoamine receptors by antidepressants appears to increase brain-derived neurotrophic factor (BDNF) transcription. The time required to synthesize neurotrophic factors has been proposed as an explanation for this delay of antidepressant effects.

It is curious to know that drugs which inhibit the uptake or drugs that enhance uptake can have antidepressant response. So possibly, there is a common mechanism in them leading to antidepressant action. The exact reason why does it happen is not known. Drugs like amineptine and tianeptine can actually increase the uptake of neurotransmitters in presynaptic neurons. Probably, increased accumulation can lead to rupture of vesicles and this can lead to antidepressant response.

Inhibition of 5-HT2A receptors in both animal and human studies is associated with substantial antianxiety, antipsychotic, and antidepressant effects.

What Goes Inside the Neurons When SSRIs Act: Implications for Therapeutic Response

SSRIs have been described here as a model. The therapeutic response in major depression from SSRIs (2–3 weeks) may be due to a progressive desensitization of somatodendritic serotonin autoreceptors in the midbrain (raphe nucleus). It has also been postulated that serotonin is a neuromodulator of several neurophysiological pathways, including dopamine and noradrenaline.

Serotonin also modulates neurotrophic factors, intracytoplasmic phosphorylations, nuclear genes expressions, etc. Several drugs may have similar mechanisms (**Fig. 7.2**). Drugs of varied classes that have reuptake blocking action can also act upon presynaptic receptors (**Fig. 7.3**).

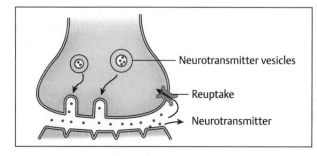

Fig. 7.2 Drugs like venlafaxine, desvenlafaxine, and milnacipran have mechanism similar to that of tricyclic antidepressants (i.e., blocking reuptake of serotonin and noradrenaline). Milnacipran is not used to treat depression. It is used for the treatment of fibromyalgia. However, it is effective in a small number of patients.

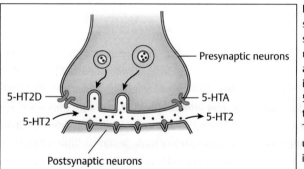

Fig. 7.3 Antidepressants block reuptake of serotonin and noradrenaline and that may stimulate resynaptic 5-HT1D and 5-HT1A receptors on somatodendritic synapses which act as autoreceptors. This may increase cAMP inside presynaptic neurons. Later on, the 5-HT receptors undergo downregulation and this correlates with antidepressant response. These and many more molecular mechanisms underlie the delays that antidepressants have in starting their pharmacological actions.

Therapeutic activity of SSRIs may finally result in a complex modulation and homeostasis between monoaminergic neurotransmission and neuronal plasticity and perhaps that is why it takes such a long time to develop.

Molecular Pharmacology of SSRIs[7-9]

Initially, SSRIs increase the synaptic levels of serotonin and hence stimulate a large number of postsynaptic receptors. Presynaptic 5-HT1A and 5-HT7 receptors on cell bodies of raphe nuclei are stimulated. This may reduce synthesis of serotonin. However, upon prolonged treatment, there is a downregulation of these inhibitory presynaptic receptors leading to a rise in synaptic levels of serotonin. Downregulation of 5-HT2A can cause stimulation of serotonergic mechanisms via serotonergic heteroreceptors. Also, there is increased clearance of serotonin transporter responsible for terminating action of serotonin. Overall, these are serotonin boosting drugs.[7]

Ultimately, SSRIs increase cAMP signaling and there is also an increase in phosphorylation of cAMP binding response transcription factor (CREB). Increase in tropic factors such as BDNFs occurs. With sustained treatment, increase in neurogenesis of dentate gyrus of hippocampus and subventricular zone occurs. In animal studies at least, it has been seen that some behavioral effects of SSRIs are mediated via increased neurogenesis in hippocampus either via neurotropic tyrosine kinase (TrKB) or BDNF.

These neurotropic effects make antidepressants like tricyclic antidepressants (TCADs) have neuroregenerative properties. Notably, antidepressants of SSRI class do not have many of these properties.

Although SSRIs like fluoxetine are the most successful treatment for depression, there seems to be a number of limitations: Fluoxetine type of drugs lack agonistic activity upon catecholaminergic receptors. SSRIs have no effect on other catecholamines such as norepinephrine or dopamine. There may be increase in expression of autoreceptors upon presynaptic receptors as a result of prolonged treatment. This can lead to reduced norepinephrine. Perhaps this is the reason for slightly increased chance of suicide noted in some studies. It has been proposed that 5-HT2 antagonist such as olanzapine could circumvent these disadvantages. Studies are underway to explore the effects of mirtazepine and olanzapine to treat refractory cases in depression.

Pharmacokinetics

Antidepressants are lipid soluble agents; hence, they are well absorbed by oral route. First-pass metabolism is high. They form inactive metabolites. Nefazodone ($t_{1/2}$ = 2 h) is shortest-acting antidepressant and hence requires frequent dosing. Fluoxetine forms a long-acting metabolite named norfluoxetine and has a half-life of 7 days. Usually, long half-life of fluoxetine is advantageous, but it could be problematic in case of overdose. SSRIs are enzyme inhibitors, and fluvoxamine is a potent enzyme inhibitor and has maximum chances of drug interactions.[6] Sertraline and citalopram have lowest possibility of drug interactions and in fact are referred drugs when patients are taking multiple drugs. Citalopram is a good choice in poststroke depression.[14] Nefazodone and venlafaxine are enzyme inhibitors. In the TCAD group, imipramine is a potent enzyme inhibitor.

Uses of Antidepressants

Antidepressants have several clinical uses apart from the treatment of depressive disorders (**Box 7.2**). There may be considerable variations among individuals of the dose at which optimal response occurs. **Imipramine** has been the *drug of choice* for nocturnal enuresis. Imipramine has long been used to control bed-wetting in children

Box 7.2: Uses of antidepressants

- Unipolar and bipolar depression.
- Organic mood disorders.
- Schizoaffective disorder.
- Anxiety disorders:
  ◊ Obsessive compulsive disorders.
  ◊ Panic.
  ◊ Social phobias.
  ◊ Posttraumatic stress disorder.
- Premenstrual dysphoric disorder.
- Impulsivity associated with personality disorders.

(older than 6 years) by causing contraction of the internal sphincter of the bladder.

Ephedrine and desmopressin are alternatives. Desmopressin is increasingly becoming drug of choice for this condition and is preferred nowadays. Imipramine could also be used in elderly who are admitted in hospitals. However, anticholinergic activity associated with this drug can contribute to side effects, for example, hallucinations.

Imipramine is used in major depression as well. It also has some additional indications like chronic pain syndromes, especially pain of diabetic neuropathy and migraine prophylaxis.

Imipramine is a commonly used drug in India for diabetic neuropathy. It is noteworthy that TCADs have ability to block sodium channels in damaged peripheral nerves. That means they have membrane stabilizing (local anesthetic) effects. They have been shown to cause repair of damaged peripheral nerves. Diabetic neuropathy is a common chronic complication of both type-1 and type-2 diabetes. Loss of myelination and axonal degeneration are its prominent features. Hyperglycemia has been identified to be the key contributor to the development of diabetic neuropathy. Some patients may have deficiency of neurotropic factors. There is evidence available that in the absence of neurotropic support, there

can be axonal degeneration and demyelination. Regeneration can be difficult in these situations.

Imipramine was tried initially as an antipsychotic drug but failed. Later on, it was introduced as an antidepressant. It has a strong serotonin reuptake inhibiting action and also has antihistaminic, analgesic, and anticholinergic activities. Multiple activities make it useful for treatment of a variety of disorders. It has a unique activity of increasing BDNF in hippocampus. Notably, hippocampus becomes shrunk in major depressive disorders due to reduced neurogenesis. Dose ranges from 25 to 300 mg in resistant cases. Pediatric cases are started with 10 mg daily doses.

Fluoxetine was the first SSRI available, and it has a long half-life, slow onset of action, and can cause sexual dysfunction, anxiety, insomnia, and agitation. Despite its limitations, it remains a popular drug. Fluoxetine is used in patients with remitting and relapsing depression due to its long duration of action. It is given in morning as the drug has potential to cause insomnia. It should be given with meals to reduce nausea. Food does not interfere with its absorption and is protein bound.

Given orally, fluoxetine is almost completely absorbed. Due to hepatic first-pass metabolism, the oral bioavailability is less than 90%. Fluoxetine has a long half-life of 2 to 7 days, whereas the half-life of its metabolite norfluoxetine ranges between 4 and 15 days. This long half-life of fluoxetine may be advantageous when the patient omits a dose since drug concentrations decrease slightly. That is why it is used. On the other hand, in the case of fluoxetine nonresponse, long washout periods are necessary before switching the patient to a TCAD or an MAOI to avoid drug interactions or the development of a serotonin syndrome.[2] Long half-life has made it an attractive alternative as an antidepressant for weekly treatment (90 mg once weekly). Long-acting metabolite norfluoxetine makes it longer acting. The drug takes around a month to achieve steady state and takes an equal duration for discontinuation of pharmacological effect. Therefore, a washout period of same duration should be given for flushing out pharmacological action to avoid any potential drug interaction. It has enzyme inhibiting tendencies; therefore, there is a potential for drug interactions. In the treatment of depression, the drug is started in dose of 20-mg capsule once a day. It can be increased to 80 mg/day. Advantages and disadvantages of fluoxetine are summarized in **Table 7.1**.

Fluoxetine is the drug of choice for the following conditions:

- Premenstrual tension:
    ◊ This can be very disruptive and is a monthly dysphoric disorder affecting over 3% of female population. Fluoxetine in doses of 20 to 60 mg can treat dysphoria. In the year 1999, fluoxetine was the first drug approved for this disorder.
- Premature ejaculation:
    ◊ Fluoxetine can delay ejaculation and has been used with success in treatment of premature ejaculation. Lately, combinations of dapoxetine and sildenafil have become popular. Patients should be encouraged to take up weight loss programs as the problem is more common in patients who are overweight.
- Dysthymia.
- Cyclothymia.
- Bulimia:
    ◊ Weight loss has been reported after long-term use of these drugs. Fluoxetine has been shown to disrupt "binge-purge" cycle in these patients. Discontinuation of drug treatment can lead to rebound in many patients.
- Kleptomania.
- Paraphilias.
- Seasonal affective disorder (treatment of choice is phototherapy).

SSRIs, in general, are *drugs of choice* for obsessive-compulsive disorder (OCD). **Sertraline** can be preferred because of its safety. Sertraline was the second SSRI to be approved and has a low risk of toxicity, has few interactions, and is more selective and potent than fluoxetine (**Table 7.2**). The drug has a weak enzyme inhibiting activity. It is a long-acting drug given in morning to avoid insomnia. Since the drug has extensive first-pass metabolism, dose is reduced in hepatic failure. It is highly protein bound and hence has the potential to cause drug interactions based upon protein binding. Early treatment with SSRIs is associated with a better treatment response compared to drugs like clomipramine.[13]

Table 7.1 Advantages and disadvantages of fluoxetine

Advantages	Disadvantages
• Long half-life, so decreased incidence of discontinuation syndromes; good for noncompliance • Initially activating so may provide increased energy • Long half-life prevents SSRI discontinuation syndrome	• Long half-life not good in patients with liver disease due to accumulation of metabolite • CYP mediated drug interactions • Initial activation may cause anxiety, insomnia, and akathisia; insomnia is more common compared to other drugs

Abbreviations: CYP, cytochrome P450; SSRI, selective serotonin reuptake inhibitor.

Table 7.2 Advantages and disadvantages of sertraline

Advantages	Disadvantages
• Weak inhibitor of CYP; drug interactions less likely	• Needs full stomach for maximum absorption
• Short half-life, so build-up of metabolites does not occur	• Gastrointestinal events are common, especially in elderly
• Less sedating compared to paroxetine	

Abbreviation: CYP, cytochrome P450.

Table 7.3 Advantages and disadvantages of fluvoxamine

Advantages	Disadvantages
• Short half-life	• Strong inhibitor of CYP 450 enzyme system, so chances of drug interactions
• Analgesic action	• Shortest half-life among SSRI group drugs
• Less sedating compared to paroxetine	• Gastrointestinal side effects occur and sedation is likely too

Abbreviation: SSRI, selective serotonin reuptake inhibitor.

Traditionally, clomipramine has been the gold standard drug for the management of this disorder. Fluoxetine has long been used. Fluvoxamine is considered to be a specific antiobsessional agent (**Table 7.3**). Fluvoxamine is the structural derivative of fluoxetine and is quite effective for OCD. The drug also treats posttraumatic stress disorder (PTSD), dysphoria, panic disorder, and social phobia.

Paroxetine is a long-acting drug and is highly protein bound. The drug has anticholinergic properties and hence can be sedative. Notably, other SSRIs can cause insomnia. The drug has enzyme inhibiting property; hence, it can cause increase in plasma levels of many drugs. Paroxetine became the third SSRI available, and is more selective than fluoxetine. Paroxetine is highly effective in reducing anxiety and PTSD as well as OCD, panic disorder, social phobia, premenstrual dysphoric disorder, and chronic headache.

Citalopram is another long-acting SSRI. Among the SSRIs, the drug has the least chance of causing drug–drug interactions. Thus, the drug is particularly likely to be useful in elderly to whom many drugs are being given at same time. Also, elderly using many other antidepressants need close monitoring.[11] It has a labelled use in premenstrual syndrome. Citalopram is well absorbed orally and is used to treat major depression, social phobia, panic disorder, and OCD. This has become a popular antidepressant. Other indications for commonly used antidepressants are given in **Table 7.4** and doses are described in **Table 7.5**.

Clomipramine is structurally a TCAD but exerts inhibitory effects on 5-HT reuptake. The drug forms desmethyl clomipramine as the active metabolite and is classified as a mixed 5-HT and norepinephrine (NE) reuptake inhibitor. It is used to treat OCD, depression, panic disorder, and phobic disorders.

Clomipramine had been a popular drug in the past, and the drug is not used due to several autonomic side effects. It is, however, considered to be gold standard drug for OCD. Fluvoxamine is considered to be a specific drug for patients with OCD. With the introduction of SSRIs, safety

Table 7.4 FDA approved indications for commonly used antidepressants

Condition	Drug
Obsessive-compulsive disorder	All drugs except fluoxetine
Social phobia	Sertraline, paroxetine
Bulimia	Fluoxetine
Generalized anxiety disorder	Paroxetine, escitalopram
Premenstrual dysphoric disorder	Fluoxetine, paroxetine, sertraline

Table 7.5 Dosages of commonly used antidepressants

Name	Dose (mg)
Amitriptyline	50–300
Doxepin	75–150
Imipramine	75–150
Nortriptyline	25–150
Fluoxetine	20–80
Citalopram	20–40
Paroxetine	20–50
Sertraline	50–200
Escitalopram	10–20
Mirtazapine	15–45
Trazodone	150–400
Bupropion	150–450

Table 7.6 Advantages and disadvantages of venlafaxine

Advantages	Disadvantages
Minimal drug interactions	Increase in blood pressure (10–15 mm Hg)
Short half-life	Gastrointestinal events with immediate release formulations
Fast renal clearance, good in elderly	Taper needed as bad discontinuation syndrome can occur after 2 weeks
	QT prolongation and sexual side effects occur

of antidepressants has increased remarkably. These drugs have little or no anticholinergic, antihistaminic, and beta adrenergic receptors. SSRIs are tolerated very well by even elderly and those with heart disease. Notably, elderly patients are prone to side effects of TCADs or MAOIs, for example, postural hypotension.

Venlafaxine and **duloxetine** block the reuptake of serotonin and norepinephrine and can be used in patients with depression and chronic pain syndromes (**Table 7.6**). Venlafaxine is also particularly effective in patients who have failed to respond to SSRIs. Venlafaxine is also a mixed 5-HT and NE reuptake inhibitor which also inhibits the reuptake of dopamine. At dosages <150 mg/day, venlafaxine is a potent inhibitor of serotonin reuptake and, at medium to higher doses, is an inhibitor of norepinephrine reuptake.

The drug produces improvements in psychomotor and cognitive function. Importantly, SSRIs are not very effective in patients who have pain syndromes. TCADs are also good drugs for depression and chronic pain syndromes. Duloxetine has a dual mechanism, that is, serotonergic and adrenergic. Till the dose of 75 mg/day, it has serotonergic action and then at doses above this, adrenergic actions become prominent. In very high doses, it also inhibits dopamine uptake.

Therefore, the drug has a variety of side effects. Specially, it is prone to increased blood pressure. When used in combination with mirtazapine, it can reduce peripheral serotonergic side effects of this drug.

Trazodone blocks postsynaptic 5-HT2A and 5-HT2C receptors. Nefazodone is more potent in this regard. Nefazodone is a unique antidepressant that resembles a TCAD as an inhibitor of 5-HT and NE reuptake but has no therapeutic superiority over TCADs and SSRIs. That means the drug has equal efficacy. 5-HT2A receptor is intimately linked to 5-HT1A receptor, which is important in anxiety, violent behavior, and depression. These also block reuptake of serotonin in the same manner as by SSRIs. Nefazodone has been associated with hepatotoxicity, including rare fatalities and cases of hepatic failure requiring transplantation. Hence, during therapy with nefazodone, liver function monitoring may be needed.

Trazodone is the drug of choice for depression with impotence as the drug brings about penile erection. Both trazodone and nefazodone are effective anxiolytics as well. Indeed, their anti-anxiety effects are evident earlier compared to their antidepressant effect. Trazodone is free from anticholinergic or cardiac side effects seen typically with TCADs. However, sedation is high. It is also the drug of choice for depression with psychomotor retardation. This is due to its brain activating properties. It is noteworthy that brain activating properties are also seen with desipramine and nortriptyline. **Trazodone** is an inhibitor of serotonin reuptake and blocks serotonin receptors as well. It is a brain activator. Sustained erection as a side effect can develop (priapism). The drug is markedly sedating; hence, driving and use of heavy machinery need to be prohibited. **Vilazodone** is a new drug of this class, which blocks the reuptake of serotonin and is a partial agonist of 5-HT1A receptors.

Tobacco smoking is the leading cause of preventable morbidity and mortality in the world. There are nearly 1 to 3 billion users of nicotine and tobacco products worldwide (population equivalent to India or China) while approximately 5 million of them die from smoking-related disease every year. Cigarette smoking is a highly addictive behavior. Nicotine replacement products are widely employed and recommended by the World Health Organization. Bupropion is the drug of choice for smoking cessation and is contraindicated in epilepsy. It is also used in prevention of seasonal affective disorder. It is a brain stimulant and is used to promote weight loss and improve symptoms of attention deficit hyperactivity disorder (ADHD). Multiple mechanisms of actions associated with this drug make it a useful drug for a variety of indications. **Varenicline** is a nicotinic receptor agonist and is also used for the same purpose. It appears to have minimal side effects. Recent studies have shown that combination therapies are more effective than the monotherapies for quitting.[4]

Mirtazapine is a tetracyclic piperazinoazepine and is a drug with unique chemical structure. It has both antianxiety and antidepressant action. Importantly, both mirtazapine and venlafaxine have low incidence of sedation, autonomic side effects, and cardiotoxicity. The drug blocks presynaptic alpha 2 adrenergic receptors and thus increases release of norepinephrine. It also has serotonin and histamine blocking activity. However, it has no anticholinergic action. Sedation and weight gain are common side effects. At high dose, however, due to increase in noradrenergic activity, sedation is less common. Lack of anticholinergic activity may be a particular advantage clinically in elderly as they will not experience side effects such as urinary retention, palpitation, and constipation. A number of studies have suggested that the treatment of major depressive disorder with antidepressants enhancing both noradrenergic and serotonergic neurotransmission may result in higher response or remission rates than treatment with antidepressants selectively enhancing serotonergic neurotransmission. Mirtazapine can be advantageous in patients with depression having sleep difficulties. Low doses of trazodone (50–100 mg) have also been used widely both alone and concurrently with SSRIs or SNRIs to treat insomnia. Advantages and disadvantages are given in **Table 7.7**.

Duloxetine is considered to be the drug of choice for painful diabetic neuropathy and has also been approved for fibromyalgia. SSRIs are in general good choices in depression associated with fibromyalgias.[15] Notably, in the past, TCADs were the most commonly prescribed drugs.[9] It has also been tried in stress incontinence and generalized anxiety disorders. Like many drugs of this class, it has been used in fibromyalgia. It is a dual inhibitor of reuptake of serotonin and norepinephrine. The drug has also been useful in back pain. Recent evidence indicates that the

drug has usefulness in many conditions (see the following text). It does not seem to offer any specific advantage in treatment of depression compared to other antidepressants. It is generally used in doses of 30 to 60 mg/day. Advantages and disadvantages of duloxetine are summarized in **Table 7.8**.

It is well tolerated and side effects are minimal at therapeutically relevant dosages. The drug also does not have clinically significant drug interactions. It has been proposed that this drug has direct effect on pain rather than the effects being a result of relief of underlying depression.

Bupropion is an inhibitor of dopamine and norepinephrine reuptake. Bupropion has virtually no direct effects on the serotonin system. Unlike the SSRIs, bupropion does not cause sexual side effects. It does not block muscarinic, histaminergic, or adrenergic receptors.

Bupropion is used for smoking cessation. Importantly, it is free from sexual side effects. It also has no anticholinergic, sedating, or orthostatic side effects. Central nervous system

Table 7.7 Advantages and disadvantages of mirtazapine

Advantages	Disadvantages
• Different mechanism of action provides good augmentation to SSRIs	• Dyslipidemia occurs in many patients
• Can be used as a hypnotic also, as the drug has antihistaminic and sedative effect	• Highly sedative
• Fast renal clearance, good in elderly	• Weight gain

Abbreviation: SSRIs, selective serotonin reuptake inhibitors.

Table 7.8 Advantages and disadvantages of duloxetine

Advantages	Disadvantages
• Treats physical symptoms of depression	• CYP2D6 and CYP1A1 inhibitor, drug interactions likely
• Lesser increase in blood pressure compared to venlafaxine	• Capsule cannot be broken as contents are not stable in stomach
• Fast renal clearance, good in elderly	• Dropout rates may be higher
	• QT prolongation and sexual side effects occur

(CNS) stimulation however does occur leading to insomnia and decrease in seizure threshold. The drug is hence avoided in epilepsy. It is a potent enzyme inhibitor and is therefore likely to increase plasma levels of drugs given concomitantly. It has a short half-life and is given many times a day. The drug, however, is available as a sustained release formulation. Findings support the use of bupropion as a sole or coprescribed antidepressant, particularly if weight gain or sexual dysfunction are, or are likely to be, significant problems.[12]

Mianserine is a mirtazapine analog and is used less commonly nowadays. Periodic blood counts may be needed.

Amoxapine is a metabolite of loxapine, an antipsychotic drug. It is particularly effective in psychotic depression. Recent evidence suggests that the use of fluoxetine and olanzapine is effective for treatment of psychotic depression. Importantly, this combination is safer compared to use of amoxapine that causes extrapyramidal side effects.

Selective Serotonin Reuptake Inhibitors

SSRIs have been available for the past two decades and basically allow for more serotonin to be available to stimulate postsynaptic receptors. They are available to treat depression, anxiety disorders, ADHD, obesity, alcohol abuse, childhood anxiety, etc.

SSRIs are most commonly used antidepressants nowadays. The drugs act by blocking the presynaptic serotonin reuptake and treat both anxiety and depressive symptoms.

Pharmacokinetics[7-12]

All SSRIs are orally active and long-acting drugs. This allows them once daily doses. The drugs of this class are metabolized by CYP2D6 and drugs like fluoxetine are prodrugs forming long-acting metabolite. SSRIs like fluvoxamine have potent enzyme inhibiting activity and can block activation of tamoxifen leading to increase in level of parent molecule. Metabolism of drugs like warfarin may be blocked and hence plasma level may be elevated.

Fluoxetine is metabolized to norfluoxetine and hence is long acting. This is the very reason for preferring this drug in remitting and relapsing depression.

Uses

SSRIs are used in the treatment of major depression, dysthymia, OCD, panic disorder, bulimia nervosa, and social phobias. SSRIs are also effective in the treatment of bipolar depression, premenstrual dysphoric disorder, and PTSD. They have some usefulness, although not as good as TCADs, in chronic pain and impulse control disorders. SSRIs have also been used to treat borderline personality disorder.

Side Effects

Most common side effects include gastrointestinal (GI) upset, sexual dysfunction (30%), anxiety, restlessness, nervousness, insomnia, fatigue or sedation, and dizziness. SSRIs have a very little risk of cardiotoxicity in overdose. SSRIs can develop a discontinuation syndrome with agitation, nausea, disequilibrium, and dysphoria. Coma can occur in overdose.

Some patients may develop anhedonia or apathy. Nausea and vomiting are transient and are relieved by meals. Drowsiness or somnolence occurs with paroxetine. Bruxism (involuntarily grinding of the teeth) has been noted. Extremely vivid and strange dreams occur in some patients particularly when the drugs are given at night.

Akathisia caused by SSRI is common and occurs in the beginning. Stimulation of 5-HT2C receptors may contribute to the agitation or restlessness sometimes induced by serotonin reuptake inhibitors. This can be mitigated by use of benzodiazepines. Dizziness can occur with SSRIs but overall, SSRIs are safer compared to TCADs. Dizziness appears to be innocuous but is a common side effect associated with SSRIs; even with relatively safer drugs, for example, escitalopram in low doses, it can be significant. It is important to know that most side effects of SSRIs may disappear by 4 weeks due to adaptation.

SSRIs were developed for inhibition of the neuronal uptake for serotonin, a property shared with the TCADs, but without affecting the other various central neuroreceptors (i.e., histamine, acetylcholine, and adrenergic receptors) that are responsible for many of the safety and tolerability problems with TCADs. In this way, fluoxetine and other SSRIs represent a major advance over tricyclics because of their lower toxicity.

These drugs are highly selective antidepressants compared to others like tricyclic or MAOIs. A number of neurobiological effects such as increase in BDNFs, neurogenesis, and neuronal resilience have been described with these drugs. These have little or no activity upon histamine, and muscarinic or alpha receptors reflecting lack of sedation, palpitations, constipation, etc., or alpha block with these drugs. These are indicated primarily for treatment of major depression. OCDs have also been managed successfully with these drugs. In bulimia, these have been shown to have a modest loss of weight. In the treatment of generalized anxiety, nowadays, long-term treatment is best done by SSRIs. Weight gain and sexual side effects can affect compliance. Starting doses of commonly used SSRI/SNRIs are given in **Table 7.9**.

Selective Norepinephrine Reuptake Inhibitors

SNRIs have slightly greater efficacy than SSRIs and have slightly fewer adverse effects than SSRIs. Current drugs include venlafaxine and duloxetine. Mechanism of action of these drugs is very similar to SSRIs except SNRIs inhibit reuptake of norepinephrine primarily than that of serotonin. However, duloxetine works on both neurotransmitters. Side effects of SNRIs are mostly similar to SSRIs except that venlafaxine can cause hypertension.

Norepinephrine-Dopamine Reuptake Inhibitors

Norepinephrine-dopamine reuptake inhibitors (NDRIs) include bupropion as the main drug. The mechanism of action is grossly similar to SSRIs and SNRIs. However, bupropion is more potent in inhibiting reuptake of dopamine. The drug is also an α_3-β_4 nicotinic antagonist explaining its efficacy in smoking addiction. Adverse effects

Table 7.9 Commonly used antidepressants with their starting dose

Drug	Dose	Features
Citalopram	20 mg daily	Few drug interactions, QT interval can occur at dose above 40 mg
Escitalopram	10 mg daily	Faster onset of action
Paroxetine	20 mg daily	Short half-life, anticholinergic
Mirtazapine	15 mg daily	Sedation, useful in insomnia, weight gain occurs
Venlafaxine	100 mg daily	Few drug interactions
Duloxetine	30 mg daily	Useful in chronic pain
Trazodone	50 mg daily	Sedation, drug interactions
Fluoxetine	20 mg daily	Longest acting

include lowering of seizure threshold and suicidal ideas. The drug is avoided in patients with epilepsy. Bupropion does not cause weight gain or sexual dysfunction (even used to counteract the two).

Tricyclic Antidepressants

TCADs effectively relieve depression with anxiolytic and analgesic action. In the past, they have been the first choice for treatment of depression. Pharmacological properties include blocking presynaptic noradrenaline reuptake transporter and presynaptic 5-HT reuptake transporter, and postsynaptic histamine and acetylcholine receptors. Although quite effective in treating depression, they have late onset of action and can cause impaired attention, motor speed, dexterity, and memory. These are cardiotoxic and potentially fatal in overdoses.

TCADs are very effective but have potentially unacceptable side effect profile, that is, antihistaminic, anticholinergic, antiadrenergic, etc. TCADs are lethal in overdose. These drugs can cause QT lengthening even at a therapeutic serum level, so electrocardiographic monitoring is advised.

Secondary Class Antidepressants

Secondary class antidepressants are often metabolites of tertiary amines, which primarily block norepinephrine. Side effects are the same as tertiary TCADs but generally are less severe. Examples are desipramine and nortriptyline.

Tertiary Class Antidepressants

Tertiary class antidepressants have tertiary amine side chains. Side chains are prone to cross react with other types of receptors, which leads to more side effects including antihistaminic (sedation and weight gain), anticholinergic (dry mouth, dry eyes, constipation, memory deficits, and potentially delirium), and antiadrenergic (orthostatic hypotension, sedation, and sexual dysfunction). They act predominantly on serotonin receptors. Examples are imipramine, amitriptyline, doxepin, and clomipramine. They have active metabolites including desipramine and nortriptyline.[9] Many of the clinically useful antidepressants are metabolites of parent drugs.

Pharmacokinetics

TCADs are well absorbed upon oral administration and have relatively long half-lives. All are metabolized in the liver and converted into intermediates that are later detoxified. Importantly, these readily cross the placenta.

Due to their lipid-soluble nature, they have high volume of distribution. The drug has a good penetration in CNS. The drugs of this class have a high first-pass metabolism and therefore have variable blood levels in individuals. Antidepressants of this class are metabolized by hepatic microsomal enzyme system and conjugated with glucoronic acid. The inactive metabolites are eliminated in urine via kidneys.

TCADs can potentiate CNS depressants and the effect of alcohol, and that of the noradrenaline as they block its uptake; some anti-Parkinson drugs become potentiated due to blocking of dopamine reuptake, and antihypertensive action of clonidine and methyldopa gets blunted as the noradrenaline amount in the synapse increases. Given with MAOIs, there is a chance of producing a potentially serious condition called "serotonin syndrome."

Drug Interactions

Drugs of TCAD class are involved in several drug interactions:

- Potentiation of direct sympathomimetics, for example, noradrenaline.
- Reduced antihypertensive action of clonidine by preventing their transport into neurons.

- Potentiate other CNS sedatives, for example, benzodiaezepines.
- SSRIs (e.g., fluxamine) inhibit metabolism of TCAs may raise their levels.
- With monoamine oxidase inhibitors, dangerous hypertensive crisis with excitement and hallucinations.
- Phenytoin, chlorpromazine, aspirin, displace tricyclic antidepressants from protein binding and produce toxicity.
- Phenobarbitone induce metabolism and inhibit the effect of the drug.

Uses

- Depression unresponsive to commonly used antidepressants (SSRIs or SNRIs). Although they are not currently the drugs of choice, they are useful when other drugs fail.
- Panic disorder: Drugs like clomipramine and imipramine are used.
- Bed-wetting in children: Imipramine is the drug of choice. The drug works by reducing bladder contractions and is quite effective in young children.
- Treatment of migraine headaches: Amitriptyline is used.
- Chronic pain syndromes (e.g., migraine): Amitriptyline is superior to SSRIs.

Side Effects

TCADs produce a wide variety of side effects due to their nonselective nature (**Table 7.10**). **Fig. 7.4** provides pharmacological basis of the

same. Common side effects of TCADs include sedation, and anticholinergic side effects such as dry mouth and urinary retention can occur. Blurred vision can occur in elderly. Drugs like amoxapine, which have D2 blocking activity, can cause extrapyramidal side effects such as acute muscular dystonia. Autonomic side effects such as failure of ejaculation and hypotension are not uncommon. Coma, convulsions, and

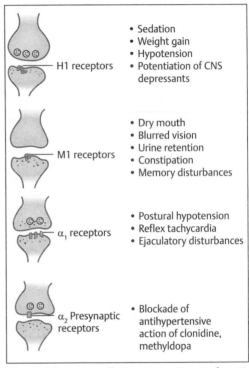

Fig. 7.4 Receptor–effector interactions of antidepressants. This diagram helps us in understanding the pharmacological basis of commonly used antidepressants and their associated side effects.

Table 7.10 Common side effects of tricyclic antidepressants

Drug	Sedation	Anticholinergic effects	Hypotension	Cardiac effects	Seizures	Weight gain
Amitriptyline	+++	+++	+++	+++	++	++
Clomipramine	++	+++	++	+++	+++	+
Desipramine	Minimal	+	+	++	+	+
Nortriptyline	+	+	–	++	+	+

cardiotoxicity can occur in overdose. Overdose of TCADs can produce profound autonomic effects such as anticholinergic and alpha-blocking effects such as hypotension. Respiratory depression, arrhythmias, shock, and hypotension can occur. Treatment is supportive and is done with sodium bicarbonate for cardiac toxicity. Benzodiazepines are used for seizures, and intravenous fluids and dopamine/noradrenaline are needed for maintaining hemodynamic stability. Mortality could still occur. Repeat prescription should be avoided until and unless necessary. This is especially true of older patients who are more sensitive to side effects of these drugs.

Anticholinergic side effects: Blockade of muscarinic M1 receptors cause several anticholinergic side effects such as dry mouth, blurred vision, constipation, urinary retention, and impotence.

Sedation: This occurs due to blockade of histamine (H1 receptors). Apart from sedation, weight gain can also occur. Weight gain may also be related to serotonin 5-HT2 receptor antagonism.

Postural hypotension: Postural drop in the blood pressure occurs due to adrenergic α receptor antagonism.

Cardiac effects: These are presumed to be due to direct membrane effects leading to cardiac arrhythmias. These side effects are more common with TCADs compared to SSRIs.

Monoamine Oxidase Inhibitors

These are long-acting, irreversible inhibitors of monoamine oxidase enzyme which degrades serotonin and noradrenaline. It is important to know that the enzyme has two isoforms: MAO-A inhibition causes antidepressant activity and MAO-B inhibition causes side effects.

These have been used since the 1950s but have a controversial past. MAOIs have potential for serious side effects and potentially fatal interactions with other drugs and food. Due to their adverse effects, several drugs that are selective inhibitors are being developed. Highly selective MAO-A inhibitors are much safer than irreversible MAOIs and their side effects are minimal. Examples include brofaromine, pirlindole, toloxatone, and moclobemide.

MAOIs are nowadays used rarely, although these have historically been the first antidepressants discovered. These have been considered specifically for refractory depression in recent times. Drugs of this class are of two types: MAO-A and MAO-B inhibitors. MAO-A enzyme degrades mainly serotonin and norepinephrine, while MAO-B degrades dopamine. MAO-A inhibitors include isocarboxazid, moclobemide, and tranylcypromine. Selegiline is an MAO-B inhibitor and is a safer alternative. Patch of selegiline has recently been approved.

MAOIs bind irreversibly to monoamine oxidase, thereby preventing inactivation of biogenic amines such as norepinephrine, dopamine, and serotonin, leading to increased synaptic levels. These drugs are very effective for depression but have toxic side effects. Side effects include orthostatic hypotension, weight gain, dry mouth, sedation, sexual dysfunction, and sleep disturbance. Hypertensive crisis can develop when MAOIs are taken with tyramine-rich foods (like cheese, beer, wine, meat, etc.) or sympathomimetics. Serotonin syndrome can develop if MAOI is taken with medicines that increase serotonin or have sympathomimetic actions. Serotonin syndrome symptoms include abdominal pain, diarrhea, sweats, tachycardia, hypertension, myoclonus, irritability, and delirium. This can lead to hyperpyrexia, cardiovascular shock, and death. To avoid this, one would need to wait for 2 weeks before switching from an SSRI to MAOIs. The exception to this rule comes in case of fluoxetine where one would need to wait for 5 weeks because of long half-life.

This happens due to its long-acting metabolite (norfluoxetine).

Tyramine is a dietary constituent of many foods and when antidepressants of this class are given with foods such as beer, wine, cheese, and meat, a dangerous hypertensive crises known as "cheese reaction" can develop. Moclobemide is a reversible drug; hence, it is not likely to have cheese reaction. It is treated by intravenous injection of phentolamine (alpha blocker). Because of this restriction on diet and other side effects such as hypotension (due to alpha block), their popularity has reduced. Moreover, drug groups such as SSRIs have become extremely popular nowadays. However, MAOIs are nowadays indicated for "neurotic depression" or "atypical depression." Sudden discontinuation of MAOIs should be avoided. Overdose can be potentially fatal and can cause seizures, agitation, and hyperthermia. Due to their reduced popularity, overdoses have become less common.

Side Effects of Antidepressants

Antidepressants have several side effects. The newer ones are relatively free from the side effects compared to older ones. However, older ones have several clinical uses in special situations.

Sedation

Most common side effect of TCADs is sedation. SSRIs, however, produce insomnia. Tricyclic drugs are given at bed time so that their sedation potential helps in correcting insomnia occurring due to depression. Desipramine and nortriptyline produce minimum sedation; hence, they are commonly used in patients with depression and hypersomnia. Drugs, like modafinil, that have brain activating properties have been uled to counteract antidepressant induced sedation. Depression-induced fatigue and lack of energy can also improve with this drug.

Gastrointestinal Afflictions[8-12]

GI upset is common with SSRIs. SSRIs lack significant anticholinergic side effects; hence, constipation is uncommon. Nausea is the most common manifestation. However, loose stool and abdominal pain can also occur. Paroxetine has anticholinergic activity; therefore, this drug does not cause much of GI upset. It is important to know that GI side effects are common reasons to discontinue these medications in early course of disease. Nausea is less common at starting dose of 20 mg/day. Starting with low dose and increasing it gradually can prevent nausea and vomiting. Drugs such as ondansetron can also be given if vomiting develops. Mirtazapine, a serotonin antagonist, is also an alternative drug having potential to treat nausea and vomiting associated with SSRI therapy. SNRIs may have a greater chance of causing nausea compared to SSRIs.

Anxiety

SSRIs produce akathisia (a form of anxiety) especially in the beginning of the treatment. This can be reduced by benzodiazepines. Anxiety thus is an important side effect of SSRIs. About 10 to 20% patients report restlessness, jitteriness, and agitated behavior. Reason could be that SSRIs affect serotonergic pathways diffusely in the brain and this could bring about CNS arousal. For this reason, drugs like fluoxetine should be taken in morning and not at bedtime. Patients may have to be given benzodiazepines, for example, clonazepam 0.5 mg twice a day, lorazepam 0.5 mg twice a day, or alprazolam 0.25 mg twice daily, early in course of therapy to deal with anxiety and restlessness. It is noteworthy that paroxetine may cause sedation, while rest of the SSRIs have potential to cause insomnia.

Vascular

Hypertension is a side effect associated with venlafaxine. MAOIs and tricyclics can cause hypotension due their alpha blocking side effects. Overdose of MAOIs can cause prominent hypotension.

Sexual Side Effects

All SSRIs have adverse sexual side effects on long-term basis leading to anorgasmia (females) and impotence (males). Around 30 to 40% of patients may experience sexual side effects and this can reduce compliance as well. Although adaptation to sexual side effects occurs in some patients, this may take a long time before it appears. This can be reduced by giving cyproheptadine half an hour before sexual intercourse. Cyproheptadine blocks serotonin receptors and can reduce the ill influence of serotonin on the male reproductive organs. Sildenafil can also be used. Mirtazapine is free from sexual side effects. Bupropion and yohimbine have also been tried. Decreasing the dose and increasing the treatment gap can also reduce their frequency. Withholding short-acting SSRIs, for example, paroxetine, can be useful in some. With long-acting drugs like fluoxetine, such approach becomes useless.

Weight Gain

Weight gain occurs commonly with TCADs. SSRIs can promote weight loss. Weight gain occurs due to antihistaminic properties of TCADs. Effect of SSRIs on weight is biphasic. Bupropion can also produce weight loss. However, bupropion does not cause sedation or anticholinergic side effects. Mirtazapine and trazodone produce prominent weight gain.

Switchover

It means converting a depression patient into mania. This may be a particular concern in adolescents and may require monitoring. Although FDA has put a black box warning in this regard, still studies done in a period after the warning have failed to find an increased risk of suicide in this population. It has been said that rare emergence of treatment-emergent suicidal thoughts is not a good enough reason to withhold treatment with SSRIs. Adverse effects seem particularly bothersome in case of paroxetine in children. Therefore, it may seem wise to try different agent before trying out this one in children.

Cardiotoxicity

Cardiotoxicity occurs with amitriptyline, and it manifests in the form of tachycardia and arrhythmias in overdose. Maprotiline produces prominent cardiotoxicity. Nefazodone has anticholinergic activity (maximum with amitriptyline and doxepin). Among the SSRIs, maximum anticholinergic property is seen with paroxetine.

Seizures

Antidepressants reduce seizure threshold. This side effect is seen mainly in overdose. Bupropion is particularly likely. The drug is contraindicated in epilepsy. Maprotiline can also provoke seizures. The drug has norepinephrine reuptake blocking activity and no anticholinergic activity.

Hepatotoxicity

This has been reported with nefazodone and duloxetine. Incidence is extremely low but increases when levels of aminotransferases rise to three times of their basal limit. It may make a clinical sense to monitor these drugs in patients with preexisting liver disease or those drugs which undergo extensive hepatic metabolism.

Extrapyramidal Symptoms

Loxapine is a prodrug and has antipsychotic nature. The drug produces a metabolite that has antidepressant activity (amoxapine). Prolonged use of this drug has been associated with extrapyramidal symptoms (e.g., tardive dyskinesia).

Serotonin Syndrome

Serotonin syndrome occurs at high doses or when combined with other drugs, an exaggerated response can occur. Serotonin syndrome is due to increased amounts of serotonin. The condition alters cognitive function, autonomic function, and neuromuscular function and is potentially fatal.

This is a combination of hyperreflexia, myoclonus, hypertension, and hyperthermia. This occurs when SSRIs are used with MAOIs or two SSRIs are used together in high dose. Condition can improve in 24 hours after stopping the offending drug, but it may continue. Benzodiazepines, cyproheptadine, and beta blockers are useful for treatment. External cooling is done. Acid–base balance is corrected if needed.

It is noteworthy that serotonin syndrome should be prevented as it may have potentially fatal outcome. Causative agents (e.g., SSRIs) should immediately be stopped. Use of cyproheptadine, a serotonin antagonist, in dose of 16 mg/day is advised. Dantrolene may also be used. External cooling is required.

Drug Interactions[13–15]

Risk of serious drug interactions with SSRIs is fairly limited. However, still some clinically important ones may be noted with others and deserve a mention. Drugs like citalopram, escitalopram, mirtazapine, and venlafaxine are less likely to be involved in clinically significant drug interactions. Bupropion, duloxetine, modafinil, and sertraline have intermediate potential, and drugs like nefazodone, fluoxetine, and fluvoxamine have powerful potential. Some noteworthy interactions are as follows:

- Drugs like warfarin, heparin, and nonsteroidal anti-inflammatory drugs (NSAIDs) can potentiate SSRIs induced thrombocytopenia. Use with caution or avoid this combination.
- Metabolism of drugs such as propafenone and encainide can be inhibited by drugs such as fluvoxamine or fluoxetine due to their enzyme inhibiting properties. Sertraline can be used in such situations.
- MAOIs are not normally combined with SSRIs/TCAD due to fear of serotonin syndrome. An adequate washout period is necessary if switchover is needed.
- Drug interactions are quite likely with paroxetine, fluoxetine, and fluvoxamine as these may increase plasma levels of drugs metabolized by CYP1A2, CYP2C19, and CYP2D6.
- SSRIs have enzyme inhibiting activity leading to increase in their plasma levels. However, escitalopram is most selective of them all and does not have enzyme inhibiting activity. Likewise, paroxetine is also less likely to be involved in drug interactions compared to other SSRIs.
- Doses of trazodone should be lowered when used with microsomal enzyme inhibitors.
- SSRIs are inhibitors of CYP2D6 isoforms and this can potentially increase plasma levels of TCADs and class IC antiarrhythmics, for example, propafenone.
- Nefazodone can inhibit metabolism of protease inhibitors in HIV positive cases; hence, possible toxicity can occur.

SSRIs Discontinuation Syndrome

It may be less of a problem compared to many other antidepressants. However, sudden discontinuation of these drugs can cause malaise, headache, and nausea. This is particularly true for short-acting drugs such as paroxetine, sertraline, and fluvoxamine. Commonly, a flu-like presentation within a week of stopping SSRIs can occur. It may be prudent to taper short-acting drugs rather than stopping them abruptly.

With discontinuation of any SSRI, the onset of withdrawal symptoms occurs within a few days and can persist for 3 to 4 weeks. Symptoms include disequilibrium, GI problems, flu-like symptoms, sensory disturbances, and sleep disturbances.

Tricyclic Antidepressant Discontinuation Syndrome

Sudden discontinuation can lead to laziness, headache, lack of energy, nightmares, and GI symptoms. There can be sudden increase in cholinergic activity, leading to diarrhea, sweating, anxiety, and piloerection. To avoid these problems, the drugs of this class should gradually be stopped.

Tricyclic Antidepressant Poisoning

These drugs have a high degree of anticholinergic activity. Therefore, in overdose, these could cause coma, convulsions, and cardiotoxicity. Death from overdose is not uncommon. One of the usual ways in which such an eventuality can be prevented is by not indiscriminately repeating these drugs. That means, they should be prescribed only in short supply. A 1.5-g dose of imipramine or amitriptyline is enough to be lethal in many patients. Ventricular tachycardia, fibrillation, and seizures are sometimes seen in overdose.

Treatment involves cardiac monitoring, airway support, and gastric lavage. Sodium bicarbonate is often administered to uncouple the TCAD from cardiac sodium channels. Charcoal and supportive measures are used. Intravenous injection of sodium bicarbonate ensures pH between 7.4 and 7.5. Life-threatening toxicity can be managed by using physostigmine, a cholinergic agent. However, it should not be used routinely due to its tendency to cause respiratory depression.

Monoamine Oxidase Antidepressant Poisoning

These are uncommon type of poisonings nowadays due to less common usage of these drugs in modern medicine. Overdose may cause hypotension. However, consumption of tyramine containing products can cause cheese reaction leading to a dangerous rise in blood pressure. Any unabsorbed drug from stomach should be removed by gastric lavage. Phentolamine is the drug of choice (alpha blocker). Never use beta blockers as they can block beta receptors leaving alpha receptors free (unopposed vasospasm).

Clinical Pharmacology of Antidepressants[12–27]

- Most effective intervention for achieving remission and reducing relapse is a medication. Combined treatment modalities may be required, for example, psychotherapy and medications.[5] Efficacy is defined as 50% or more improvement on standard assessment tools such as Hamilton depression rating scale. SSRIs are very effective in the treatment of depression, but apart from depression, they have a useful role in panic attacks, OCDs, generalized anxiety disorders, PTSD, etc. However, they have little role in pain syndrome. On the contrary, TCADs are very effective there for a number of reasons, for example, increase myelination in damaged nerves and reduce degeneration by increasing BDNFs.

- Side effects and drug safety are major reasons of selecting an antidepressant. Dropout and reduced compliance are cause for concern. Patients need to be explained about the latency of onset of action of many antidepressants (therapeutic delay). Patients may be called frequently during the course of treatment, especially during first month or so. In long-term compliance studies, weight gain and sexual dysfunctions have been most important reasons for reduced compliance. Weight gain commonly occurs due to TCADs, MAOIs, and mirtazapine. It is least problematic in case of bupropion and fluoxetine. Likewise, sexual side effects are seen commonly with SSRIs and MAOIs. Nefazodone, mirtazapine, and bupropion are least problematic in this regard. Novel antidepressants such as agomelatine do not have sexual side effects. It should be remembered that optimal dose is the dose of a drug that has minimal side effect and produces best therapeutic response. First assessment of the patient regarding therapeutic response should only be made after 4 weeks.

- Efficacy of SSRIs and TCADs in depression is equal. Reason for selecting SSRIs and other newer antidepressants is their safety and tolerability.

- Avoid TCADs in patients with serious cardiovascular diseases as their overdose can be fatal; desipramine has the greatest risk. It is noteworthy that a short supply for say 10 days should be prescribed rather than giving a 3-month supply. This will reduce drug availability among patients and reduce chance of intentional overdose.

- Geriatric patients will require a low dose and slow upward titration (start low and go slow). This is because a lot of concurrent medications are being taken, hepatic and renal functions are reduced, and fat-to-muscle ratio is increased leading to accumulation of drugs. Citalopram, sertraline, and escitalopram are best-tolerated antidepressants for elderly. Fluoxetine should be avoided due to its anticholinergic and very long half-life. Likewise, TCADs and

MAOIs are poorly tolerated in elderly and hence can be second line and third line, respectively.

- Indian patients may require lower than usual dose of drugs due to slow metabolism (pharmacogenetic differences). Genetic testing chips are available at many centers around the world to pick and choose which patients are likely to have a better response to these medicines.

- Most antidepressants have a lag period of 4 to 6 weeks; hence, there will be a delay in producing therapeutic response. Therefore, acutely agitated patients or those who are overtly suicidal can be considered for electroconvulsive treatment. However, some patients can respond before 4 weeks and others may need longer than 8 weeks also. So, final assessment about treatment response should be made after 2 months as stated earlier. Increase in the drug dose or switching the drug to another class is reasonable alternative if patients fail to respond. If a patient becomes stabilized at a particular dose, it should be maintained for 6 to 12 months. Long-term maintenance therapy should be considered for those who have had three or more episodes of severe depression in last 5 years.

- Antidepressants are not recommended as monotherapy in "bipolar patients" as there is a possibility of "switch." That means, patients have a risk of suicide due to occurrence of hypomanic or manic episodes as underlying depression gets treated. Data establishing a clear link between antidepressants and suicide in general are lacking. In children and adolescents, especially in the early course of disease, the possibility of suicidality (suicidal behavior) should be kept in mind. Because of this, patients and caregivers are warned to look for signs and symptoms such as worsening anxiety, insomnia, agitation, and suicidal thoughts early in course of disease.

- Newer drugs used for depression, for example, SSRIs and SNRIs, have advantage of being safer in overdose and have fewer side effects and drug interactions. Therefore, these are used more commonly compared to TCADs or MAOIs. Most of the clinical guidelines of professional psychiatric associations consider newer antidepressants to be the frontline drugs for treatment of depression. However, if older ones are available for clinical use and patients cannot afford the newer ones due to higher costs older ones can be used. Older patients have reduced ability to metabolize drugs of these classes; therefore, lower than normal doses should be used. Careful monitoring of side effects should be done in this population.

- SSRIs are the drugs of choice for mild to moderate depression. Their main advantage is that these do not cause cardiovascular or anticholinergic side effects. Moreover, these are well tolerated in cases of overdose. Moreover, SSRIs have shorter half-life (fluoxetine is an exception); therefore, their side effects disappear early. Moreover, these do not participate in major cytochromal enzyme-dependent drug interactions. Highly selective SSRIs such as escitalopram may have slightly higher efficacy compared to other SSRIs due to their ability to allosterically modulate the binding site of serotonin transporters. Some SSRIs are preferred in given situations more than the others, for example, sertraline in cardiac disease patients, fluvoxamine or sertraline for those with OCDs, and fluoxetine for relapsing depression. Depression in Parkinson's disease is treated by sertraline.

- Some TCADs are useful in special situations: Clomipramine (OCD), amoxapine (psychotic depression), desipramine (cocaine withdrawal), and nocturnal enuresis (imipramine).

- MAOIs are considered to be third-line antidepressants after SSRIs and TCADs/atypical antidepressants. Side effects include postural hypotension and signs and symptom of catecholamine excess. Hypertensive crises can occur (blood pressure > 180/120).

- Agomelatine is a new melatonin receptor agonist that can be used in unipolar depression. Recall that melatonin receptor agonist is also used in initial insomnia. Ongoing trials show that the drug offers an important alternative for the treatment of depression, combining efficacy, even in the most severely depressed patients, with a favorable side-effect profile. The drug is generally given in dose of one 25-mg tablet at night. The dose can be increased to 50 mg daily after 2 weeks. It can be given when tapering SSRIs or SNRIs. Liver function tests are recommended in patients at baseline.

- In long-term treatment of anxiety disorders, SSRIs are now preferred. In short-term or acute treatment, benzodiazepines are drugs of choice. Although drugs like buspirone have the advantage of being nonsedative and selective, efficacy of benzodiazepines makes them preferred in acute situations. Since benzodiazepines have tendency to cause tolerance, addiction, dependence, and withdrawal upon long-term use, SSRIs have emerged as drugs of choice for long-term treatment of these disorders. SSRIs are free from abuse and withdrawals; therefore, they are now the main drugs. A recent meta-analysis has shown that fluoxetine and sertraline are better than other drugs in terms of therapeutic response.

- A patient should be evaluated after 2 months of antidepressant treatment. About three-fourths will show clinical improvement. If there is none, then patients should be referred to a mental health specialist after checking compliance.

- Patients should be educated about the possible side effects of antidepressants and against use of alcohol. Patients with depression and pain respond better to TCADs or duloxetine compared to other medications. Those with arrhythmias and coronary artery disease (CAD) respond better to SSRIs compared to TCADs.

- One of the most important points which need to be kept in mind is to prescribe antidepressants based upon side effect profile. For example, for those with sedation potential, for example, mirtazapine/TCADs could be given to patients of depression with insomnia. Likewise, for those with oversleepiness, a brain stimulating drug such as nortriptyline or desipramine could be chosen. Those experiencing too much fatigue could be treated by selegiline or bupropion. Similarly, those with significant anxiety accompanying depression should be treated with SSRIs as these have excellent antianxiety activity.

- Since patients with depression may have suicidal thoughts, the amount of drug to be dispensed should be limited, else fatal suicides could occur.

Starting Treatment

- Antidepressant efficacy is similar, so selection is based on past history of a response, side effect profile, and coexisting medical conditions. There is a delay typically of 3 to 6 weeks after a therapeutic dose is achieved before symptoms improve.

If no improvement is seen after a trial of adequate length (at least 2 months) and adequate dose, either switch to another antidepressant or augment with another agent.

- Nowadays, SSRIs are the mainstay for treatment of depressive disorders. If no background information about the patient is available, then it is wiser to start someone with an SSRI, for example, sertraline, at a low dose, for example, 25 mg/day. The dose can then be increased to 200 mg depending upon the therapeutic response.

- Among the older antidepressants, a drug with brain activating properties such as desipramine will be appropriate. The drug is started in dose of 50 mg once daily and increasing it to 150 mg. Mood worsening and suicidal ideas should be looked into in case that happens; a prompt change in response in terms of increasing dose or change of medication should be done.

- Psychotic depressant needs a drug like amoxapine or antipsychotics such as olanzapine. SSRI and olanzapine combinations can be used in their usual doses. Mifepristone, a new glucocorticoid antagonist, has a good activity in psychotic depression.

- Major depression with atypical feature with seasonal onset (seasonal affective disorders) can be treated with MAOI or with SSRIs. Nonpharmacological measures such as phototherapy could be used in seasonal affective disorders.

- Augmentation with dextroamphetamine and methylphenidate has been used for short-term treatment of depression in medically ill and geriatric patients. They have a rapid onset and do not have many side effects in the short term. However, long-term treatment is avoided. They are given in two doses, early in morning with breakfast so as to avoid interference with sleep due to their stimulant nature. They also work as adjunctive treatment for refractory patients.

Choosing an Appropriate Antidepressant[8]

- Among antidepressants, citalopram, sertraline, venlafaxine, mirtazapine, bupropion, and duloxetine have minimal drug–drug interactions.
- Paroxetine and fluoxetine have most drug interactions. Try to avoid the two drugs with older persons. Fluoxetine has anticholinergic activity too, which is capable of producing cognitive dysfunction and worsening glaucoma and benign prostatic hyperplasia.
- Venlafaxine, duloxetine, fluoxetine, and bupropion are most activating; sertraline is slightly activating; citalopram is neutral; paroxetine is mildly sedating; and mirtazapine and trazodone are very sedating.
- Paroxetine may cause mild anticholinergic effects and mirtazapine causes more pronounced effects.
- Mirtazapine (moderate) and trazodone (high) have higher rates of orthostatic hypotension.

- SSRIs have an increased risk of bleeding, hyponatremia (SIADH), and osteoporosis, which could be problematic in special risk groups.
- Older age (>75 years), lesser severity of disease, late onset depression (≥60), first episode, and anxious depression and associated executive dysfunction may be associated with poor response to antidepressant. Special features of antidepressants help to choose best antidepressants for the given situations (**Table 7.11**).

Treatment of Refractory Depression

Treatment-resistant depression may be related to polymorphisms in the promoter region of the serotonin transporter gene (5-HTTLPR) or dysregulation of noradrenergic systems.[3] MAOIs are considered to be effective for certain types of refractory depression; electroconvulsive treatment is the method of choice.

Augmentation of antidepressants with lithium, thyroxine, or olanzapine has been a popular way of treating this form of depression. Magnesium has been an investigational drug. Treatment-resistant depression with psychosis, for example, delusional depression, is treated by electroconvulsive therapy.

Table 7.11 Clinically important features of commonly used antidepressants

Antidepressant	Feature
SSRIs	Sexual dysfunction, headache, GI upset, tremors, and exacerbation of anxiety
TCAD	Overdose may be lethal; alpha blocking effects can cause hypotension and sexual dysfunction; cardiac conduction abnormalities likely
Venlafaxine	Blood pressure may increase
Mirtazapine	Sedation, weight gain
Nefazodone	Hepatic failure risk
Bupropion	Increased risk of seizures
Duloxetine	Monitor liver functions; risk of liver toxicity

Abbreviations: GI, gastrointestinal; SSRIs, selective serotonin reuptake inhibitors; TCAD, tricyclic antidepressant.

As a general notion, most "treatment-resistant" depressed patients have received inadequate therapy. Several issues need to be considered in patients who have not responded to treatment as listed in **Box 7.3**.

The current antidepressant may be stopped, and a trial initiated with an agent of unrelated chemical structure.

Alternatively, the current antidepressant may be augmented by the addition of lithium, liothyronine, or an atypical antipsychotic.

A third approach is to use two different classes of antidepressants concurrently. The combination of an SSRI and MAOI should not be used.

Pharmacoeconomic Considerations

- Drug costs account for about 10 to 12% of the direct costs of treating depression. When evaluating the costs of treatment, more must be considered than the cost of medications alone. Several studies have shown that the SSRIs are a more economical approach to treatment of depression when all treatment costs are considered.

- A recent evaluation found that both nefazodone and fluoxetine were cost effective when compared with imipramine,

with nefazodone being slightly more cost effective than fluoxetine. Additional, longer term studies in more diverse populations are needed before judgments can be made regarding which of the newer antidepressants offers a cost-effectiveness advantage.

Evaluation of Therapeutic Outcomes

- Several monitoring parameters, in addition to plasma concentrations, are useful in managing patients. Patients must be monitored for adverse effects, remission of previously documented target symptoms, and changes in social or occupational functioning. Regular monitoring should be assured for several months after antidepressant therapy is discontinued.

- Patients given venlafaxine and those given TCADs concurrently with adrenergic neuronal blocking antihypertensive should have blood pressure monitored regularly.

- Patients older than 40 years of age should receive a pretreatment electrocardiogram (ECG) and it should be performed periodically.

- Patients should be monitored for emergence of suicidal ideation after initiation of any antidepressant.

- In addition to the clinical interview, psychometric rating instruments allow for rapid and reliable measurement of the nature and severity of depressive and associated symptoms.

- Patients should be monitored closely for relapse or recurrence if the brand of antidepressant is changed.

Failure of Antidepressants

Several reasons are now being elucidated for the failure of antidepressant responses. One of the important reasons is the polymorphism of the genes that encode for drug metabolizing enzymes.

Box 7.3: Checklist of treatment refractory patients
• Is the diagnosis correct?
• Does the patient have a psychotic depression?
• Has the patient received an adequate dose and duration of treatment?
• Do adverse effects preclude adequate dosing?
• Has the patient been compliant with the prescribed regimen?
• Was treatment outcome measured adequately?
• Is there a coexisting or pre-existing medical or psychiatric disorder?

Polymorphisms of select genes encoding iso-enzymes of cytochrome P-450, responsible for metabolism of popular antidepressant drugs, namely, CYP2C19, CYP2D6, CYP1A2, and CYP3A4/5, are being explored.[3] It has been suggested that for optimal response, the nature of these genes will have to be kept in mind.[10]

Recent Advances

- AmpliChips are now available in many countries that can determine therapeutic response to a particular drug in a particular case. This is like as we do in microbiology (sensitivity and testing of antibiotics). It is assumed that a particular isoform that is relevant in a particular case metabolizing a particular drug could one day be identified, and we shall be able to use the best possible drug for an individual case in most accepted doses.

- Monitoring of prefrontal electroencephalogram (EEG) is also being considered as one of the diagnostic modalities that could be considered for possible use in knowing the therapeutic response.

- Polymorphism in serotonin transporters located in presynaptic neurons (SERT) has been studied to know which patients are likely to experience the side effects to particular drug. In the experimental assays done so far, some positive predictive values of these tests have been found.

- Vortioxetine is a new antidepressant that addresses cognition of depression patients more reliably compared to other drugs. A number of other drugs such as sertraline, citalopram, escitalopram, duloxetine, and desvenlafaxine have been found to improve cognition.[16,17]

References

1. Papakostas GI, Homberger CH, Fava M. A meta-analysis of clinical trials comparing mirtazapine with selective serotonin reuptake inhibitors for the treatment of major depressive disorder. J Psychopharmacol 2008;22(8):843–848

2. Bilbao Garay J, Mesa Plaza N, Castilla Castellano V, Dhimes Tejada P. Serotonin syndrome: report of a fatal case and review of the literature. Rev Clin Esp 2002;202(4):209–211

3. Reimherr F, Amsterdam J, Dunner D, et al. Genetic polymorphisms in the treatment of depression: speculations from an augmentation study using atomoxetine. Psychiatry Res 2010;175(1-2):67–73

4. Smith SS, McCarthy DE, Japuntich SJ, et al. Comparative effectiveness of 5 smoking cessation pharmacotherapies in primary care clinics. Arch Intern Med 2009; 169(22):2148–2155

5. Blier P, Ward HE, Tremblay P, Laberge L, Hébert C, Bergeron R. Combination of antidepressant medications from treatment initiation for major depressive disorder: a double-blind randomized study. Am J Psychiatry 2010;167(3):281–288

6. Knadler MP, Lobo E, Chappell J, Bergstrom R. Duloxetine: clinical pharmacokinetics and drug interactions. Clin Pharmacokinet 2011;50(5):281–294

7. Schatzberg AF, Cole JO, DeBattisa C. Antidepressants. In: Manual of Clinical Psychopharmacology. Washington DC and London: American Psychiatric Publishing Inc.; 2010;37–167

8. Levenson JL. Psychopharmacology. In: Textbook of Psychosomatic Medicine. Washington DC and London: American Psychiatric Publishing Inc.; 2011:957–1021

9. Rico-Villademoros F, Slim M, Calandre EP. Amitriptyline for the treatment of fibromyalgia: a comprehensive review. Expert Rev Neurother 2015;15(10):1123–1150

10. Jeleń A, Sałagacka A, Balcerczak E. Characterisation of selected molecular mechanisms influencing pharmacokinetics and pharmacodynamics of antidepressants. Postepy Hig Med Dosw 2015;69:753–762

11. Tham A, Jonsson U, Andersson G, Söderlund A, Allard P, Bertilsson G. Efficacy and tolerability of antidepressants in people aged 65 years or older with major depressive disorder—a systematic review and a meta-analysis. J Affect Disord 2016;205:1–12

12. Patel K, Allen S, Haque MN, Angelescu I, Baumeister D, Tracy DK. Bupropion: a systematic review and meta-analysis of effectiveness as an antidepressant. Ther Adv Psychopharmacol 2016;6(2):99–144

13. Varigonda AL, Jakubovski E, Bloch MH. Systematic review and meta-analysis: early treatment responses of selective serotonin reuptake inhibitors and clomipramine in pediatric obsessive-compulsive disorder. J Am Acad Child Adolesc Psychiatry 2016; 55(10):851–859.e2

14. Tan S, Huang X, Ding L, Hong H. Efficacy and safety of citalopram in treating post-stroke depression: a meta-analysis. Eur Neurol 2015;74(3-4):188–201

15. Walitt B, Urrútia G, Nishishinya MB, Cantrell SE, Häuser W. Selective serotonin reuptake inhibitors for fibromyalgia syndrome. Cochrane Database Syst Rev 2015; (6):CD011735

16. What is new about antidepressants? https://www.karger.com/Article/FullText/48894 5#:~:text=Vortioxetine%20is%20said%20 to%20improve,found%20to%20improve% 20similar%20cognitive (Accessed online on September 7, 2020)

17. Cognitive impairment in depression: recent advances and novel treatments. https://www. dovepress.com/cognitive-impairment-in-depression-recent-advances-and-novel-treatment-peer-reviewed-article-NDT (Accessed online on September 7, 2020)

CHAPTER 8

Antipsychotics

Vikas Dhikav

Clinical Case Example

- A 21-year-old male, college student, with symptoms consistent with schizophrenia, is admitted because of profound psychotic symptoms. He is treatment-naïve, and if one plans to start an antipsychotic, what baseline blood work would you obtain? Which drug to start with?

Answer: Many atypical antipsychotics can cause dyslipidemia, transaminitis, and elevated blood levels, and there is a class risk of diabetes unrelated to weight gain; so, you need the following: Lipid profile, fasting blood sugar, liver function tests, and complete blood count. Risperidone can be a good option.

He is likely to experience akathisia, which is not uncommon with risperidone. Given he is very ill, reducing the dose may not be the best choice; so, likely treat with an anticholinergic agent or propranolol. One needs to treat akathisia because it is associated with an increased risk of suicide.

Psychosis[1–3]

As per the World Health Organization (WHO), neuropsychiatric illnesses account for a major disease burden, more than cancers and cardiovascular diseases. Psychosis is a common psychiatric illness and contributes to significant caregiver and societal burdens. Schizophrenia contributes to a major part of this disease burden.

Psychosis is an abnormal mental condition in which the patients lose touch with "reality." Patients may appear to be poorly kempt, may behave awkwardly, and respond to inappropriate and unreal stimuli.

Psychosis is a thought disorder characterized by disorganized speech, loss of touch with reality, and delusional ideas. Patients with psychosis, of which schizophrenia is the most common

example, have poor self-care and at times are even violent.

Patients often experience abnormal voices coming to their ears (auditory hallucinations). These may be highly suspicious (delusional thinking) and, rarely, could become aggressive also. There are two different kinds of features seen in psychosis commonly known as positive and negative symptoms. The former are probably the manifestations of dopamine excess, while latter are seen due to hypoglutaminergic state.

Types

Schizophrenia is the most commonly seen condition responsible for psychotic episodes. It could be divided into many subtypes, for example, if emotional state of the patient is highly incoherent or out rightly silly, it is known as hebephrenic schizophrenia. Likewise, excited patients or those with rigidity of muscles are known as catatonic schizophrenia. If symptoms are not specific, it is known as undifferentiated schizophrenia.

Symptomatology

Delusions are fixed, false, and firm beliefs that are rigid and do not change even if there is an evidence of contrary. For example, patient may have suspicious or hostile attitude toward family members and would doubt them as well. Hallucinations are perceptions without stimuli and can be auditory, tactile, or visual. Typically, patients keep hearing abnormal voices coming to their ears which are giving a day-to-day account of what they are doing, how, and when. These are often derogatory and are known as "third person hallucinations." This is because, typically, there are two imaginary persons who keep speaking to the patient and "pass comments" on his actions/ behavior. Patients are quite troubled by them. Catatonia is an immobile state accompanied by motor manifestation of schizophrenia. Abulia is lack of will, while avolition means lack of motivation. In general, schizophrenia is considered as a "split" mind. These patients are indecisive, incoherent, and, rarely, violent. Delusions and hallucinations of auditory type constitute a core of schizophrenic patients' symptomatology (**Box 8.1**).

Clinically, patients may be indifferent with regard to self-care. At times, appearance can be bizarre. Language may appear to be fragmented

Box 8.1: Features of psychosis
• Delusions.
• Hallucinations.
• Catatonia.
• Abulia.
• Avolition.

with invention of new words, which is known as neologism, apart from verbigeration (repetition of senseless or purposeless words), and echolalia (repeating words spoken by others). Emotional state is flat (no expression). Thought contents may be paucity of thoughts or delusional thinking of persecutory nature. Bizarre perceptions, for example, anesthetic hallucinations (like "burning in brain" or "blood flowing" in the brain) can occur.

Schizophrenia is the most common disorder of thought and has affected 1% of world population. The disorder has an onset in adolescence or early adulthood. It is a heterogeneous disorder and is associated with positive and negative symptoms. WHO has listed schizophrenia as 1 of the top 10 causes of disability worldwide.

Drugs effective against various types of psychotic behavior are known as antipsychotic drugs. These are also known as neuroleptic drugs as they supposedly "grip the nerves" and "set them right." This results in suppression of motor activity and improvement of emotional expression. Antipsychotic agents have been known to treat patients of psychosis in both acute phase and to prevent relapse.

Antipsychotic Drugs[1-8]

Traditionally, antipsychotics have been divided into two different types: Typical and atypical. The former are typified as dopamine-2 (D2) receptor blockers, while the latter block serotonin receptors (5-HT2). It has been said that development of atypical antipsychotic represents an important therapeutic advance in treatment of psychosis. This is shown by improvement in quality of life of these patients and better performance in social context. Better safety profile with equal or better efficacy of these agents may be the reason behind this.

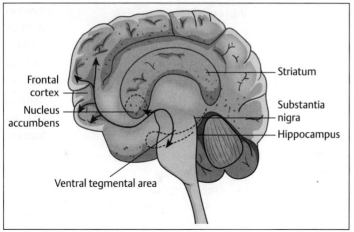

Fig. 8.1 An overactivation of dopaminergic transmission in mesolimbic system has been held responsible for occurrence of positive symptoms of schizophrenic psychosis. The loop-like structure shown in this figure is also known as limbic system ("emotional brain").

Pathophysiologically, an overactivation of dopaminergic systems in mesolimbic areas has been identified among many other neurochemical abnormalities (**Fig. 8.1**).

Similarly, hypoglutaminergic state in frontal lobe has been correlated with refractory forms of schizophrenia. That is why, nowadays, augmentation with NMDA agonist is being evaluated. This hypothesis is strengthened by the fact that NMDA antagonists such as ketamine or phencyclidine are able to produce psychotic manifestations. Disease often begins in adolescent and follows a remitting and relapsing course.

Mechanism of Action

Traditionally, older antipsychotics, also known as typical ones, act by blocking dopaminergic transmission (D2 blockers). New ones (atypical) act by blocking 5-HT2 or dopaminergic receptors (D4). Mesolimbic and mesocortical systems have been focused prominently for explaining the antipsychotic activity of D2 blockers. **Fig. 8.2** compares the older and newer drugs with regard to their mechanisms of actions.

Recent evidence has confirmed the role of limbic system hyperdopaminergic activity in generating positive symptoms of schizophrenia.

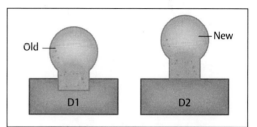

Fig. 8.2 Older drugs or conventional antipsychotics bind to dopamine-2 (D2) receptors very tightly, while the newer drugs have a loose binding. Hence, the conventional drugs produce extrapyramidal symptoms (EPS), while newer drugs have a significantly lesser risk of producing the same.

Recent evidence suggests that muscarinic and glutaminergic actions can also play some role in conferring antipsychotic activity. **Fig. 8.3** displays the general mechanism of action of antipsychotics, and **Fig. 8.4** explains the multitude of actions produced by antipsychotics.

When antipsychotics are started, then classic manifestations of psychotic behavior are reduced (**Box 8.2**). There are a variety of drugs available with diverse pharmacological actions (**Box 8.3**).

The newer drugs, as stated earlier, act by blocking dopamine receptors or 5-HT2A/5-HT2C. Newer drugs such as aripiprazole (D2) and ziprasidone (D1) are partial agonists. This represents

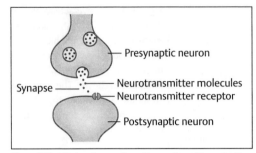

Fig. 8.3 Mechanism of action of antipsychotics. Note that older antipsychotics are dopamine-2 (D2) receptor blockers, while the newer ones block D4 or 5-HT2A. Clinical Antipsychotic Trials in Intervention Effectiveness (CATIE trial) has indicated that atypical antipsychotics are safer than the older ones.

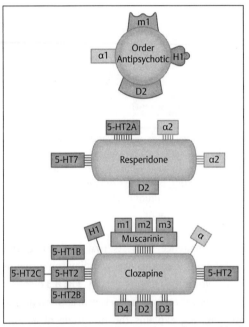

Fig. 8.4 Typical antipsychotics drugs block dopamine-2 (D2) receptors in mesolimbic system to produce pharmacological effects, while the atypical drugs block 5-HT2A/D2 receptors. In addition to this, several receptor systems are blocked by both the groups, producing adverse effects.

a newer thinking in this area. It is assumed that blockade of D2 receptors in mesolimbic area is responsible for relief of positive symptoms of schizophrenia, while block of same receptors in basal ganglia leads to extrapyramidal symptoms

---

Box 8.2: Clinical effects of antipsychotics

- Calming down of patients.
- Reduced response to delusional stimuli.
- Less agitation.
- Decreased hostility.
- Decreased social isolation.

Box 8.3: Classification of antipsychotic drugs

Older antipsychotics (1st generation):
- **Phenothiazines.**
- **Aliphatic chain:**
  ◇ Chlorpromazine.
  ◇ Prochlorperazine.
- **Piperazine:**
  ◇ Fluphenazine.
- **Piperidine:**
  ◇ Thioridazine.
  ◇ Mesoridazine.
- **Butyrophenones:**
  ◇ Haloperidol.
  ◇ Droperidol.
  ◇ Penfluridol.
  ◇ Flupenthixol.

Newer drugs (atypical antipsychotics—2nd generation antipsychotics):
- Clozapine.
- Olanzapine.
- Risperidone.
- Sertindole.
- Quetiapine.
- Aripiprazole.
- Ziprasidone.
- Paliperidone.
- Iloperidone.
- Asenapine.

(EPS). **Fig. 8.5** provides details of blockade of which dopaminergic system is pharmacologically needed and blockade of which leads to adverse effects.

Likewise, blockade of D2 receptors in tuberoinfundibular pathways leads to endocrinal alteration with antipsychotics. Conventionally, it has been thought that atypical antipsychotics

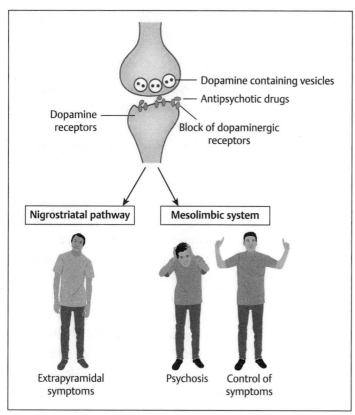

Dopamine containing vesicles

Antipsychotic drugs

Dopamine receptors

Block of dopaminergic receptors

Nigrostriatal pathway

Mesolimbic system

Extrapyramidal symptoms

Psychosis

Control of symptoms

Fig. 8.5 The relief of psychotic symptoms is related to blockade of dopamine receptors in the mesolimbic system. The block of same receptors in the nigrostriatal tract is related to generation of extrapyramidal symptoms (EPS).

are free from the problem of hyperprolactinemia. However, drugs like risperidone commonly cause endocrinal alteration (increased prolactin).

Clozapine has been the first drug that was virtually free from the extrapyramidal system. The drug blocks D4 and 5-HT2A receptors rather than D2 unlike typical antipsychotics. Importantly, 5-HT2A receptors are presynaptic in location and hence are inhibitory. Block of these receptors in mesocortical areas leads to relief of negative symptoms, while release of dopamine in basal ganglia decreases the likelihood of EPS. Drugs of aliphatic or piperidine chain class have lower potency, while that of piperazine group have high potency. Low-potency drugs produce more of autonomic side effects, while high potency produces EPS.

Pharmacokinetics

Oral absorption of these drugs is excellent, but they have high first-pass metabolism. Therefore, bioavailability is low. Their metabolites are pharmacologically inactive and are eliminated unchanged. Volume of distribution is high due to high-lipid solubility. Drugs are highly protein-bound and accumulate in tissues with high blood supply, for example, brain. Thioridazine forms mesoridazine as an active metabolite, which is also used as an independent antipsychotic drug. Chlorpromazine is shortest acting, while penfluridol is the longest. Pharmacological effects of most of the drugs last for at least 24 hours and, therefore, permit once-a-day daily administration. Most antipsychotics have a measurable plasma concentration immediately, following intramuscular (IM) administration.

105

Pharmacological Actions

Antipsychotics produce a variety of pharmacological effects. Newer and older differ in terms of producing these effects.

- **Anticholinergic**

  Drugs like chlorpromazine have a wide variety of actions such as blockade of muscarinic receptors. This is responsible for side effects such as dry mouth, palpitation, and urinary retention. Conventional antipsychotics are significantly anticholinergic.

- **Antihistaminic**

  Typical antipsychotics have antihistaminic properties that contribute to their sedation and weight gain-causing ability. Conventional antipsychotics have significant antihistaminic actions.

- **Antidopaminergic**

  Most typical antipsychotics have such properties; therefore, these are able to produce relief of psychosis and related symptoms. Block of dopamine-1, 2, and 3 are responsible for their pharmacological action. However, as stated earlier, the main pharmacological effect is due to blockade of D2 receptors. Importantly, dopamine blockade is the basis of "dopamine hypothesis." Blockade of dopamine receptors is responsible for galactorrhea also.

- **Alpha-blockade**

  Alpha-receptors are mainly vascular receptors and, therefore, are responsible for side effects such as hypotension, tachycardia, etc. However, presence of alpha-receptors in salivary glands (alpha-2) causes salivation and leads to incontinence in urinary bladder. Since some alpha-receptors are also present in the brain, especially alpha-2, their stimulation can lead to reduction of release of neurotransmitter such as norepinephrine. This can contribute to sedation.

Uses of Antipsychotics[8–18]

1. **Chlorpromazine** is used in treatment of hiccups and heat stroke apart from psychotic disorders. Benzodiazepines (BZDs) and several anticonvulsants have also been used. Chlorpromazine is the most studied and appears to be the drug of choice for hiccups and heat stroke. Increments of 25 to 50 mg oral/intravenous (IV)/IM are effective in 80% of the cases. To avoid or minimize hypotension from the agent, preloading the patient with 500 to 1,000 mL of IV fluid is advised. Another major tranquilizer, haloperidol, is effective at doses of 2 to 5 mg as well for the same indications. Metoclopramide has been used successfully at a dose of 10 mg every 8 hours for treatment of vomiting with or without hiccups. Historically, this has been one of the most popular drugs with several uses (**Box 8.4**). The drug is used in a wide range of doses in case of psychotic disorders (25–800 mg/d). There is a risk of seizure provocation and photosensitivity with the drug. Granulocyte count may need monitoring.

Box 8.4: Uses of chlorpromazine
• Acute schizophrenia.
• Chronic psychosis.
• Drug-induced psychosis (e.g., amphetamine-induced).
• Severe aggression.
• Tetanus.
• Refractory nausea and vomiting.
• Delirium (low doses).

Chlorpromazine is the first of the typical antipsychotic class drug used worldwide. Its efficacy has been documented for over half a century. The drug has an array of pharmacological effects, for example, D2 blocking, anticholinergic, alpha-blocking, and antihistaminic effects accounting for myriad effects that it produces clinically. It is an antipsychotic drug with a good deal of antianxiety properties. Although it has now been superseded by newer and atypical antipsychotic drugs, in India, it is still a commonly used antipsychotic at peripheral centers. It has been the most popular low-potency antipsychotic drug. Although it has been a useful drug in most parts, a variety of side effects have reduced the usefulness of the drug. This is because of the broad spectrum of action of the drug.

2. **Clozapine** has been a popular drug in clinical psychiatry. However, it fell out of favor in the late 1980s, when it was associated with agranulocytosis. This requires weekly monitoring of blood counts for initial 6 months, followed later by every other week. Later, it was found that this problem occurs only when the drug is given to Jews, and it was not a general side effect (population-specific side effect). It was, therefore, reintroduced in the year 2000. Till then, it has regained its clinical utility as a preferred drug in many situations. For example, it is the drug of choice for treatment of refractory schizophrenia, schizophrenia with negative symptoms, and patients bothered by extrapyramidal symptoms. It is commonly regarded as the "gold standard" for treatment of refractory patients. Importantly, one-third patients of schizophrenia do not respond adequately to conventional

antipsychotics. Most experts agree that at least two different antipsychotics at adequate therapeutic doses should be tried before using clozapine. A recent meta-analysis suggested that although clozapine is superior for treatment-refractory disorder, but if there is no response by 6 months, then drugs with lower adverse reactions should be considered.[13]

Clozapine is a dibenzodiazepine and is a D4 blocker rather than D2. It also has antihistaminic, anticholinergic, and alpha-blocking activity. The drug may also have some role in decreasing suicidality among schizophrenics. Clozapine is a dibenzodiazepine available as 25- and 100-mg tablets. An increment of 25 to 50 mg every 2 to 3 days can be made till the target dose of 300 to 600 mg is reached. Patients need to be watched out for orthostatic hypotension and agranulocytosis. It does not cause extrapyramidal side effects (EPS). Fluvoxamine can increase its plasma levels. The drug is avoided in granulocytopenia. The drug is stopped if white blood cell (WBC) count drops to 50% of patients' normal count. The patient may be restarted if the WBC count becomes normal. They should be monitored for first 3 months and then every 2 weeks or monthly. A 5% risk of seizure can occur when the dose of drug is > 600 mg daily. The drug should be stopped, and sodium valproate should be started. Apart from agranulocytosis, constipation is a common problem in clozapine-treated patients.[15]

3. **Penfluridol** is used in patients with remitting and relapsing schizophrenia. This is a highly potent antipsychotic and has been in clinical use since the

last four decades or so. Extremely long half-life results in measurable plasma concentrations, even after the use of single oral dose. The drug is equipotent compared to haloperidol and pimozide. It is mainly indicated in chronic forms of schizophrenia; even for this indication, atypical antipsychotics are increasingly replacing it. It is given as oral tablets given on weekly basis.

4. **Ziprasidone** and **aripiprazole** have antianxiety activities. While selective serotonin reuptake inhibitors (SSRIs) remain the Food and Drug Administration (FDA)-approved drugs for generalized anxiety disorders, it has been seen that low-dose antipsychotic drugs are useful in SSRIs' refractory anxiety. Drugs like ziprasidone appear to be free from metabolic side effects typical of drugs such as clozapine or olanzapine. Ziprasidone is effective in both positive and negative symptoms of schizophrenia. Hyperlipidemia, weight gain, and new onset diabetes that are seen with clozapine and olanzapine are not seen with this drug. History of cardiac risk factors however should be taken when this drug is being given as it has the ability to prolong QT interval. Ziprasidone is a benzisothiazolyl piperazine derivative and a weak D2, D3 blocker. It has antagonistic activity at 5-HT2A receptors. The drug is given as a 40-mg capsule twice daily. EPS are unlikely.

5. **Aripiprazole** is a "dopamine stabilizer" and a D2 partial agonist. The drug is effective both in positive and negative symptoms of schizophrenia. The side effect profile resembles that of clozapine. The drug appears to be brain-activating rather than sedative. It has been tried in resistant depression. Lack of weight gain makes it especially attractive drug for teenage patients. Most antipsychotic drugs have antiemetic activity, while this drug can cause nausea. Aripiprazole is used at doses of 10 to 15 mg daily. The safety of doses above 30 mg has not been evaluated.

6. **Haloperidol** is the drug of choice for Gilles de la Tourette syndrome, psychosis in renal and hepatic failure, acute agitation, excitement in mania, acute schizophrenia, and tics and Huntington's disease. Quetiapine is also an alternative drug for acute manic episodes associated with mania as a monotherapy or as an adjunct to lithium or sodium valproate. In an acutely agitated patient, 10 mg IM haloperidol can quickly control the patient's agitated behaviors. The dose can be repeated as well every 3 to 4 hours. In Tourette syndrome, haloperidol has long been used. Pimozide was an alternative. However, due to issues related to cardiac safety, the drug has reduced its usefulness in this disorder. In Huntington's disease, tics are a prominent feature. Blockade of basal ganglia D2 receptors brings about symptomatic relief. With the introduction of tetrabenazine, a paralyzer of vesicular monoamine transporter (VAMT), there has been reduced usefulness of haloperidol in this disorder. Haloperidol is a high-potency antipsychotic which is used at doses of 5 to 10 mg daily.

7. **Risperidone** is a 5-HT2 and D2 blocker that appears to be almost as effective as clozapine in the treatment of refractory patients. So long, the drug is used in up to 6 mg daily doses, the drug is associated with minimal risk of extrapyramidal symptoms. Hyperprolactinemia is a significant concern and has been reported even on low dose. This is more common

with risperidone compared to any other antipsychotic drug. Long-acting preparations are available as well. A metabolite of risperidone, called paliperidone, has been introduced, and it runs low risk of diabetes, weight gain, and dyslipidemia. Risperidone has been given approval for the treatment of behavioral outburst in autism-affected children. Risperidone is a benzisoxazole class drug and an antagonist of serotonin-2A, D-2 and alpha-1 receptors. The drug is available as 0.25-, 0.5-, 1-, 2-, 3-, and 4-mg tablets (1-mg tablet is scored) and a syrup of 1 mg/mL. Initial dose is 1 mg twice daily and then increased by 1 mg every 2 to 3 days to 2 to 3 mg twice daily. A dose of 2 to 3 mg bid, many patients can be treated with 4 mg given as a single dose. In elderly, reduced dosage (1–4 mg/d) is given. Often elderly will do well at a dose of 1 mg once or twice daily.

The drug is not a very long-acting drug but still can be taken once or twice daily. Risperidone is a well-tolerated drug. Alpha-block-mediated orthostatic hypotension can occur but can be managed with slow upward titration. Risk of EPS is low, especially when the drug is used in doses below 6 mg daily. QT interval prolongation can occur. Few case reports of neuroleptic malignant syndromes are there.

8. **Olanzapine** is a potent anticholinergic, antiserotonergic, and blocker of dopamine receptors (D1, D4). It is quite effective in treating negative symptoms. An injectable form for controlling acute agitation has become available in some countries. Risk of tardive dyskinesia and acute muscular dystonia is much lower compared to haloperidol. Sedation and significant weight gain is a particular concern with the drug. Olanzapine has been extensively used for the treatment of patients with schizophrenia and bipolar disorder. Olanzapine has various affinities for multiple receptors, including D2 receptor, serotonin (5-HT2A, 5-HT2C, 5-HT6) receptors, and adrenaline (alpha$_1$), histamine (H$_1$), muscarine (M$_1$-M$_5$) receptors. Therefore, olanzapine is known as multiacting receptor-targeted antipsychotics (MARTA). Olanzapine advantages are given in **Box 8.5**.

Olanzapine is a thiobenzodiazepine available at doses of 2.5, 5, and 10 mg. Initial dose is 5 mg once daily, which is increased later to 10 mg daily. It is a long-acting drug, and metabolism may be induced in smokers and those taking carbamazepine. Metabolism may be inhibited by fluvoxamine. Sedation and dryness of mouth can occur. Orthostatic hypotension is likely. Weight gain and metabolic syndrome may need monitoring. This is especially the case in young individuals.[17]

9. **Quetiapine** is a 5-HT2 blocker which also blocks D2 receptors minimally. The drug has high affinity for alpha-adrenergic receptors. It is effective in treating both positive and negative symptoms of schizophrenia. Even at high dose, risk of EPS is not very high. Sedation and postural hypotension occur on high dose.

Box 8.5: Olanzapine advantages

- Effective in positive symptoms.
- More effective in negative symptoms than many others.
- Improves quality of life of schizophrenics.
- Reduced hospitalizations.
- Antidepressant activity.
- Reduced suicidal behavior.

Because of its association with cataract, initial ophthalmological examination and then subsequently every 6 months is recommended. It is useful both in acute and chronic forms of schizophrenia. The drug follows a linear pharmacokinetics and has a short half-life. Incidence of EPS is less compared to conventional antipsychotics.

Quetiapine is a dibenzodiazepine available in 25-, 50-, 100-mg doses as tablets. Initial dose is 25 to 50 mg once or twice daily and can be increased every 1 to 3 days to 300 to 400 mg daily. Clearance is reduced in elderly; hence, low doses are needed. It is a relatively short-acting drug with limited potential for drug interactions. Orthostatic hypotension due to alpha-block can occur. It may be effective for primary negative symptoms of schizophrenia. Weight gain is minimal, and it has no anticholinergic side effects. It does not increase serum prolactin levels.

10. **Molindone** is a dihydroindolone derivative which is used in refractory cases. Its side effects are slightly higher than that of atypical antipsychotics but lower than that of the typical group.

Drug Interactions

- Antipsychotic drugs such as chlorpromazine intensify the side effect profile of usually used CNS depressant agents, for example, BZDs and opioids.
- Chlorpromazine is an inhibitor of CYP2D6. It is notable that this enzyme isoform metabolizes majority of CNS drugs. Therefore, there is a chance of drug interactions as well.
- Chlorpromazine inhibits ether-a-go-go (hERG) potassium channels and can result

in QT interval prolongation. This can lead to a serious cardiotoxicity.

- Carbamazepine and clozapine used together can cause significant bone marrow depression.
- Carbamazepine and phenytoin used with clozapine can induce its metabolism and reduce plasma levels.
- Most drugs of antipsychotic class have CNS depressant effect and can potentiate other CNS depressants.
- Pharmacokinetics of these drugs can be significantly altered by enzyme inducers and inhibitors.
- Smoking and alcohol are potent enzyme inducers and may increase antipsychotic clearance by half. Dose will have to be increased in these patients.

Side Effects

A significant problem with the use of antipsychotics is the high incidence of side effects. Although equal in efficacy, atypical antipsychotics are associated with lesser risk of side effects. The side effects determine the overall choice, selection in subgroups, and repeat uses in given patients (**Table 8.1**).

Sedation

The most common side effect is sedation. Tolerance to sedative effect develops. Dependence to antipsychotics is minimal, and hence, there is little or no withdrawal syndrome. Chlorpromazine is a low-potency drug which produces high degree of sedation.

Autonomic Side Effects

These are very common with conventional antipsychotics like chlorpromazine, etc. Hypotension is a major issue. With newer drugs like quetiapine, there is a significant chance of hypotension, especially in elderly.

Table 8.1 Side effect profile of newer antipsychotic drugs

Side effect	Aripiprazole	Clozapine	Olanzapine	Quetiapine	Risperidone	Ziprasidone
Sedation	+	++++	++	++	+	++
Weight gain	±	++++	++++	++	++	±
Hypotension	±	++++	++++	++	++	±
Increased QT	–	–	±	++++	±	±
Increased prolactin	±	±	++	±	++++	++
EPS	±	–	+	–	++	+

Abbreviation: EPS, extrapyramidal side effects.

In elderly, this can contribute to falls and fractures, leading to mortality.

Anticholinergic Side Effects

Anticholinergic side effects are common and occur most commonly with thioridazine. Olanzapine also has anticholinergic activity. Haloperidol has minimal anticholinergic activity. These side effects include dry mouth, palpitation, fever, constipation, and lack of sweating. At times, high dose of these drugs can produce significant hyperthermia. It is important to know that all drugs that have anticholinergic property do not cause dry mouth. For example, clozapine has good deal of such activity but can cause drooling of saliva from an angle of the mouth. Importantly, most of the newer antipsychotic drugs have no significant anticholinergic properties, hence are devoid of these side effects. Clozapine, however, commonly causes constipation.

Weight Gain

It can be due to antihistaminic activity (H1) associated with antipsychotic agents. Increased appetite and reduced physical activity seem to be contributory. As per some surveys, weight gain has been replaced as a cause for concern among clinician over EPS. It can be significant and can cause increase in morbidity and mortality. It needs to be kept in mind that obesity in general is a risk factor for cardiac and vascular disorders

as well. The mechanism is not clearly understood. It can be due to antihistaminic or anticholinergic properties associated with these drugs. Antipsychotic-induced weight gain is seen within the first few months of treatment. Diet, exercise, and drugs such as topiramate or metformin can be recommended to treat this problem. Importantly, in weight-conscious people, this can affect treatment compliance as well. Molindone is the only antipsychotic drug that is associated with some degree of weight loss.

Metabolic Side Effects

Prevalence of type II diabetes among schizophrenics is twice as high as compared to general population. As type II diabetics are not always fat, weight monitoring alone may not be sufficient to predict occurrence of this important side effect. Metabolic syndrome is a complication of olanzapine, a thiobenzodiazepine and clozapine, a dibenzodiazepine. Hyperglycemia is an important component of both of them.

Around a decade back, fasting hypertriglyceridemia was noted with clozapine and olanzapine. Later, it was shown to occur with quetiapine as well. It can be a clinical consequence of insulin resistance which occurs as a result of use of antipsychotics. Such is the pharmacological association between these two that occasionally, in the treatment of insulinoma, a rare tumor of tail of pancreas; low-potency antipsychotics such as chlorpromazine are used. This is because of their actions on pancreas to reduce insulin secretion.

Weight again occurs maximally with olanzapine and is a complication of H1 antagonism. Newer antipsychotics can even produce metabolic disturbances in young patients for treatment of early psychosis. Risperidone has been reported to pose lowest risk of metabolic disturbance. In the so-called Comparison of Atypicals for First Episode (CAFÉ) study, in which olanzapine, quetiapine, and risperidone were evaluated, and whose primary outcomes have been reported elsewhere. The study lasted for 52 weeks. Olanzapine treatment has been associated with clinically meaningful weight increases, hypertriglyceridemia, insulin resistance, and diabetes mellitus. In the clinical antipsychotic trials of intervention effectiveness (CATIE), ziprasidone was associated with betterment of metabolic parameters. Studies indicate that drugs like metformin and orlistat are effective in treating obesity or metabolic syndrome associated with clozapine.[14]

Cardiac Side Effects

Cardiac toxicity remains a cause for concern in patients taking antipsychotic drugs. This is because these prolong QT interval by blocking phase-III potassium currents. Both newer and older drugs appear to be equally responsible with regard to this side effect. It is noteworthy that cardiac arrhythmia is the most common etiology of sudden cardiac death.

QT interval prolongation can occur in patients taking sertindole, ziprasidone, and quetiapine. Thioridazine can sometime produce significant cardiotoxicity, even at therapeutic dose. Ziprasidone has maximum risk of increasing QT interval. Thioridazine has anticholinergic and QT-prolonging activity, leading to potential cardiac arrhythmias. Torsade de pointes is a

clinical consequence of QT-prolonging tendencies associated with these drugs. Sertindole was withdrawn and reintroduced because of this complication. Although risk of QT prolongation and occurrence of significant arrhythmias is there, it still does not justify routine use of ECG in all patients using antipsychotic agents.

Agranulocytosis

Chlorpromazine and clozapine produce agranulocytosis. It presents as fever or sore throat. Clozapine needs discontinuation when the levels reach below 500 cells/mm^3. Although classically, clozapine is associated with neutropenia; 2nd generation drugs or newer drugs (e.g., olanzapine, risperidone, etc.) are not associated with these side effects. Chlorpromazine too can cause agranulocytosis. Clozapine has been particularly notorious in causing drop in WBC counts. The drug according to FDA carries a black-box warning for the same. It also has high risk of myocarditis, which may also require hospital admission. Moreover, the drug has a seizure-inducing risk as well (see above) which is significantly high. Therefore, all of these three side effects carry black-box warning.

EPS occur most commonly with high-potency antipsychotics such as haloperidol. Since the introduction of atypical antipsychotics such as risperidone in 1991, incidence of EPS have become less. Clozapine and thioridazine have minimal risk of EPS. Maximum risk of EPS is on second day. EPS are serious side effects and may even be permanent (**Box 8.6**).

Box 8.6: Extrapyramidal side effects
• Tardive dyskinesia.
• Akathisia.
• Acute muscular dystonia.
• Neuroleptic malignant syndrome.
• Parkinsonism.

Acute muscular dystonia is the most common EPS in children, while akathisia is most commonly seen in adults. Acute muscular dystonia occurs early (hours to days) and is commonly seen in young patients. Head and neck muscles, tongue, etc., are usually affected. Oculogyric crises or laryngospasm makes it a severe form. The former is treated with anticholinergic drugs like promethazine and trihexyphenidyl, while the latter is treated with propranolol or diazepam.

Tardive dyskinesia (**Box 8.7**) manifests as choreoathetoid movements of head and neck and is seen most commonly in elderly women after long-term treatment. These movements are repetitive, purposeless, and involuntary by nature. It may be misdiagnosed as a mental illness rather than a neurological disorder. The disorder was described in the 1950s soon after the introduction of drugs such as chlorpromazine, etc., when their use became common. Elderly men and women in particular are more prone to the development. It is seen that 50% of women after the age of 50 after 5 years develop tardive dyskinesia. The condition can be socially disabling as well.

It is treated either by diazepam or clonazepam. The exact cause is not known. Possibly, there is a supersensitivity of D2 receptors (if receptors are suppressed for far too long, then withdrawal of antagonist can increase receptor sensitivity, which is also known as upregulation). The condition is characterized by dopamine receptor supersensitivity. This is coupled to gamma-aminobutyric acid (GABA) deficiency and acetylcholine (ACh) deficiency.

Box 8.7: Ways to prevent tardive dyskinesia

- Use lowest dose for shortest duration.
- Discontinue the causative agent.
- Atypical agents have a smaller chance.
- No evidence of using concomitant anticholinergics.

Therefore, anticholinergic drugs are contraindicated. It can be improved temporarily by giving antipsychotic drugs; but in the long run, it is prudent to start the patient on atypical antipsychotics. Although it is known to occur with high frequency with typical antipsychotics, it is also likely with 2nd generation or newer drugs but with lesser frequency. Tetrabenazine, a newer dopamine-depleting agent, is the only approved treatment of tardive dyskinesia. Drugs boosting cholinergic activity in the brain such as donepezil have been tried with variable success. Early cases can benefit from botulinum toxin injections. Melatonin, high-dose vitamins (e.g., vitamin E) and antioxidants have also been tried.

Risk for tardive dyskinesia increases every year with antipsychotic treatment. Several scales such as abnormal movement scale can be used to quantify. Reducing dose or stopping antipsychotics may work.

Parkinsonism occurs when more than 80% of striatal dopamine receptors are occupied. Patients present with mask-like face, slowness (bradykinesia), and also with reduced arm movements along with walking. It generally evolves over weeks and tremors appear ("pill rolling"). Treatment involves reducing dose and anticholinergic drugs. In elderly, use of anticholinergics may cause dry mouth, palpitations, worsening of glaucoma, cognitive deficits, and also urinary retention. Drugs of this class include trihexyphenidyl, biperiden, benzatropine, diphenhydramine, etc. Amantadine is a nonanticholinergic drug used for Parkinsonism. It works by facilitating dopamine transmission.

Akathisia does not involve nigrostriatal pathway but involves "motor restlessness." Therefore, it may actually be mistaken for an exacerbation of psychotic and dose of antipsychotics increased mistakenly. Drugs like propranolol or diazepam are effective in treating it.

Neuroleptic malignant syndrome is a rare complication of antipsychotic drug treatment (1%). It presents as hyperthermia, rigidity, and autonomic instability. Due to muscular rigidity, muscles may undergo rupture, leading to increase in release of myoglobin. High dose of potent antipsychotics given parenterally could cause this life-threatening complication. Patients' acid base balance may be disrupted and admission to hospital might be necessary. Use of external cooling, 100% oxygen, and IV dantrolene sodium can give symptomatic relief. Bromocriptine too can be helpful.

Seizures

Seizure threshold is reduced by antipsychotic drugs. The risk is maximum with clozapine and is dose-dependent. Notably, the drug has also been shown to cause seizure episode in those with no prior diagnosis of seizure disorder. Bromides are used in patients with epilepsy and psychosis. Carbamazepine and phenytoin should, however, be avoided as the drugs can behave as enzyme inducers.

Ocular Side Effects

Thioridazine can produce retinitis pigmentosa-like illness. Quetiapine can produce cataract. Thioridazine has highest anticholinergic property; therefore, risk of EPS is minimal. Thioridazine is free from antiemetic property. The drug has significant cardiac toxicity as well. Since antipsychotic drugs work on a number of different receptors, hardly any major organ is spared in terms of side effects. However, they are still well-tolerated drugs and given with monitoring.

Sexual Side Effects

These side effects per se do not get enough attention. Part of the reason is that in schizophrenia, sexual health is poorly affected. More so, drugs too can be contributory. Alpha-blockade by drugs such as chlorpromazine and others can cause delayed or retrograde ejaculation.

Sexual side effects of antipsychotic drugs could be considerable. They may cause relationship issues, divorces, and serious marital discord.

Hyperprolactinemia

Blockade of D2 receptors have been known to correlate very well with the rise of dopamine levels. Risperidone can cause hyperprolactinemia of same degree to that of the usual antipsychotic drugs. Increase in prolactin levels is a known risk factor for sexual abnormalities. If this is a cause for concern, the patient could be shifted to a prolactin-sparing agent. Metabolite of risperidone, paliperidone, too can cause similar side effects. Notably, barring the exception of these two atypical drugs, none of the remaining ones show any significant tendency toward raising prolactin levels. Importantly, hyperprolactinemia is rapidly reversible when drugs are discontinued.

Use of Antipsychotics in Pregnancy

In general, antipsychotic drugs are considered to be safe during pregnancy. To date, no definitive association has been found between use of antipsychotics during pregnancy and an increased risk of birth defects or other adverse outcomes.

Antipsychotic Drug Usage

While considering a patient on antipsychotic drugs, there are few general rules that should be kept in mind. For example, the drug with minimal side effect profile should be chosen. A patient's past history of drug use, if available, is a significant predictor of good therapeutic response in future. Compliance to medications is important as many patients have delusions, and they may not wish to take the medications. In such patients, depot preparations of long-acting drugs could be considered. Dose range of these drugs is quite broad. For example, a low dose of 0.25 to 1 mg of risperidone at bedtime may be appropriate for a demented elderly, whereas a young schizophrenic will require a much higher dose (e.g., 6 mg/d) (**Table 8.2**).

Guidelines for prescribing antipsychotics:

- Monotherapy is the standard acceptable method of drug prescription. There is little or no justification for polytherapy in usual cases. Polytherapy is known to contribute to reduced compliance, increased risk of side effects, and also higher rate of drug interactions.
- Divided doses are not necessary once the patient has been stabilized on a maintenance dose, and most patients can be managed using a single dose.
- After careful monitoring, patients could be taken off the medications after 6 months of initial treatment.
- Fluphenazine or haloperidol (daconate or enanthate salts) will be useful in patients who have delusional ideas or who are

otherwise noncompliant; IM depot injections of these drugs will be able to control symptoms for about a month (range: 7–30 days). Usual dose of fluphenazine by IM injection is 25 mg every 2 weeks. Likewise, 25- to 50-mg risperidone can be given as an IM injection. In agitated and delirious patients, haloperidol can be given intravenously under ECG guidance.

- Hospitalization may be necessary for patients exhibiting grossly disorganized behavior.
- High-dose antipsychotics of low-potency drugs such as chlorpromazine are associated with high risk of EPS. However, in low dose, their anticholinergic and alpha-blocking side effects are prominent.
- CATIE, although not definitive, suggested that atypical antipsychotics are better tolerated than typical antipsychotics. It should be kept in mind that although older drugs may not have side effects such as EPS or hyperprolactinemia, they may have peculiar side effects, for example, metabolic syndrome or QTc prolongation. These side effects may limit use of atypical

Table 8.2 Doses of commonly used antipsychotic drugs. Doses may vary as per indications

Drug	Dose/d	Brand
Chlorpromazine	25–100 mg	Largactil, Megatil
Prochlorperazine	5 mg	Stemetil
Fluphenazine	1–10 mg	Prolixin
Trifluoperazine	1–5 mg	Neocalm, Trazine
Thioridazine	25–100 mg	Thioril, Milozinc
Haloperidol	5–20 mg	Halopidol
Penfluridol	20 mg	Flumap
Risperidone	1–6 mg	Respidon
Quetiapine	25–300 mg	Qutan, Quitipin
Clozapine	50–100 mg	Clozapine, Sizopin
Olanzapine	5–20 mg	Olan, Oleanz

drugs, just as hyperprolactinemia and EPS can limit use of older antipsychotics.

- Olanzapine is useful both in acute and chronic cases of psychosis. It has also been found to be useful both in adults and adolescents. Olanzapine is a thieno-benzodiazepine analog that binds to a large number of receptors such as D1, D2, D4, and 5-HT2A.

- Clozapine is preferred in refractory cases. However, the drug can produce myocarditis; hence, it is avoided in patients with cardiac failure. Risperidone is as effective as clozapine in refractory cases. Clozapine alpha-2 blocker, therefore, can produce excessive salivation and urinary incontinence. Clozapine-induced hyper-salivation affects a mean of approximately 30% patients and is a troublesome adverse effect that leads to massive compliance problems in patients with schizophrenia. A recent study has shown that moclobemide, a reversible inhibitor of monoamine oxidase, can be used to treat this problem.

- It should be kept in mind that compliance is a big issue in schizophrenic patients. Roughly, one-third patients take their medications regularly, one-third take partially, and other one-third do not take medicines at all. Steps should, therefore, be taken to ensure good compliance.

- All patients with acute onset of a chronic psychotic disorder are given atypical antipsychotics nowadays. Moreover, those who are treatment-refractory are also given similar kind of drugs. Patients with tardive dyskinesia or any other kind of extrapyramidal symptom are also given antipsychotic drugs. There should, however, be no urgency in switching one patient who is already stable on the pharmacological doses of a conventional antipsychotic drug.

- Clozapine needs weekly monitoring of blood counts. Metabolic side effects may also require special monitoring.

- Clozapine is the treatment of choice for treatment-refractory patients (defined as those cases who have not responded to haloperidol in 7 mg/d or equivalent dose of other antipsychotic). However, clozapine should not be used as a drug of first choice in these patients due to the need of weekly monitoring of blood counts.

- In patients with comorbid psychiatric disorders, or those with substance abuse, atypical antipsychotics are better compared to typical ones.

- Most antipsychotics have antiemetic activity (except thioridazine). Importantly, this pharmacological effect is seen even at low dose.

- Risperidone and aripiprazole have been used for treatment of bipolar disorders in adolescents. Pharmacological effect of risperidone on prolactin may need to be monitored in younger population.

- Side effects of antipsychotic agents such as EPS, anticholinergic side effects, and hypotension due to alpha-blockade are more common in elderly patients.

Clinical Pharmacology of Psychotic Disorders

- **Initial therapy of schizophrenia:**
  - ◊ The goals during the first 7 days are:
    - □ Decreased agitation.
    - □ Hostility.
    - □ Anxiety.
    - □ Aggression.
    - □ Normalization of sleep and eating patterns.
  - ◊ After 1 week at a stable dose, a modest dosage increase may be considered. If

there is no improvement within 3 to 4 weeks at therapeutic doses, then an alternative antipsychotic should be considered. However, the assessment should be done only at the end of 3 to 4 weeks. An earlier assessment could lead the clinician to a false conclusion about therapeutic failure.

◊ Larger daily doses to more severely symptomatic patients may not be highly beneficial. It is wiser to start with a lower dose, particularly so in Asian patients, as lower than usual doses may be effective. However, in partial responders who are tolerating the antipsychotic well, it may be reasonable to titrate above the usual dose range. Some patients will definitely need a high dose. Even in some elderly, adequate sedation and calmness is not achieved until high dose of antipsychotics are used.

◊ In general, rapid titration of anti-psychotic dose is not recommended. This may lead to EPS. Moreover, sedation in the beginning can be considerable.

◊ Intramuscular antipsychotic admin-istration can be used to calm agitated patients. However, this approach does not improve the extent of response, time to remission, or length of hospitalization. This is often used in emergencies. Additionally, those with remitting and relapsing disorder could gain from weekly or monthly administration. Finally, this mode of administration can be useful in poorly compliant patients also. Patients who have paranoidal ideas, IM administration of long-acting antipsychotic could be valuable.

◊ IM lorazepam, 2 mg, as needed in combination with the maintenance anti-psychotic may actually be more effective in controlling agitation than using additional doses of the antipsychotic. This is more effective in older pat-ients with dementias and behavioral and psychological disturbances of dementias (BPSD). Antipsychotics are currently recommended for patients of dementia with severe symptoms.[11] Too frequent and too long-time usage of antipsychotics in dementias can contribute to worsening of cognition as well.[12]

• **Maintenance therapy:**

In the 2nd and 3rd weeks, the following goals should be kept in mind:

◊ Socialization.

◊ Mood.

◊ Self-care.

These would respond progressively as the insight of the patient about the illness start coming. Improvement in formal thought disorder will be slow to come by and may need 6 to 8 weeks. Chlorpromazine equivalent of 300 to 600 mg will be needed. Second-generation antipsychotics are in usual doses could be used as well. They have equal or more efficacy but better safety for most of the patients. However, they are expensive.

Dose titration may continue every 1st to 2nd week if symptom improvement is not satisfactory. A different drug/dosage change should be done in case of no response.

Once started, medications should be given for at least 1 year after remission of psychotic episode. Long-term treatment, however, could be needed in many patients.

Tapering of an Antipsychotic

Drugs should be tapered slowly before disconti-nuation; however, there is a mild withdrawal. However, in most cases, it would appear as a rebound cholinergic withdrawal. In general, when switching from one to another drug, the first should be tapered and discontinued over 1 to 2 weeks after the second antipsychotic is started.

Treatment-Resistant Schizophrenia

Clozapine is the drug of choice for treatment-refractory patients in randomized clinical trials. Symptomatic improvement often occurs slowly in resistant cases as opposed to those with treatment-responsive states. Up to two-third cases may improve in 6-month treatment with clozapine. Side effects include orthostatic hypotension and agranulocytosis. For orthostatic hypotension, the drug is titrated more slowly than other antipsychotics. Usual starting dose is 12.5 mg at bedtime, increased to 25 mg twice daily after 3 days. The target is to achieve a dose of 300 mg daily in an increment of 25 to 50 mg every 3 days.

Augmentation of Antipsychotics

Combination of nonantipsychotic with antipsychotic could be useful. Likewise, combination of antipsychotics could also be considered at the higher risk of side effects. Responders would improve rapidly, and if there is no improvement, the augmenting agent should be discontinued. Mood stabilizers could be useful as augmentation agents (**Box 8.8**).

Augmentation agents may improve labile affect and agitated behaviors. Divalproex combined with risperidone or olanzapine is useful. Combination of first-generation and second-generation antipsychotics or combination of two second-generation antipsychotics has

Box 8.8: Augmentation agents
• Carbamazepine.
• Valproate.
• Lithium.

been suggested. However, evidence about the same appears to be conflicting, leaving this to the discretion of individual psychiatrist or neurologist. If a series of combinations fail, then a time-limited combination trial may be given. If there is no improvement within 6 to 12 weeks, one of the drugs should be tapered and discontinued.

SSRIs have been combined with older antipsychotics, improving negative symptoms. SSRIs have also been used for obsessive-compulsive symptoms that worsen or arise during clozapine treatment.

Propranolol, pindolol, and nadolol have been used for antiaggressive effect. These are effective in organic aggressive syndromes such as dementias. Authors have a good experience with propranolol in BPSD. Propranolol 20 mg should be given to access the tolerability. Beta-blockers are evaluated for their safety with regard to heart rate. If it dips below 60, then do not give this drug. Likewise, if the patient develops breathing difficulty, avoid the drug. It might be precipitating asthmatic episode in this patient. A dose of 20 mg twice a day or thrice a day would be sufficient in most cases in the beginning. The dose can be increased to 60 mg/day every 3 to 5 days to a maximum of 480 mg. A total of 6 to 8 weeks may be needed for evaluation of full therapeutic response. Dose in elderly patients should be kept toward lower side, especially in those with cognitive disorders. This is because they can slow down cognition.

Pharmacoeconomics

Traditional antipsychotics are inexpensive but have the high risk of side effects. The better side effect profile of newer agents has made them popular. More so, the cost of total health care is not significantly different in many studies, notwithstanding the high cost of newer antipsychotics. First-generation agents have been shown to have pharmacoeconomic advantages but second-generation agents are better in terms of their safety.[16]

Recent Advances

- Use of antipsychotics of atypical type has been associated with a higher rate of mortality.
- Asenapine is a new atypical antipsychotic developed for schizophrenia and bipolar disorders.
- Bifeprunox is a new partial dopamine and serotonin agonist and can cause nausea and vomiting as side effect. Other antipsychotics have antiemetic properties. The drug otherwise has a low incidence of side effects.

References

1. Patel JK, Buckley PF, Woolson S, et al; CAFE Investigators. Metabolic profiles of second-generation antipsychotics in early psychosis: findings from the CAFE study. Schizophr Res 2009;111(1-3):9–16
2. Einarson A, Boskovic R. Use and safety of antipsychotic drugs during pregnancy. J Psychiatr Pract 2009;15(3):183–192
3. Henderson DC, Fan X, Copeland PM, et al. Aripiprazole added to overweight and obese olanzapine-treated schizophrenia patients. J Clin Psychopharmacol 2009; 29(2):165–169
4. Kreinin A, Miodownik C, Libov I, Shestakova D, Lerner V. Moclobemide treatment of clozapine-induced hypersalivation: pilot open study. Clin Neuropharmacol 2009; 32(3):151–153
5. Ching H, Pringsheim T. Aripiprazole for autism spectrum disorders (ASD). Cochrane Database Syst Rev 2012;5(5):CD009043 Review
6. Praharaj SK, Jana AK, Goyal N, Sinha VK. Metformin for olanzapine-induced weight gain: a systematic review and meta-analysis. Br J Clin Pharmacol 2011;71(3):377–382
7. Crossley NA, Constante M, McGuire P, Power P. Efficacy of atypical v. typical antipsychotics in the treatment of early psychosis: meta-analysis. Br J Psychiatry 2010;196(6): 434–439 Review
8. Komossa K, Rummel-Kluge C, Schmid F, et al. Quetiapine versus other atypical antipsychotics for schizophrenia. Cochrane Database Syst Rev 2010; (1):CD006625 Review
9. Deng C, Weston-Green K, Huang XF. The role of histaminergic H1 and H3 receptors in food intake: a mechanism for atypical antipsychotic-induced weight gain? Prog Neuropsychopharmacol Biol Psychiatry 2010;34(1):1–4 Review
10. Leucht S, Kissling W, Davis JM. Second-generation antipsychotics for schizophrenia: can we resolve the conflict? Psychol Med 2009;39(10):1591–1602
11. Tampi RR, Tampi DJ, Balachandran S, Srinivasan S. Antipsychotic use in dementia: a systematic review of benefits and risks from meta-analyses. Ther Adv Chronic Dis 2016;7(5):229–245
12. Wolf A, Leucht S, Pajonk FG. Do antipsychotics lead to cognitive impairment in dementia? A meta-analysis of randomised placebo-controlled trials. Eur Arch Psychiatry Clin Neurosci 2017;267(3):187–198
13. Siskind D, McCartney L, Goldschlager R, Kisely S. Clozapine v. first- and second-generation antipsychotics in treatment-refractory schizophrenia: systematic review and meta-analysis. Br J Psychiatry 2016 (e-pub ahead of print). doi:10.1192/bjp.bp.115177261
14. Zimbron J, Khandaker GM, Toschi C, Jones PB, Fernandez-Egea E. A systematic review and meta-analysis of randomised controlled trials of treatments for clozapine-induced obesity and metabolic syndrome. Eur Neuropsychopharmacol 2016;26(9):1353–1365
15. Shirazi A, Stubbs B, Gomez L, et al. Prevalence and predictors of clozapine-associated constipation: a systematic review and meta-analysis. Int J Mol Sci 2016;17(6):E863

16. Grover S, Sarkar S. Antipsychotic trials in schizophrenia from India: a systematic review and meta-analysis. Indian J Pharm Sci 2015;77(6):771–779

17. Galling B, Roldán A, Nielsen RE, et al. Type 2 diabetes mellitus in youth exposed to antipsychotics: a systematic review and meta-analysis. JAMA Psychiatry 2016; 73(3):247–259

18. Schozphrenia: synthetic strategies and recent advances in drug design. Available at: https://www.ncbi.nlm.nih.gov/pmc/articles/PMC6072500/. Accessed September 7, 2020

Antimanic Agents

Vikas Dhikav

Clinical Case Examples

Case 1

- A 35-year-old lady, schoolteacher by profession, was hospitalized with her first episode of mania, and she had no previous history of a depressive episode. She has no history of drug or alcohol/smoking and no significant medical issues. What medication would you like to start?

Answer: Given her first presentation was a manic episode, statistically, she will do better on lithium. Make sure to do a pregnancy test, serum creatinine, and thyroid-stimulating hormone (TSH) levels prior to initiation of treatment. Discuss with her what she will use for birth control during the treatment due to fear of Ebstein's anomaly. You start her at 300 mg twice daily, which is the average starting dose. When she comes to see you after a week, she complains about stomach irritation and some diarrhea. What do you think is going on and what should you do?

Gastrointestinal (GI) irritation including diarrhea is common, particularly early in the treatment regimen. Encourage the patient to drink adequate fluid, leave at current dose, and see if side effects resolve.

Case 2

- A 27-year-old male is admitted secondary to a manic episode. In reviewing his history, you find he has five to six manic or depressive episodes a year. He has also struggled on and off with alcohol abuse. What medication would you like to start?

Answer: Valproate would be a good choice because patient is a rapid cycler (four or more depressive or manic episodes/year) and because of comorbid ethanol abuse.

One can start with 250 mg twice daily and titrate to 500 mg twice daily. His serum valproate level is within therapeutic range. It is not unusual for patients on anticonvulsants to experience an increase in liver function tests (LFT), and as long as they do not more than triple, no change in therapy is indicated. Continue to monitor over time every 3 to 6 months as the situation demands.

Mania

The dictionary meaning of the word "mania" is a *mental illness marked by periods of great excitement or euphoria, delusions, and over activity.*

Episodes of mania and depression alternating in the same patient are collectively known as *bipolar disorder.* Psychiatric intervention is needed when mood swings are severe and disrupt life of the patient and/or family. The estimated population prevalence is about 4% worldwide. The *Diagnostic & Statistical Manual* of diagnostic criteria needs at least one manic, hypomanic, or mixed episode to be able to diagnose bipolar disorder. Bipolar disorders are diagnosed by clinical history. Generally, they are suspected in young individuals presenting with irritability, expansive mood, flight of ideas, grandiosity, hypomania, and distractibility.

Bipolar I is severe and interferes with activity of daily living; hence, hospitalization is common. *Bipolar II* may have hypomanic or full manic episodes but severe episodes are not common.

Cyclothymia is a milder form of bipolar II or bipolar spectrum disorder. "Rapid cycling" needs four or more episodes in a 1-year period and is a special category of bipolar disorder needing particular treatment. The diagnostic criteria for bipolar disorders are given in **Box 9.1**.

Biological Basis[1-6]

There is a genetic influence that plays a decisive role in the pathogenesis of bipolar disorders. There are biochemical changes in neurotransmitters in the brains of patients with bipolar disorders and these include noradrenaline, serotonin and dopamine. Metabolites of these neurotransmitters are enhanced in the cerebrospinal fluids (CSF).

Public Health Importance

Bipolar disorder is a serious mental disorder, and it is estimated that 1 out of 4 to 5 individuals commit suicide from inadequate or no treatment during its depressive phase. Onset of illness occurs in the late teens or around 25 years. If untreated, bipolar disorder often results in loss of approximately 10 years of life, 15 years of activity, and around 10 years of normal health. Several drugs are useful for the treatment (**Box 9.2**).

Box 9.1: Diagnostic criteria for bipolar disorders

Mania: 1 week of the following symptoms (4 days for hypomania)

- Elevated, expansive, and irritable mood, with at least three of the features given below:
  ◊ Inflated self-esteem or grandiosity.
  ◊ Decreased need for sleep.
  ◊ Increased talkativeness.
  ◊ Flight of ideas.
  ◊ Distractibility.
  ◊ Psychomotor agitation.
  ◊ Indulgence in pleasure activity.
- Depressive episode (2 weeks of five symptoms):
  ◊ Depressed mood/irritability in children.
  ◊ Anhedonia.
  ◊ Appetite changes.
  ◊ Sleep changes.
  ◊ Psychomotor agitation/retardation.
  ◊ Fatigue or decreased energy.
  ◊ Worthlessness/guilt.
  ◊ Decreased concentration/indecisiveness.
  ◊ Suicidal ideas.

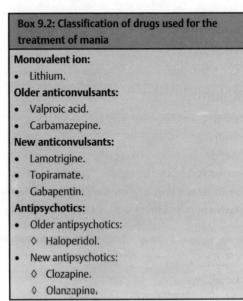

Box 9.2: Classification of drugs used for the treatment of mania

Monovalent ion:
- Lithium.

Older anticonvulsants:
- Valproic acid.
- Carbamazepine.

New anticonvulsants:
- Lamotrigine.
- Topiramate.
- Gabapentin.

Antipsychotics:
- Older antipsychotics:
  ◊ Haloperidol.
- New antipsychotics:
  ◊ Clozapine.
  ◊ Olanzapine.

Treating Bipolar Disorders

A number of drugs as per a very large meta-analysis of >10,000 patients have been found to be useful and include aripiprazole, asenapine, carbamazepine, cariprazine, haloperidol, lithium, olanzapine, paliperdone, quetiapine, risperidone, tamoxifen, valproate, and ziprasidone.[7] Drugs like quetiapine, lamotrigine, paroxetine, lithium, olanzapine, aripiprazole, and divalproex sodium have been found to be particularly useful for the depressive phase. Most trials were identified for quetiapine and lamotrigine.[8,9] Meta-analysis of placebo-controlled trials demonstrated the efficacy of lithium, valproate, and lamotrigine as maintenance therapy for the prevention of relapse in bipolar disorder.[10] Adequate efficacy exists for lithium or antidepressants in treatment of unipolar affective disorder.[11,12] In the treatment of acute mania, haloperidol or diazepam is often used to control excitement. From the limited data available, there seems no difference in overall efficacy of treatment between haloperidol and olanzapine or risperidone in acutely manic patients.[11,12] Lithium has been shown to reduce suicidality but is associated with occurrence of new episodes upon discontinuation.[13]

Lithium

This is a monovalent ion. Although the drug was discovered way before chlorpromazine and other drugs like imipramine were introduced in psychiatry, it was not accepted until the 1970s due to its toxicity. With the advent of methods which could study its pharmacology better, its acceptability increased.

History of Usage of Lithium[14]

Lithium was discovered by James Cade, an Australian psychiatrist, in the year 1949. In the 1920s, it was used as a sedative, hypnotic, and anticonvulsant. In the 1940s, it was investigated as a salt substitute for heart disease patients.

The tolerability of lithium was poor, as many people died from toxicity. The doctors at that point in time decided that maybe it was not such a good idea to use lithium in their practice.

No one believed his findings when he first proposed that this drug could be used as a mood stabilizer. This is because the drug was obtained from soil, and no one was convinced that something obtained from soil could actually be used in treatment of a psychiatric disorder.

In 1949, experiments with animals led to lethargy and use for acute mania. The drug, after reviewing evidence of its efficacy, was formally endorsed as a part of psychiatric drug treatment armamentarium in the 1970s by the American Psychiatric Association.

Mechanism of Action

Traditionally, it has been believed that lithium interacts with Na^+ and K^+ and is substituted for them in the body, as it may behave as an imposter for these ions. It may also duplicate the actions of calcium and phosphate. Effects may be mediated by Na^+/K^+-ATPase as this is one important cellular homeostatic enzyme that controls cellular excitability.

Mood-stabilizing effects may be related to dopamine receptor supersensitivity or increase in the presynaptic uptake of noradrenaline. The drug also increases metabolism of dopamine and noradrenaline; hence, it may reduce hyperactivity associated with mania.

Uptake and synthesis of serotonin is increased in presynaptic neurons. This is due to increase in tryptophan uptake in the serotonergic neurons. This effect is potentiated by selective serotonin reuptake inhibitors (SSRI). This action helps lithium in treating refractory depression. Actions on acetylcholine (e.g., increase in its synthesis) contribute toward its antimanic effects by increasing choline uptake.

Hyperactivity of mania is perhaps reduced by stimulating GABAergic activity by increasing conversion of glutamate to GABA.

In addition, the drug has been shown to have interaction with beta-adrenergic receptor coupled with secondary receptor system in the brain neurons. This may downregulate beta-adrenergic receptors in much the same way as antidepressants do. This may also explain the delay that lithium needs in stabilizing mood of manic patients.

Modern theory about the mechanism of action of the drug is as follows: Lithium is believed to interact with membrane phospholipids. The drug acts by inhibiting phosphoinol biphosphate (PIP_2) recycling in the brain. This stabilizes the excessive neurotransmission, as the neuronal response to inositol triphosphate (IP3) is reduced. **Fig. 9.1** provides details of mechanism of action.

Lithium has no psychotropic effect on nonbipolar patients. It affects nerve membranes, multiple receptor systems, and intracellular 2nd messenger impulse transduction systems.

The drug also interacts with multiple receptors, for example, serotonin which has the potential to regulate central nervous system (CNS) gene expression, stabilizing neurons without associated multiple gene expression change.

Upon entry into the cells, lithium interacts with G-proteins, modulates activity of cAMP, and decreases inositol, which decreases calcium and stabilizes cellular membranes of neurons via CREB. This leads to decrease in neuronal firing. Lithium also upregulates neuroprotective proteins and promotes neuroregeneration at some places in the brain.

Even as a simple ion, lithium has complex effects on multiple transmitter systems and mood stabilizing attributes. This is due to the latter's effect in reducing a neuron's response to synaptic input, thereby stabilizing the membrane.

Pharmacokinetics

Given orally, the drug is well-absorbed and has a half-life of 20 hours. The peak plasma levels reach in 3 hours, and the drug is fully absorbed in

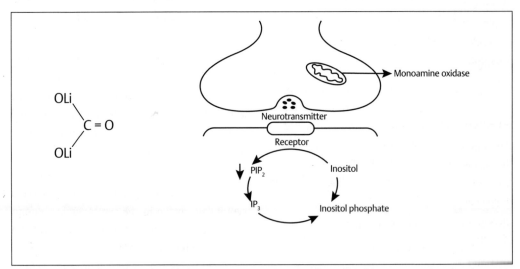

Fig. 9.1 Lithium was used as table salt prior to introduction in psychiatry. The drug was introduced in the 1970s amidst the suspicion of whether it will work, which proved to be wrong later. Based upon the available evidence, it appears that lithium acts presynaptically on the receptors on serotonin secreting neurons in the brains and blocks the reuptake of serotonin. The drug blocks the secondary messenger system as well.

8 hours. Efficacy of lithium correlates with blood levels; hence, the blood levels are frequently monitored. Lithium crosses the blood–brain barrier (BBB) slowly and incompletely. Lithium is a widely distributed drug.

Lithium takes approximately 2 weeks to reach a steady state within the body. Half of the oral dose is excreted in 18 to 24 hours while the rest happens within 1 to 2 weeks. Because of its resemblance to sodium chloride, when Na$^+$ intake is lowered or loss of excessive amounts of fluid occurs, blood levels may rise and create intoxication.

Pharmacokinetic features of lithium are as follows:

- No metabolism, eliminated unchanged.
- Almost completely reabsorbed via proximal tubules; dehydration leads to increased levels.
- Excretion is reduced in elderly but increased in pregnancy.
- Half-life is 24 hours; steady state achieved in 5 days.

Antipsychotics (e.g., haloperidol) or benzodiazepines (e.g., diazepam) may be required initially (1 week) to control excitement in manic patients. Absorption is increased in presence of meals. The drug is not a protein-bound one and is eliminated unchanged by kidneys.

Predictors of Response to Lithium

Lithium is one of the few drugs in psychiatry and neurology which has a very good therapeutic response. There are several predictors of good response. Following are some of the good and bad predictors of therapeutic responses to lithium therapy.

Good predictors of therapeutic response to lithium therapy are as follows:

- Past response.
- Euphoric mania or classical type.

- Mania-depression-euthymia sequence.
- No psychosis.
- No rapid cycling.

Poor predictors of therapeutic response to lithium therapy are as follows:

- Mixed mania (adolescents).
- Irritable mania.
- Secondary mania, for example, geriatric patients.
- Psychotic symptoms.
- Rapid cycling.
- Depression-mania-euthymia sequence.
- Comorbid substance abuse.

Uses of Lithium[12–14]

- Lithium is used in the treatment of acute mania as well as for prophylaxis of bipolar disorder. The drug is more effective during the manic phase compared to the depressive phase. It is often combined with antidepressants during the depressive phase. One should be aware of manic phase being triggered when antidepressants are used with lithium.
- Lithium is used for schizoaffective disorders as well. As an augmentation agent, it has been used with antidepressants which have not responded adequately or those patients with schizophrenia who have failed on antipsychotics.
- It has been tried in borderline personality disorders and intermittent explosive disorder.

Lithium is used in doses of 300 to 1,200 mg in divided doses; a single dose of 1,200 mg can also be used. Dose should be increased till a level between 0.8 and 1.2 meq/L can be achieved. Therapeutic effects may take about a month to develop. The drug is contraindicated in pregnancy, as it is a category D drug (high risk). The drug may not work in about 25% patients,

125

and these refractory patients may have some pharmacogenetic reasons for this response.[4] Lithium is an effective treatment for reducing the risk of suicide in people with bipolar disorders. Lithium may exert its antisuicidal effects by reducing relapse of mood disorder.[5]

Side Effects

Majority of the patients treated with lithium therapy will experience some side effects. Side effects of lithium therapy relate to plasma concentration levels; so, constant monitoring is the key. Higher concentrations (>1.0 meq/L) produce bothersome effects, and higher than 2 meq/L can be serious or fatal. A useful mnemonic of the side effects of lithium is as follows:

L = Leukocytosis.

I = Increased urination.

T = Tremors.

H = Hypothyroidism.

I = Increased thirst.

U = Underperformance of memory.

M = Mother's teratogenicity: Ebstein's anomaly.

Side effects of lithium therapy often occur when the levels are more than 1.2 meq/L. Side effects start with nausea, vomiting, diarrhea, and fine tremors. Polyuria and polydipsia occur perhaps due to antidiuretic hormone (ADH) resistance caused by lithium. This condition is similar to that of diabetes insipidus. This is a reversible condition.

The most common side effect is GI upset. The drug can be taken with meals to avoid the side effects. In addition, the dose can be lowered as many of the peak plasma level-related side effects can be significantly reduced by lowering the plasma levels (by using lower dosage). Slow-release formulations can be used or night-time use can salvage many patients who experience

side effects. Lithium citrate is less irritating to gastrointestinal tract (GIT) compared to lithium carbonate.

Tremors will usually respond to lowering of the dosage but in some cases propranolol 20 mg twice daily may be needed. Patients experiencing acne may be given topical antibiotic (e.g., clindamycin). Some cases of psoriasis or exacerbation of it have been noted.

Polyuria with early lithium therapy often resolves on its own, but in some cases, it may be persistent, needing treatment. Once daily bedtime dose of lithium can be an effective solution to tackle this problem. Renal failure is rare.[6] Fluid intake should be adequate, and patients should be given lowest effective dose. Those who experience persistent polyuria, polydipsia can be helped by a diuretic, for example, thiazide (hydrochlorthiazide 25–50 mg daily). The dose of lithium should be reduced by 50% if this is done to prevent increased lithium reabsorption that occurs during thiazide therapy. Thiazides can increase sensitivity of ADH onto the receptors. It is important to note that patients experience nephrogenic diabetes insipidus due to lithium-induced impairment of adenylate cyclase mechanisms at collecting ducts. Amiloride is an alternative to hydrochlorothiazide and it does not change the levels of lithium as hydrochlorothiazide does (amiloride-5–10 mg twice daily).

Increase in calcium and magnesium and lowering of phosphate are a manifestation of increase in the levels of parathyroid hormone produced by lithium. These actions can occur even at therapeutic levels of lithium. These changes can affect bone mineralization.

The same mechanisms explain the impairment of functions of thyroid gland produced by lithium due to interference in the action of TSH. Thyroid disturbances can occur in up to one-third of patients treated with lithium. This is not a contraindication for use of lithium and can easily be treated by levothyroxine.

ECG changes, atrioventricular (AV) nodal blocks, or rarely a new onset cardiac arrhythmia can occur during lithium therapy.

Changes in dopaminergic receptors can explain changes in the probatin levels too.

Weight gain is common, which is reflected in increase in food intake and decrease in carbohydrate metabolism due to decrease in release of insulin. Hyperglycemia may occur. Enzymes of glycolysis may be inhibited.

Symptoms of neurological impairments, for example, concentration or memory disturbances, can be helped by using lower dosages. Sedation, lethargy, or incoordination of gait also improves by the same. Long-term treatment has been associated with cognitive impairment with no evidence of improvement.[9]

Ataxia and incoordination of gait can occur in overdose. Some of the common and serious side effects are listed in **Box 9.3**.

Toxicity[10–14]

Toxic effects of lithium are seen when the levels are above 1.5 meq/L; at a level above 2.0 eq/L, life-threatening side effects are seen. Drowsiness, tremors, nausea, vomiting, diarrhea, and ataxia occur, and patients also experience vertigo and confusion. At a level > 2.5 meq/L, seizures occur with clonic movements along with arrhythmia, coma, and circulatory collapse. Rapid steps to reduce serum levels are necessary by immediate discontinuation of lithium therapy. Best method of treatment is hemodialysis and use of anticonvulsants (e.g., diazepam or lorazepam). Progressive clinical deterioration or severe toxicity is the indication of hemodialysis rather than absolute levels of lithium.

Box 9.3: Common and serious side effects of lithium therapy

- Common side effects:
  ◊ GI distress.
  ◊ Polyuria/polydipsia.
  ◊ Sedation-lethargy.
  ◊ Cognitive (memory, concentration difficulties).
  ◊ Weight gain.
  ◊ Poor coordination, tremor.
  ◊ Acne.
  ◊ Psychomotor impairment.
- Serious side effects:
  ◊ Renal:
    □ Nephrogenic diabetes insipidus.
    □ Tubular interstitial nephritis.
  ◊ Hypothyroidism.
  ◊ Psoriasis.
  ◊ Cardiac:
    □ Flat T waves in ECG.
    □ Sinus node dysfunction.
    □ Tachycardia.
  ◊ Lithium toxicity:
    □ Nausea, vomiting, diarrhea, delirium, ataxia, stupor in overdose.
    □ Treatment: Dialysis if lithium levels > 3.0 meq/L.
  ◊ Correct fluid–electrolytes imbalance.

Monitoring

Plasma level of lithium needs monitoring as the drug has narrow therapeutic index:

- Safe prophylactic level = 0.6 to 0.8 meq/L.
- Safe therapeutic level = 0.8 to 1.2 meq/L.
- Toxic levels (toxicity begins at) = 1.2.
- Toxic levels (toxicity becomes established) = 1.5 meq/L.
- Toxic levels (hemodialysis is needed).

Dose

The drug is used as lithium carbonate which is given as 300 mg three times a day. Maximum dose is 2,100 mg/day. Once started, lithium is given for about 1 year and then slowly tapered.

Drug Interactions (Fig. 9.2)

- Loop diuretics and thiazides can reduce the plasma levels of lithium and hence increase toxicity of lithium.
- Angiotensin-converting enzyme (ACE) inhibitors and nonsteroidal anti-inflammatory drugs (NSAIDs) can also increase its plasma levels.
- Certain drugs due to their diuretic activity may decrease levels of lithium. Theophylline, aminophylline, caffeine, etc., are common drugs increasing renal clearance of lithium. Increased dietary sodium and sodium bicarbonate and diuretics such as carbonic anhydrase inhibitors (acetazolamide) and osmotic diuretics (mannitol) may increase renal clearance and hence decrease plasma levels.
- Neurotoxicity is a frequent consequence of lithium toxicity, and a number of medications will enhance the risk of lithium neurotoxicity. These medications include methyldopa, typical antipsychotics, carbamazepine, phenytoin, and calcium channel blockers. Close monitoring for symptoms of neurotoxicity is recommended. These symptoms include tremor, disorientation, confusion, ataxia, and headaches. Action of neuromuscular blocking agents, especially succinylcholine, is enhanced.
- Given with haloperidol, confusion, ataxia, and reflexes may exacerbate in some patients.
- Tardive dyskinesia is more likely with typical antipsychotics and lithium combination.

Starting Lithium

Lithium is the drug of choice for prophylaxis of bipolar affective disorder. The drug decreases frequency and severity of both mania and depression in majority of the patients. One could start lithium in doses of 300 to 600 mg and in divided doses and do baseline investigations like renal, thyroid function tests and electrocardiogram. If a drug interaction is

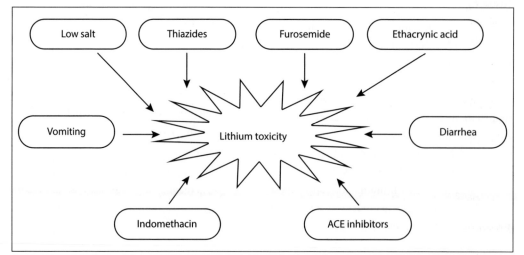

Fig. 9.2 Low-salt diet and drugs of diuretic class (e.g., thiazides, loop diuretics such as furosemide and ethacrynic acid) can precipitate lithium toxicity. The same is likely with nausea, vomiting, and diarrhea, as these conditions favor the reabsorption of lithium. Certain drugs like nonsteroidal anti-inflammatory drugs (NSAIDs) can reduce renal clearance of lithium and also cause toxicity.

suspected, it may be wise to get frequent blood levels done. The dose could be increased to 300 to 900 mg/day every 5 to 7 days till the final therapeutic response is achieved. Rapid cyclers respond poorly to this drug. Lithium is also good for prophylaxis of unipolar depression. Most cases of bipolar patients can be managed with lithium alone.

Other Agents in Acute Mania

There is an increasing trend of using atypical neuroleptics as monotherapy or as adjuvant. Acute manic symptoms of agitation and psychosis may be treated initially with these agents. Olanzapine, risperidone, and aripiprazole have been found to be useful with benzodiazepines. High-potency benzodiazepines could also be used in acute phase as adjuvants. Intramuscular injection of olanzapine or haloperidol could be used for acute behavioral control. Clonazepam could be an alternative for acute behavioral symptoms. Main benefit of using benzodiazepines is lack of extrapyramidal side effects. Olanzapine can also be used for maintenance phase of bipolar disease. List of the Food and Drugs Administration (FDA) approved agents in treatment of bipolar disorders is as follows:

- Aripiprazole.
- Asenapine.
- Carbamazepine.
- Lamotrigine.
- Lithium.
- Olanzapine.
- Risperidone.
- Valproate.
- Quetiapine.

Pretreatment Starting Workup

Baseline tests such as renal function (blood urea nitrogen, creatinine, electrolytes, urine examination) tests, thyroid functions tests (T3/T4/TSH), pregnancy test (if woman), and electrocardiogram for patients older than 40 years may be needed. Body weight and relevant medical history should be noted. The drug is started in dose of 300 to 600 mg/day divided doses and the levels are done in 5 days. Increase in dose can occur to 300 to 900 mg/day every 5 to 7 days.

Compliance

Relapse rate is high regardless of withdrawal being gradual or acute, suicide risk backup episodes are often worse than original symptoms, so treatment is often life-long. Weight gain, less energy, and productivity are common reasons of noncompliance. Patients tend to feel disease has resolved, and they no longer need medication.

Combination therapy with lithium and antiepileptics may demonstrate better protection against relapse, greater therapeutic efficacy, and studies support this as a rule rather than an exception.

Uses

Lithium is the *drug of choice* for acute mania. It is also used for prophylaxis of bipolar disorder.

Contraindications

The drug should be avoided in sick sinus syndrome due to tendency of lithium to produce AV nodal block. Lithium is ineffective in rapid cyclers, and these patients are treated by sodium valproate. Carbamazepine is an alternative drug.

Sodium Valproate

Valproate was approved as a mood stabilizer in 1996. Traditionally, it has been used as an antiseizure drug. The drug acts by increasing GABA levels, and pharmacological effects are known to occur in 2nd messenger system as well as Prot-Kinase-C. The drug is an effective antimanic, which fights bipolar depression as well. The drug is safer than lithium.

Pharmacokinetically, it is 80 to 95% protein-bound. The drug is metabolized by CYP 450 which is an enzyme inhibitor; hence, there is a significant risk of drug interactions. The half-life of valproate is 10 to 15 hours.

The therapeutic effect starts within 2 days and the levels are 50 to 125 mg/L. The drug is started in oral loading 20 to 30 mg/kg/day. Elderly and hypomania may respond to lower doses.

Common side effects include GI distress, sedation at high doses, liver transaminase elevation, tremors, hair loss, weight gain, increased appetite, thrombocytopenia (especially in elders), neural tube teratogenicity, and craniofacial abnormality (in pregnancy). Tremors can be managed with dose reduction or by use of propranolol. Leukopenia and thrombocytopenia occur, and dose reduction can restore platelet counts. Coagulopathies, endocrine abnormalities, amenorrhea, polycystic ovaries, hypothyroidism, and hypocortisolemia are less common side effects.

Idiosyncratic hepatic failure is rare but life-threatening side effects persist. It presents as lethargy, anorexia, nausea, vomiting, jaundice, bleeding, edema, etc. The risk is highest in children below 2 years of age. Importantly, the risk is very low in children above 10 years or in adult psychiatric patients. Acute hemorrhagic pancreatitis has been reported. Bone marrow suppression can occur.

Drug Interactions

- Protein-bound drugs such as amino-salicyclic acid, phenobarbitone, carbamazepine, warfarin, etc., may increase free valproic acid.
- Sodium valproate is an enzyme inhibitor and hence can increase plasma levels of other drugs metabolized in liver.
- Valproate may increase levels of liver-metabolized drugs such as tricyclic antidepressants, phenobarbitone, lamotrigine, and phenytoin.

Starting Sodium Valproate

Proper medical history and baseline medical investigations should be done before starting this drug. Complete blood count (CBC), LFT, and the patient may be screened for blood or pancreatic disorders. Patients could be warned about hepatic, pancreatic, hematologic, and teratogenic risks. The patients could be loaded orally at a dose of 20 mg/kg/day. Plasma level could be checked and kept as 50 to120 µg/mL. Monitoring of LFT and CBC can be done. The predictors of good therapeutic response to anticonvulsants are as follows:

- Mixed mania (adolescents).
- Irritable mania.
- Secondary mania (geriatric).
- Psychotic symptoms.
- Rapid cycling.
- Depression-mania-euthymia.
- Comorbid substance abuse.

Carbamazepine

Carbamazepine has conventionally been used in epilepsy. However, due to observations made about three decades back, the drug elevated the moods of patients treated with epilepsy. Additionally, cognition seemed to improve, and it was thought that the drug had psychotropic properties.

Carbamazepine was approved by FDA in trigeminal neuralgia in the late 1960s, and temporal lobe epilepsy in the 1970s. The drug is an effective antimanic, and it is useful in treating refractory depression.

The drug acts by blocking sodium channels and stabilizes the cell membranes. It is noteworthy that the metabolite of carbamazepine (epoxide) has psychotropic activity. Another important feature of carbamazepine mechanism in psychiatry is that Na⁺ block is related to its psychotropic action. Decrease in release of norepinephrine and decrease in dopamine turnover are responsible for its usefulness in mania. Increase in acetylcholine synthesis and GABA stimulation aid the same actions.

The onset of antimanic action occurs in 2 weeks, and antidepressant action is seen in 4 to 6 weeks. Therapeutic levels range from 4 to 12 or 15 mg/L. The drug is an autoinducer of liver enzymes and the half-life decreases to 10 to 15 hours.

Carbamazepine is superior to lithium for rapid cycling and is regarded as a second-line treatment for mania. Correlation between therapeutic and plasma levels (estimated between 5 and 10 mg/L) and therapeutic response is very good. The drug has been used in resistant depression and alcohol withdrawal as well. Behavioral dyscontrol of panic attacks may also respond.

Side Effects

The drug is safer than lithium in terms of producing cognitive problems, weight gain, hair loss, tremor, etc.; however, neurological side effects such as diplopia, blurring of vision, fatigue, etc., occur. Sedation and ataxia are dose related.

GI side effects such as nausea, diarrhea, and dry mouth occur. Leukopenia, thrombocytopenia, and rash can occur. Some patients may have increase in liver enzymes. Rare side effects include agranulocytosis, liver failure, pancreatitis, Stevens–Johnson syndrome, and teratogenicity in pregnancy.

Beneficial effects on cognition are probably mediated by its effect on cortisol and cholecystokinin in the hippocampus.

Drug Interactions

- Carbamazepine is an enzyme inducer of CYP 450 enzymes; and hence, it may decrease its own levels and that of several other drugs such as valproate, lamotrigine, tricyclic antidepressants, prednisone, theophylline warfarin, benzodiazepines, oral contraceptives, etc.
- Metabolism of carbamazepine may be inhibited by p450 inhibitors such as acetazolamide, and calcium channel blockers such as diltiazem and verapamil. Levels of nifedipine are not affected. Danazol, erythromycin, fluoxetine, isoniazid, valproate, etc., may increase carbamazepine levels.

Starting Carbamazepine

Baseline investigations and thorough medical history should be taken. Investigations include CBC, LFT, kidney function tests (KFT), etc. Start low in the dose of 100 to 400 mg/day and then increase by 100 to 200 mg for several days twice daily. Follow complete cell count and LFT periodically.

Gabapentin

Primarily an anticonvulsant, yet also "off label," or without FDA approval for treatment of bipolar and many other anxiety, behavioral and substance abuse problems, possibly pain disorders, it is a GABA analogue. The drug is not bound to plasma proteins, not metabolized, few drug interactions. The half-life is 5 to 7 hours. The side effects include sleepiness, dizziness, ataxia, double vision, etc. The drug is started in dose of 300 mg once daily and can be used till 2,400 mg daily.

Lamotrigine

Lamotrigine has been reported effective in patients with bipolar, borderline personality, schizoaffective, and posttraumatic stress disorders. Most of the administered drug reaches plasma. Half-life is 24 hours. The drug acts by blocking the sodium channels and excitatory neurotransmitters. The drug modifies the synaptic plasticity as well.

The drug has been approved for long-term maintenance of bipolar disorders. Side effects may include dizziness, tremor, headache, nausea, rashes, etc. The drug is used in dose of 100 mg daily to 600 mg/day. Rashes are a common side effect. Some patients may develop renal stones.

Topiramate and Tiagabine

These are two newer anticonvulsants that have potential for use in the treatment of bipolar disorders. Topiramate is started in dose of 25 mg/day, and then the dose can be increased 25 to 50 mg daily till a target dose of 100 to 300 mg is achieved.

Atypical Antipsychotics

Three drugs that may be used for bipolar include clozapine, risperidone, and olanzapine. Risperidone seems more antidepressant than antipsychotic. Clozapine is effective, yet not readily used due to potential serious side effects. Olanzapine is approved for short-term use in acute mania. Lusaridone has recently been approved for major depressive episodes in bipolar I disorders. The drug is used either as monotherapy or as adjunctive therapy with lithium or with lithium or valproate in combination. It is started in dose of 20 mg orally once daily initially and then may be increased to 80 mg daily but not to exceed 120 mg/day.

Drugs under Development

- **Tamoxifen:** This is selective estrogen receptor modulator and a protein kinase C inhibitor. It is noteworthy that lithium

too has interaction with protein kinase C pathway. The drug has been found to be useful as an adjunct to lithium in doses up to 200 mg.

- **Memantine:** Memantine is an NMDA receptor blocker, and the drug is approved for use in Alzheimer's disease. Decreased locomotor activity of this drug is being exploited for use in mania in doses between 20 and 30 mg/day.
- **Valnoctamide:** This is an analogue of valproic acid which has less teratogenicity, making it suitable for women with child-bearing potential. The drug is used in doses between 600 and 1,200 mg/day.

Current Status

Lithium is a widely recommended treatment for bipolar disorders around the world and has 60 to 80% success in reducing acute manic and hypomanic states. However, the issues in noncompliance due to side effects and relapse rate with its use precludes its use as the best option in many patients. During manic episodes, antipsychotics or benzodiazepines, the latter can be quite sedating in the beginning. During depressive episodes, temporary coadministration with antidepressants may be needed. As a whole, lithium is considered to be the gold standard mood stabilizer, but antiepileptics are also currently being used.

References

1. Antimanic-Mood Stabilizers. Lithium & Anticonvulsants. www.academicpsychiatry. org/htdocs/.../powerpoint./slideUC3mood-stablizers.ppt (Downloaded on 14th June 2016)
2. CNS Neurosciences & Therapeutics. Lithium: Still a Major Option in the Management of Bipolar Disorder. Available at: www.

simhandl.at/downloads/licht-lithium2012. pdf. Accessed October 27, 2020

3. Drugs Used to Treat Bipolar Disorder. Available at: wings.buffalo.edu/aru/PSY402C16.ppt. Accessed October 27, 2020

4. Oedegaard KJ, Alda M, Anand A, et al. The pharmacogenomics of bipolar disorder study (PGBD): identification of genes for lithium response in a prospective sample. BMC Psychiatry 2016;16:129

5. Cipriani A, Hawton K, Stockton S, Geddes JR. Lithium in the prevention of suicide in mood disorders: updated systematic review and meta-analysis. BMJ 2013;346:f3646 Review

6. Bschor T, Bauer M. Side effects and risk profile of lithium: critical assessment of a systematic review and meta-analysis. Nervenarzt 2013;84(7):860–863

7. Yildiz A, Vieta E, Leucht S, Baldessarini RJ. Efficacy of antimanic treatments: meta-analysis of randomized, controlled trials. Neuropsychopharmacology 2011;36(2): 375–389

8. Vieta E, Locklear J, Günther O, et al. Treatment options for bipolar depression: a systematic review of randomized, controlled trials. J Clin Psychopharmacol 2010;30(5): 579–590 Review

9. Wingo AP, Wingo TS, Harvey PD, Baldessarini RJ. Effects of lithium on cognitive performance: a meta-analysis. J Clin Psychiatry 2009;70(11):1588–1597

10. Beynon S, Soares-Weiser K, Woolacott N, Duffy S, Geddes JR. Pharmacological interventions for the prevention of relapse in bipolar disorder: a systematic review of controlled trials. J Psychopharmacol 2009; 23(5):574–591

11. Cipriani A, Smith K, Burgess S, Carney S, Goodwin G, Geddes J. Lithium versus antidepressants in the long-term treatment of unipolar affective disorder. Cochrane Database Syst Rev 2006;(4):CD003492

12. Cipriani A, Rendell JM, Geddes JR. Haloperidol alone or in combination for acute mania. Cochrane Database Syst Rev 2006;(3):CD004362

13. Young AH, Newham JI. Lithium in maintenance therapy for bipolar disorder. J Psychopharmacol 2006; 20(2, Suppl):17–22 Review

14. Psychiatric Times. New Drug Developments for Bipolar Mania. Available at: https://www.psychiatrictimes.com/view/new-drug-developments-bipolar-mania. Accessed October 27, 2020

Drugs for Anxiety and Insomnia

 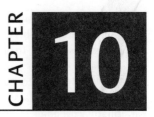
Vikas Dhikav and Kuljeet Singh Anand

> "Doctors who treat the symptom tend to give a prescription, but doctors who treat the patient are more likely to offer guidance."
>
> – J. Apley 1978

Clinical Case Example

- This is the case of a 55-year-old diabetic man with hypertension (160/90 mm Hg) and painful diabetic neuropathy, with a history of previous depressive episodes and one suicide attempt. He meets current criteria for a major depressive episode with anxiety disorder. He has been treated with paroxetine, sertraline, and bupropion. His depression improved slightly with each of these drugs but never remitted. What would you like to treat him with?

Answer: Given his hypertension, one should not choose venlafaxine. Tricyclic antidepressant (TCAD) can help with neuropathic pain and depression; however, it is not a good choice, given the side effect profile and lethality in overdose. Duloxetine is a good choice since it has an indication for neuropathic pain, depression, and anxiety. Three birds get killed with one stone here! However, one should keep in mind that duloxetine is a CYP2D6 and CPY1A2 inhibitor and has potential drug–drug interactions.

Sedatives and Hypnotics[1-3]

Sedative is a drug that produces calmness, clinically treating agitation, and *hypnotic* produces sleep. The difference between the sedative and the hypnotic is that of the dose, that is, sedatives become hypnotics at higher doses.

Benzodiazepines (BZDs) are the most commonly used drugs for this purpose. These are so named because they contain a benzene ring attached to two diazepine molecules containing nitrogen groups.

History

Alcohol has been the oldest known sedative since time immemorial. In the bygone era, people used to prefer alcohol over water due to its purity. However, its inebriant effects soon became a social hazard and water started gaining popularity. Toxic drugs, for example, bromides, paraldehyde, and chloral hydrates have been used as sedatives and hypnotics in the past. Nowadays, with the arrival of better drugs, these drugs have been replaced.

Barbiturates were introduced in early 1900 and became very popular sedatives and hypnotics. However, their addiction ability and narrow therapeutic range made them unpopular.

Before the1960s, BZDs were not used; instead, barbiturates were the mainstay drugs. Later, with the development of BZDs, things changed. Barbiturates went into disfavor due to narrow therapeutic index, drug interactions, low efficacy, and fatalities in overdoses.

The early 1960s witnessed the arrival of chlordiazepoxide, the extremely popular sedative and hypnotic of BZD class introduced by Starnbach. Although initially touted as a drug that was free from abuse liability, dependence and abuse soon became apparent. The investigator had to issue a warning later that unscrupulous use could lead to development of abuse. Till now, almost a population half the size of India's has taken BZDs for various indications worldwide.

Biochemical Basis of Anxiety

There is an increase in noradrenergic derives in patients with generalized anxiety disorders, more so in those with acute panic. Drugs like yohimbine that are alpha-2 blockers of presynaptic type can cause increase in noradrenaline release and can provoke anxiety. Likewise, clonidine, an alpha-2 agonist of presynaptic sympathetic receptors, can reduce the release of noradrenaline and has useful antianxiety properties.

Serotonin is another neurotransmitter implicated. BZDs can reduce firing of serotonergic neurons in midbrain raphae nuclei and are very effective antianxiety agents. This action of reducing serotonin activity may be related to the gamma-aminobutyric acid (GABA)-stimulating actions of BZDs. Drugs like buspirone that stimulate presynaptic 5-HT1A receptors can bring about relief of anxiety.

GABA is third major neurotransmitter that plays a role in anxiety. Reduced GABA derivatives have been noted in anxiety disorders, which is why GABA potentiating drugs have effective antianxiety responses. Drugs like bicuculine which block GABA receptors provoke anxiety; likewise, drugs that block GABA synthesis too have similar effects. It should be noted that primary action of BZDs on GABA receptors perhaps helps reducing serotonin and noradrenergic activity responsible for their antianxiety effects.

What Causes Anxiety?

Interactions of several neural pathways occur to produce symptoms of anxiety. These include the reward center in the ventral tegmental area of the midbrain, septohippocampal and amygdale-hippocampus-hypothalamus of the medial temporal lobes. Alterations in the parahippocampal area of medial temporal lobes and inferior frontal cortex have been found in patients with obsessive compulsive disorders (OCD). Notably, these become normal after treatment with clomipramine. There is a supersensitivity of serotonin receptors seen in anxiety, and this becomes normal after treatment with selective serotonin reuptake inhibitors (SSRIs). Increase in cerebrospinal levels of 5-HT or its metabolites have been found, and these abnormalities become normal after treatment with drugs.

Structure Activity Relationship

About 30 years back, it was thought that the BZD nucleus was a prerequisite toward the antianxiety effect. With the arrival of non-BZD (Z drugs such as zolpidem, etc.), this has changed. Now, it has been thought that subunits of $GABA_A$ receptors, when stimulated, will have sufficient antianxiety effect.

135

Neuropharmacology of Sleep

Sleep is a state of passive central nervous system (CNS) depression produced by inhibition of neuronal connections in reticular formation. Locus coeruleus projections of noradrenaline are involved in maintaining cortical arousal. GABA and cholinergic pathways are important in rapid eye movement (REM) sleep. Serotonin plays a vital role in sleep patterns. Lesions of dorsal noradrenergic bundles can cause hypersomnia. BZDs act on the raphae nucleus and locus coeruleus. They prolong the stage II of non-REM sleep and suppress REM sleep.

Drugs for Anxiety and Insomnia

Box 10.1 lists the common drugs used in the treatment of anxiety and insomnia.

Functional Classification

The action of all BZDs are qualitatively similar, but there are prominent differences in selectivity and time course of effect. For this reason, different members of BZD groups are used for different therapeutic purposes. BZDs exert relatively selective anxiolytic (antianxiety), hypnotic (sleep promoting), muscle relaxant, and anticonvulsant (antiepileptic) effects. An overview of drugs that are used for such indications is as follows:

- *Hypnotics*:
    ◇ Flurazepam.
    ◇ Flunitrazepam.
    ◇ Nitrazepam.
    ◇ Midazolam.
    ◇ Triazolam
- *Anticonvulsive (antiepileptic)*:
    ◇ Clonazepam.
    ◇ Clorazepate.
    ◇ Diazepam.
    ◇ Lorazepam.
- *Central muscle relaxants*:
    ◇ Diazepam.

Box 10.1: Common drugs for treating anxiety and insomnia

- **BZDs:**
    ◇ **Ultrashort:**
        □ Midazolam.
    ◇ **Short:**
        □ Triazolam.
        □ Temazepam.
    ◇ **Intermediate:**
        □ Alprazolam.
        □ Estazolam.
        □ Lorazepam.
    ◇ **Long-acting:**
        □ Diazepam.
        □ Chlordiazepoxide.
        □ Clonazepam.
        □ Clorazepate.
        □ Clobazam.
- **Non-BZDs:**
    ◇ Zolpidem.
    ◇ Zopiclone.
    ◇ Zaleplon.
    ◇ Indiplon.
- **Azapirones:**
    ◇ Buspirone.
- **Sedative H1-blockers:**
    ◇ Hydroxyzine.
- **Nonselective beta-blockers:**
    ◇ Propranolol.
- **SSRIs:**
    ◇ Fluoxetine.
    ◇ Escitalopram.
- **Antipsychotics:**
    ◇ Quetiapine.
    ◇ Risperidone.

Mechanism of Action

These drugs act by stimulating GABA$_A$ receptors and act as allosteric modulators. Facilitation of GABA transmission is a prominent pharmacological action induced by these drugs.

GABA is the most abundant inhibitory transmitter in the brain and spinal cord. GABA-ergic neurons are distributed widely in the brain and spinal cord. GABA controls the state of excitability in all brain areas and the balance between excitatory inputs (mostly glutamatergic) and the inhibitory GABA-ergic activity is maintained. If the balance swings in favor of GABA, then sedation, amnesia, and muscle relaxation occurs, and ataxia appears. Nervousness and anxiety are reduced. Experimental evidence suggests that even the mildest reduction of GABA-ergic activity elicits arousal, anxiety, restlessness, insomnia, and exaggerated reactivity, as per the experimental evidence.

Most drugs used in insomnia act as agonists at the GABA$_A$ receptor and have effects other than their direct sedating action, including muscle relaxation, memory impairment, and ataxia, which can impair performance of skills such as driving. Clearly, those drugs with onset and duration of action confined to the night period will be most effective in insomnia and less prone to unwanted effects during the day. Those with longer duration of action are likely to affect psychomotor performance, memory, and concentration; they will also have enduring anxiolytic and muscle-relaxing effects.

Several other drugs like barbiturates, alcohol, propofol, thiopentone, and steroidal anesthetic agents, for example, pregnanolone also bind to same receptors. Importantly, GABA$_B$ agonists such as baclofen do not bind to GABA$_A$ receptors. Drugs of related class such as zolpidem, zaleplon, zopiclone, and indiplon bind to alpha-1 receptors, which are also known as omega-1 or benzodiazepine1 (BZD1) receptors. As per Paul Ehrlich's principle of selectivity, the drugs binding to the receptors selectively are safer; hence, non-BZDs are safer compared to BZDs. **Fig. 10.1** and **Table 10.1** provide details of mechanism of

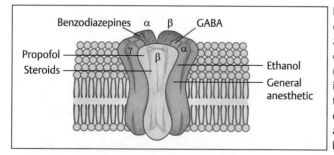

Fig. 10.1 Benzodiazepines (BZDs) receptors are pentameric structures with an ion channel that allows passage to chloride ions. Drugs binding to them (BZDs) have muscle-relaxant, motor-impairing, and anxiolytic-like properties thought to be mediated by α2, α3, and/or α5 subunits 2. Anticonvulsant activity and amnesic properties are thought to be mediated by α1 receptors subunit 2.

Table 10.1 Type of BZD receptors, location, and their pharmacological actions

Type of receptors	Location	Action
Type-I	Most common throughout CNS	Sedation and tolerance
Type-II	Hippocampus, striatum, spinal cord, medulla	Antianxiety action
Type-III	Cerebellar granule cells	Ataxia, incoordination, impair motor performance

Abbreviations: BZDs, benzodiazepines; CNS, central nervous system.

action of BZDs, receptors, and the drugs binding to the same.

BZDs increase frequency of opening of this channel. Barbiturates have GABA-mimetic actions, which means these drugs could stimulate the receptors. Non-BZDs (e.g., Zolpidem) stimulate alpha-1 subunit, which are also known as omega-1 receptors. Since these drugs stimulate only one subunit, they are highly selective and hence safer. BZDs also decrease uptake of adenosine in coronary arteries. That is why BZDs dilate coronaries. **Fig. 10.2** describes

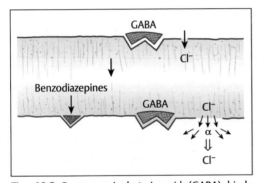

Fig. 10.2 Gamma-aminobutyric acid (GABA) binds to the GABA$_A$ receptors and increases the opening to enhance passage of chloride ions. The same response is enhanced multiple folds when benzodiazepines (BZDs) bind to the same receptors.

what happens to the GABA$_A$ receptor when GABA or BZDs bind to the same. **Table 10.2** provides details of the sites where such actions occur.

Treating Anxiety and Panic

Selecting one BZD over the other or being comfortable with one could be an individual choice of the treating clinician. A recent Cochrane Database Systemic Review concluded that there are little differences among BZDs in terms of treatment of anxiety disorders.[4] For short-term treatment of anxiety disorders, with or without agoraphobias, propranolol is as good as BZDs.[6] In the treatment of anxiety disorders, like panic disorder, generalized anxiety disorders and social phobias, SSRIs, TCADs, cognitive behavioral therapy, and psychodynamic therapies are effective apart from BZDs.[7] In addition, melatonin has been shown to be effective in reducing preoperative anxiety.[8] A combination of antidepressants and BZDs may be needed in patients with depression along with comorbid anxiety.[9] Agomelatine is effective in generalized anxiety.[10] Since repeat prescription and unscrupulous BZD usage can be an issue in older people, supervised withdrawal is indicated.[11]

Table 10.2 Pharmacological actions of BZDs and their therapeutic effects as per the brain areas

Location	Pharmacological action	Status
Amygdale, orbitofrontal cortex, insula, cerebral cortex	Antianxiety effect	Used most commonly to alleviate anxiety
Hippocampus	Mental confusion, memory impairment, antiepileptic action	Memory impairment (anterograde amnesia) is a common side effect. BZDs are used as add on antiepileptic agents
Spinal cord, brain stem, cerebellum	Muscle tone reducing effect	Not used as muscle relaxants commonly; however, in spasms of skeletal muscles, drugs like diazepam are useful
Ventral tegmental area, nucleus accumbens	Dependence and abuse	Very big problem in clinical practice; unscrupulous usage in developing countries like India contributes to dependence and abuse

Abbreviation: BZDs, benzodiazepines.

Dexmedetomidine, an alpha-2 agonist, has been used for sedation in ICUs.[12] Atypical antipsychotics are useful for severe anxiety disorders.[13] BZDs are quite effective for treating anxiety of alcohol withdrawal and have protective effect in seizures.[14] SSRIs are effective in children and adolescents with anxiety disorders.[15]

Neuropharmacology of Benzodiazepines

BZDs act at the limbic, thalamic, and hypo-thalamic levels of the brain and spinal cord. Neuroanatomically, the amygdala, orbitofrontal cortex, and insula are associated with the production of behavioral responses to fearful stimuli and central mediation of anxiety and panic, which are inhibited by BZDs. The hypo-function of $GABA_A$ receptors activity may sensi-tize the amygdala to anxiogenic responses. It is thought that the BZDs may reset the threshold of the amygdala to a more normal level of responsiveness.

Pharmacokinetics

These are lipid-soluble drugs and hence have excellent absorption and tissue distribution (**Box 10.2**). The drugs are extensively metabolized. Lipid solubility varies 50-fold among them-selves. However, their first-pass metabolism is high in general. Although these are metabolized by cytochrome P450 (CYP) enzymes, their

---

Box 10.2: Salient features of benzodiazepines pharmacokinetics

- Well absorbed orally.
- Pith peak plasma concentration achieved in 1 hour.
- Diazepam, chlordiazepoxide, clorazepate, clorazepate biotransformed to pharmacologically active intermediates.
- Long-lasting BZDs degraded to active intermediates.

---

metabolism is neither induced nor inhibited. Midazolam, flurazepam, triazolam, and diazepam are highly lipid-soluble drugs. Hence, these drugs have a rapid onset of pharmacological effect.

BZDs enter the circulation at very different rates that are reflected in the speed of onset of action, for example, alprazolam is rapid and oxazepam is slow. The liver metabolizes them, usually to inactive metabolites, but some compounds produce active metabolites with long $t_{1/2}$, which greatly extends drug action, for example, chlordiazepoxide, clorazepate, and diazepam.

Rate of absorption and distribution are major parameters of pharmacological responses rather than half-life alone in case of BZDs. They are usually effective within couple of weeks; occasionally, the onset of action may be delayed by 6 weeks. There is no evidence that increasing the dose or duration of these drugs beyond this period is effective.

Hepatic metabolism accounts for metabolism of most of the BZDs. Correlation between the plasma half-life and duration of action is poor. This is because of the active metabolites such as desmethyldiazepam, which may often extend the duration of action of drugs of this class. Metabolites of some drugs like chlordiazepoxide can increase the duration of action till 60 hours or more.

BZDs are metabolized by CYP enzyme system. Lorazepam, oxazepam, and temazepam are meta-bolized outside liver; hence, these are safe in liver disease and among the elderly. Metabolites are eliminated via renal mechanisms. An additional reason because of which these are preferred in elderly is that these are metabolized by conju-gation as opposed to oxidation, which most BZDs are metabolized by. With age, oxidative capacity of liver is reduced, while that of conjugation is retained.

Both diazepam and chlordiazepoxide form long-acting metabolites such as desmethyldiazepam and chlordiazepoxide. Long duration, which is partly due to active metabolites, makes them particularly useful for alcohol withdrawal. After discontinuation of these drugs, their rate and extent of accumulation depends upon elimination half-life and clearance.

Midazolam is an ultrashort-acting BZD having half-life less than 1 hour. It undergoes redistribution responsible for its short duration of action.

Triazolam is a short-acting BZD having half-life of 2 hours. Alprazolam is an intermediately acting drug with a half-life of 15 hours. Chlordiazepoxide, flurazepam, flunitrazepam, and diazepam are long-acting drugs belonging to this category.

It is important to know that their clearance become less in old age and those with liver diseases. Therefore, their dosage should be accordingly lowered in these groups of patients.

Uses of Individual Benzodiazepines

BZDs are extensively used for generalized anxiety disorders and acute panic, and used as muscle relaxants, sedatives, hypnotics and anticonvulsants (**Box 10.3**). Doses are described in **Table 10.3**. Drug-induced anxiety or medical disorders causing anxiety should be excluded

before starting the BZDs. Several drugs like theophylline, aminophylline, amphetamines, cocaine, cyclosporine, and tacrolimus can produce significant anxiety.

Midazolam

Midazolam is the drug of choice for sedation in short procedures. Since midazolam is a BZD, which is rapidly acting and shares the class effect of respiratory depression and hypotension, this should be kept in mind while administering the drug via intravenous (IV) injection. The drug is IV administered as 1 to 2 mg over 2 minutes; if narcotic premedication/other CNS depressants are used, patients will require less dosage of midazolam. Safety and ease of administration by a variety of routes make this drug a preferred choice.[5]

Box 10.3:   Therapeutic uses of benzodiazepines
• Sedative-hypnotic.
• Anxiolytic.
• Panic disorder.
• Generalized anxiety disorder.
• Muscle relaxants.
• Anticonvulsants.
• Alcohol withdrawal.
• Premenstrual syndrome.
• Psychoses.
• Adjunct in mania of bipolar disorder.

Table 10.3   Daily doses of some of the common BZDs and doses equivalent to 5-mg diazepam

Drug	Daily dose	Dose equivalent to diazepam (5 mg)	Elimination half-life
Alprazolam	0.25–4 mg	0.5 mg	10–20 h
Clonazepam	2–8 mg	0.25 mg	20–60 h
Diazepam	5–30 mg	5 mg	100 h
Flunitrazepam	0.5–2 mg	1 mg	20 h
Lorazepam	2–4 mg	1 mg	15 h
Oxazepam	40–90 mg	15 mg	5–25 h
Buspirone	15–30 mg	15 mg	10 h

Abbreviation: BZDs, benzodiazepines.

Triazolam

Triazolam is a short-acting antianxiety drug, and rebound anxiety can occur due to its short duration of action. This is typically known as "daytime anxiety." The drug is given in doses of 0.25 to 0.50 mg at bedtime. However, a dose of 0.125 mg may be sufficient for some patients (e.g., low body weight and elderly).

Alprazolam

Alprazolam has been the drug of choice for acute panic attacks, generalized anxiety disorders, and agoraphobia. Some physicians favor selective SSRIs/TCADs in acute panic attacks. This is because the drugs require a large dose in this condition and sedation thus produced can limit its usefulness.

Alprazolam is a fast-onset BZD that provides quick relief of acute anxiety. Alprazolam has a relatively short duration of action and multiple dosing throughout the day is required. It is associated with less sedation but a high incidence of interdose anxiety recurrence. Dependence and withdrawal could be problems with this drug. Since SSRIs and other antidepressants are effective in anxiety disorders, alprazolam is less commonly used as a first-line drug for the treatment of anxiety disorders. Alprazolam is used in dose of 0.25 to 2 mg twice or thrice daily. Among the elderly, the dose is reduced by half. Repeat prescriptions should be avoided too. The clinical duration of action is short despite moderate serum half-life.

Lorazepam

Lorazepam is an intermediately acting drug with a half-life of 15 hours. The drug does not produce any active metabolite. Metabolism is not P450 dependent and will only be affected when hepatic dysfunction is severe. The inactive glucuronide is renally excreted. It is the BZD of choice in patients with serious or multiple medical conditions. It is the only BZD available in intramuscular (IM) form with rapid and complete absorption. Its metabolism is not affected by age.

These properties make it ideal for alcohol withdrawal or in a patient with liver dysfunction or among the elderly. Since the half-life is relatively short, accumulation with multiple dosing usually does not occur. The IM form is useful in rapid control of agitation, resulting from psychosis, or drug-induced agitation. It is also widely used orally as per need basis as an adjunct to fixed doses of antipsychotic medication.

Lorazepam is used in anxiety disorders, alcohol withdrawal, and in the treatment of acute psychotic agitation. The drug is available as 0.5-, 1-, and 2-mg tablets, and 2 mg/mL, 4 mg/mL solution for IV or IM use. The drug is used at doses of 2 to 4 mg as a single daily dose before bedtime for anxiety. Elderly patients do well on half the dosage.

This is the only BZD available in IM formulation that has rapid, complete absorption. The usual dose is 0.5 to 6 mg/day given in divided doses. For alcohol withdrawal, 0.5 to 2 mg every 2 to 4 hours can be given up to a maximum of 10 mg/day.

Clonazepam

Clonazepam has a rapid onset and provides prompt relief. Clonazepam, with its long half-life, may be substituted for shorter acting BZDs, such as alprazolam, in the treatment of BZD withdrawal and panic disorder. Its long half-life allows for once-a-day dosing. Clonazepam is approved as an anticonvulsant. It is also used in panic disorders, social phobia, and general anxiety. The drug is useful in acute treatment of mania to control excitement. It is available as 0.5-, 1-, and 2-mg tablets. The drug is used at doses of 0.25- to 10-mg divided dose twice or thrice daily.

Initial dose should not exceed 1.5 mg/day divided into three doses. The dose may increase in increments of 0.5 to 1 mg every 3 days until seizures are controlled or until side effects appear. The maintenance dose should be individualized but should not exceed 20 mg/day. The initial dose in panic disorders may be 0.25 mg twice daily and may increase to target dose of 1 mg/day after 3 days; for some, it may increase in increments of 0.125 to 0.25 mg twice daily every 3 days until panic disorder is controlled or until side effects appear. Dose should not exceed 4 mg daily.

Clorazepate

Clorazepate is a long-acting BZD prodrug metabolized to desmethyldiazepam in the gastrointestinal tract (GIT) and absorbed in the active form. This drug accumulates with multiple dosing and over time. Because clorazepate is metabolized by CYP isoenzymes, metabolism can be slowed in the elderly or those with hepatic impairment. If used for anxiety, once-a-day dosing may be possible. The drug is used in anxiety disorders at doses of 7.5 to 15 mg twice or thrice daily. Dose can be increased up to a maximum of 90 mg/day. The drug is avoided in elderly due to its long half-life.

Oxazepam

Oxazepam is a safe hypnotic for older people. Zolpidem is an alternative drug. Oxazepam is used at doses of 10 to 20 mg daily. Dose in those with hepatic impairment or elderly should be kept at 10 mg once daily.

Zolpidem

Zolpidem is among the most commonly used non-BZDs nowadays, which is structurally unrelated to BZDs but acts in much the same manner. The drug however binds to (subtype 1) $GABA_{A1}$ receptors. It is useful for the short-term treatment of insomnia. The drug primarily is a sedative (rather than an anxiolytic). Zolpidem is rapidly absorbed in the GIT following oral administration, and a small part is metabolized

as first-pass metabolism in the liver. The peak plasma levels are reached in 1 hour.

The drug produces sedation and promotes good sleep without anxiolytic, anticonvulsant, or muscle-relaxant effects seen with BZDs. Long-term use can cause memory impairment, although less likely compared to BZDs. Flumazenil is reported to reverse memory impairments and overdoses and is reported to improve memory and learning, thus suggesting a possible role of endogenous BZDs in memory functions. The adverse effects include drowsiness, dizziness, and nausea at therapeutic doses. Severe nausea and vomiting may occur in overdoses. The drug is safe in older adults and has metabolism in the liver. No active metabolites are formed; hence, unusually long duration effects (e.g., hangover) are minimally likely.

Zolpidem has a reputation for causing only a low incidence of abuse and dependence; however, when taken for prolonged periods of time, dependence can develop, resulting in withdrawal upon discontinuation. The drug is used in dose of 5 to 10 mg once daily. In elderly patients, who are the biggest likely users, the dose should be kept at 5 mg once daily as there is no evidence of usefulness of higher doses. Zolpidem is used for short-term treatment of insomnia like other members of its class such as zaleplon, eszopiclone, etc. Zolpidem has minimal antianxiety effect. One of the main reasons of popularity of Z drugs (e.g., zolpidem andzopiclone) is that they have reduced potential compared to members of BZD class for tolerance, addiction, dependence, or rebound insomnia.

Zaleplon/Zopiclone

Zaleplon and zopiclone are non-BZD agonists that act at the $GABA_{A1}$ receptors to exert actions similar to BZDs but have short half-lives. Only one-third of an orally administered dose reaches the plasma, and most of that undergoes first-pass metabolism. The drugs are half as potent as zolpidem. Both improve sleep quality without rebound insomnia and little chance of developing dependency.

Diazepam

Diazepam is not only the most rapidly absorbed BZD but also a long-acting drug. Due to its long half-life (100 h), it may accumulate with multiple dosing. Diazepam is metabolized by CYP enzymes; hence, the metabolism can be slowed in the elderly and patients with hepatic impairment. If used for anxiety, once-a-day dosing may be possible. The drug is used in anxiety and alcohol withdrawal. It is available as 5- and 10-mg tablets and 5 mg/mL solution for IV use. IM administration is not recommended due to erratic absorption and painful injections. The drug is often given in status epilepticus at doses of 2 to 5 mg IM/IV; may repeat in 3 to 4 hours in mild-to-moderate seizures; for those patients with repetitive or severe seizures, 5 to 10 mg IM/IV; may repeat in 3 to 4 hours as well. The detailed uses are listed in **Box 10.4**.

Chlordiazepoxide is a long-acting BZD which accumulates with multiple dosing. Because this drug is metabolized by CYP isoenzymes, drug interactions are likely. Metabolism is slow in the elderly and patients with hepatic disease. The onset of action is slower compared to diazepam

Box 10.4: Uses of diazepam
• Endoscopic sedation.
• Muscle spasms.
• Preoperative medication.
• Relief of anxiety before cardioversion.
• Picrotoxin poisoning.
• Convulsions of tetanus.
• Status epileptics.
• Alcohol withdrawal.
• Febrile seizures (intrarectal).

and the drug is a longer acting; hence, once daily dose is possible. Chlordiazepoxide is used for chronic anxiety and alcohol withdrawal. The drug is available as 5-, 10-, and 25-mg tablets and given at doses of 5 to 25 mg once or twice daily. In the treatment of alcohol withdrawal, the dose used is 25 to 50 mg every 2 to 4 hours (maximum 400 mg/d) as per need basis. Usual dose range is 10 to 100 mg/day. Due to its long duration, the drug is avoided in elderly.

Flunitrazepam

Flunitrazepam has some forensic application. This drug is not used clinically but used by people with criminal mentalities to perform "date rape."

Nitrazepam

Nitrazepam does not interfere with REM sleep; therefore, this does not lead to REM rebound upon discontinuation. The drug is used at doses of 5 to 10 mg.

Side Effects

Sedation

Sedation is the most common side effect. Although this decreases with passage of time, it could be incapacitating in the beginning. At low doses, symptoms can include sedation, drowsiness, ataxia, lethargy, mental confusion, motor and cognitive impairments, disorientation, slurred speech, etc.

Memory Impairment

Anterograde amnesia occurs and this could contribute to impaired learning. Long-term usage can simulate a full-fledged picture of dementia. This is usually the case with alprazolam. Falls could occur in people taking these drugs due to impaired coordination. Inhibition of learning behaviors, academic performance, and psychomotor functioning could persist long after treatment is discontinued.

Hangover

Hangover is common with long-acting BZDs such as diazepam, chlordiazepoxide, etc., and these should be substituted with short-acting drugs such as estazolam or newer non-BZDs such as zolpidem, if needed. Long-acting agents taken at bedtime can result in daytime sedation the following day.

Psychomotor Dysfunction

At high doses, mental and psychomotor dysfunction can progress to hypnosis.

Rebound Insomnia

Short-acting drugs taken at bedtime can result in both early-morning wakening and rebound insomnia the following night.

Respiratory Depression

Respiration is not seriously depressed unless BZDs are taken concurrently with another CNS depressant (i.e., alcohol). However, acute overdose can lead to respiratory depression.

Tolerance, Addiction, and Dependence

Addiction, tolerance, and dependence occur upon regular use. Time-dependent decrease in pharmacological effects of BZDs can occur. The neurochemical basis of tolerance is unclear but varying rates for different behavioral effects can contribute. These include sedative and psychomotor effects which diminish within

few weeks. Memory and anxiety effects persist despite chronic use. Cross-tolerance with alcohol and other sedatives and hypnotics can occur. Tolerance to the BZDs is a major issue on long-term administration.

With long-term administration, tolerance develops to sedative-hypnotic action. However, no tolerance develops to the antianxiety and antiepileptic action. Cross-tolerance to barbiturates and other CNS depressants develops.

Common side effects of benzodiazepines are summarized in **Box 10.5**.

Overdose

BZDs impair hypoxic derive. This is in contrast to phenobarbitone, which depresses both hypoxic and neurogenic derive in overdose and can cause potentially fatal respiratory depression.

Withdrawal of Benzodiazepines

Negative reinforcement of withdrawal is a major deterrent to discontinuing use; hence, patients continue to use BZDs for a long period of time. Anxiety of withdrawal may be difficult to distinguish between preexisting and rebound. Patients may have insomnia, fatigue, headache, muscle twitching, tremor, sweating, dizziness, tinnitus, difficulty concentrating, nausea, depression, abnormal perception of movement, irritability of mood, etc., during withdrawal. Several predictors have been identified (**Box 10.6**).

Box 10.5: Side effects of benzodiazepines
• Diminished psychomotor performance.
• Impaired reaction time.
• Loss of coordination, decreased attention.
• Ataxia.
• Falls.
• Excessive daytime drowsiness.
• Confusion.
• Amnesia.
• Increase of existing depressed mood.
• Overdose, rarely lethal.

Box 10.6: Predictors of benzodiazepines withdrawal
• High potency like alprazolam, lorazepam, and triazolam more likely.
• Higher daily doses.
• Rapid tapering.
• Panic disorder.
• Comorbid substance dependence/abuse.
• Personality pathology, for example, neurotic or dependent.
• Abrupt discontinuation.

After long-term usage (>3 mo) of BZDs, if BZD administration is stopped, then patients may experience anxiety, headache, and tremors. GI upset can occur. Long-lasting drugs are less likely compared to short-acting drugs like temazepam and triazolam. In severe cases, delusional ideas and seizures can occur. Slow tapering is needed.

General Rules of Prescribing Benzodiazepines

- Choosing BZDs should be based upon the past response to the drug or family history or medical conditions and concomitant drug usage.
- Half-life of BZD is very important consideration as these drugs are given less frequently, have less serum fluctuations, and have less severe withdrawal. However, they have greater chance of accumulation and daytime sedation.
- The initial dose should be low and gradually increased (remember start low and go-slow rule).
- Be aware of tolerance and dependence. A regular use beyond 3 weeks is associated with development of tolerance and dependence; hence, there is a risk of withdrawal too.
- Tolerance develops to the sedative effects quickly; a cross-tolerance with alcohol and other CNS depressants also occurs.
- Avoid diazepam and chlordiazepoxide in patients with liver disease or else there is chance of hepatic encephalopathy.

Special Issues in Benzodiazepine Therapy

Benzodiazepines in Elderly

Short-lasting BZDs are not converted to active intermediates; they are metabolized directly into inactive products and eliminated via urine. The elderly have a reduced ability to metabolize long-acting BZDs and their active metabolites; hence, the drugs become unusually long-acting. Lipid-soluble BZDs like chlordiazepoxide, diazepam, etc., cross the blood–brain barrier (BBB) quickly and have rapid onset of action. They persist longer in high fat-to-lean body mass; hence, obese and elderly will have longer action. Start low and go slow is a useful principle of using BZDs in old age.

Drug Interactions of Benzodiazepines

Pharmacokinetic Interactions

BZDs are additive with other CNS depressants. They are metabolized by CYP enzyme system, and their levels may be increased by SSRIs and other potent enzyme inhibitors like ketoconazole, itraconazole, antibiotics like erythromycin, etc. It should be noted that the CYP enzyme functions is impaired in elderly or liver failure; hence, there lies the possibility of increased pharmacological effects.

Similarly, drugs metabolized by CYP3A4 such as triazolam, midazolam, alprazolam, carbamazepine, quinidine, terfenadine, erythromycin, disulfiram, and cimetidine too can increase BZD levels.

Pharmacodynamic Interactions

- CNS depressants metabolized by CYP2C9 such as diazepam, TCADs, warfarin, phenytoin, etc., may exaggerate BZD action due to additive action.
- All BDZs potentiate the effects of alcohol, and all are likely to exacerbate breathing difficulties where this is already compromised, for example, obstructive sleep apnea.
- BZDs potentiate the action of opioid analgesics or alcohol or other CNS depressants like barbiturates.

Benzodiazepine Abuse

BZD abuse is very common in developing countries like India. Two patterns of abuse have been identified: Recreational abuse (nonmedical use) which is common in young people to get high or self-medication (quasi-therapeutic use). BZDs are often used for long-term drug. Repeat prescriptions are very common among elderly, which is the second most common type of abuse.

Treatment

It is challenging to treat BZD abuse. Patients may be young or old. A delicate handling with good history taking and empathy may help solve the issue.

Traditionally, tapering method is used. Alternatively, substitution and tapering can also be used. Anticonvulsants (decrease electrical excitation in the limbic system) could be used as first-line too. The examples include carbamazepine, gabapentin, or valproic acid. Alternatively, phenobarbital, chlordiazepoxide, or clonazepam could be tried as well. One has to calculate equivalent dose and provide the same in the divided doses. One will have to add the dose as per need basis during the first week as there are chances of withdrawal during tapering. After dose becomes stabilized, gradually reduce the BZD dose by 10% of starting dose. Slow tapering assures good treatment success, and one should hold for some time to stabilize. Frequent visits should be avoided. Last doses are the most difficult to eliminate and then one can slow down and reduce very slowly. Complete elimination may vary from one patient to another. Reliable follow-up is needed. Supportive therapy for depression, hypertension, etc., should go on simultaneously.

Current Therapeutic Status

BZDs are good for immediate symptom relief, especially in anxiety disorders. They provide faster symptom relief than SSRIs for panic deciders as well. Long-acting, low-potency ones like clonazepam or chlordiazepoxide are preferred. These drugs are best used for exacerbations of anxiety or short-term treatment of insomnia. Long-term use, however, should be discouraged. In absence of genuine medical indication, BZDs should not be used for a period beyond 1 week.

Benzodiazepines in Pregnancy and Lactation

BZDs and their metabolites can freely cross the placental barrier and accumulate in fetal circulation. Administration during the first trimester can result in fetal abnormalities. There are malformation reports with diazepam. Administration in third trimester can result in "floppy-infant syndrome." BZDs are also excreted in the breast milk and can result in sedation in the suckling baby.

Benzodiazepines Withdrawal

Withdrawal of the BZDs can be problematic but is often mild to moderate in intensity. Mostly, it manifests as GI upset, diaphoresis, and increase in heart rate and blood pressure. Tremor, lethargy, dizziness, headaches, restlessness, insomnia, irritability, and anxiety occur in some patients. Others may experience depersonalization and perceptual disturbances. Tinnitus, delirium, panic, hallucinations, and abnormal muscular movements also occur.

Rarely, it may manifest as seizures, delirium, confusion, or psychosis. During the withdrawal phase, triggering of depression, mania, and OCD can occur. Most of the long-term users experience significant withdrawal. However, it can be insignificant if the use was confined to less than 2 weeks.

Treatment

Slow tapering of BZDs is suggested. If the patient has used them for a period > 30 days, then psychotropic medications such as carbamazepine, valproic acid, trazodone, and imipramine can be prescribed. Cognitive behavioral therapy could be effectively used in treating panic or anxiety. Following are the predictors of BZD withdrawal.

Flumazenil

This is a BZD receptor antagonist (**Fig. 10.3**). This should be differentiated from beta-carbolines which are inverse agonists of BZD receptors. The drug is a specific antagonist with no action in opioid, TCAD, or barbiturate poisoning. Indeed, given in these cases, it may even worsen.

Flumazenil is a short-acting drug with a half-life of 1 hour. The drug is IV administered. It is the drug of choice for BZD poisoning. Since half-life is short and the drug undergoes prompt redistribution, it has to be repeated frequently. It also has some degree of usefulness in hepatic coma as BZDs are supposed to play an important role in its pathogenesis. Apart from

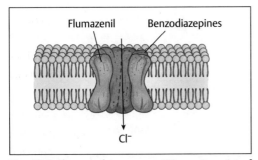

Fig. 10.3 Flumazenil is a competitive antagonist of benzodiazepine (BZD) receptors. The drug is used in BZD overdose and hastens the recovery. It can also block effect of BZDs given before anesthesia. Due to its short duration, multiple doses may be needed.

flumazenil, airway assessment and maintenance and ventilator support is needed. Nasogastric suction with activated charcoal may be given. Since flumazenil is a competitive antagonist and a short-acting drug, one may need to repeat it every hour. Care is needed in dependent patients as seizures may occur due to sudden precipitation of withdrawal.

Flumazenil is IV administered at dose of 0.2 mg over 15 to 30 seconds. If there is no response after 30 seconds, then administer 0.3 mg over 30 seconds, and if still there is no response after 1 minute, then one can repeat IV administer the dose of 0.5 mg over 30 seconds at 1-minute interval to the maximum of 3 mg/hour. In the event of resedation, which will be an issue due to short duration of action of flumazenil, one may repeat dose at 20-minute intervals if needed. Rarely, patient may require titration up to total dose of 5 mg; if there is still no response after 5 minutes, one should reconsider the cause of sedation due to BZDs.

Phenobarbitone

This is the most commonly used barbiturate. Others are lipid soluble and include pentobarbital, amobarbital, and thiopental. It is a GABA-mimetic drug as discussed previously. For this reason, phenobarbitone has a linear dose response curve (DRC) and respiratory depression, coma, and death can occur in progressively higher doses. That is why it is much more toxic in overdose compared to BZDs. For the same reason, unlike BZDs, which do not depress respiration to a significant degree (only reduce hypoxic derive, that too in overdose), barbiturates can impair both hypoxic and neurogenic derives of respiration.

Pharmacokinetics

Phenobarbitone has slow but excellent oral absorption. Only a handful is metabolized by oxidation and the rest of amount is eliminated unchanged. It has a long half-life due to slow redistribution from the brain. It has a quick onset of action within 30 minutes.

The most common side effect is sedation. Tolerance, addiction, and dependence are more marked compared to BZDs.

Uses

It is the drug of choice for epilepsy in pregnancy and is used for hemolytic anemia and jaundice in newborn. It is the most commonly used agent for hypnosedative withdrawal.

The drug is used in dose of 30 to 120 mg daily in two or three divided doses. In children, the dose is 6 mg/kg of body weight daily in three divided doses. As an oral anticonvulsant, the dose in adult is usually between 50 and 100 mg two or three times daily. In children, the dose varies between 15 and 60 mg two or three times daily.

Contraindications

- Acute intermittent porphyria (this induces key enzyme of porphyrin synthesis, named δ-amino levulinate synthetase). This can thus increase porphyrin synthesis.
- Chronic obstructive pulmonary disorder (COPD) (bronchospasm can occur).
- Asthma (bronchospasm can occur).
- Obstructive sleep apnea (respiratory depression can occur).
- Cardiopulmonary disorders (respiratory depression can occur).

Benzodiazepines versus Barbiturates

BZDs have a high therapeutic index compared to barbiturates. In hypnotic doses, they do not affect respiration and cardiovascular functions. Only in IV injection, the blood pressure may fall. BDZs cause less distortion of sleep architecture. They do not alter disposition of other drugs by microsomal enzyme induction. They have lower abuse liability compared to barbiturates, development of tolerance is milder, and psychological and

physical dependence and withdrawal syndrome are less marked comparatively.

Chloral Hydrate

This is the oldest sedative and hypnotic for clinical use. It has been used for a long time. However, due to availability of better agents, its use declined. It can displace warfarin from plasma protein-binding sites and hence can lead to bleeding.

Buspirone

Buspirone is a non-BZD, nonsedative hypnotic anxiolytic, which is considered to be a selective antianxiety drug without abuse potential (**Fig. 10.4**). Buspirone is a 5-HT1A partial agonist. It is not a very long-acting drug and does not produce any active metabolite. However, onset of action may take 2 weeks as it takes that long to achieve steady state. The drug is used in generalized anxiety disorder and also sometimes to augment the antidepressant treatment of major depressive disorders. It has also been tried in OCD. Usefulness has been reported in aggression and agitation in dementia. The drug is available as 5-, 10-, and 15-mg tablets and is used at doses of 7.5 to 60 mg daily. Usually, 15 to 30 mg is needed. Dose is reduced in elderly. Buspirone is generally well-tolerated but some patients may experience dizziness, headache, GI distress, and fatigue.

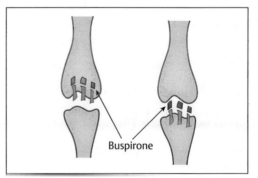

Fig. 10.4 Buspirone is a 5-HT1A partial agonist with no action on gamma-aminobutyric acid (GABA) receptors. This makes buspirone a selective antianxiety drug with no sedation.

The main clinical advantage over BZDs is that buspirone lacks the sedation and dependence associated with BZDs, and it causes less cognitive impairment. However, the efficacy is less than BZDs as it lacks the euphoria and sedation that these patients may expect with anxiety relief. The patient may be started on a BZD and buspirone for 2 weeks, followed by slow tapering of the BZD.

Nonbenzodiazepines

Zolpidem, an imidazopyridine compound, is the most commonly used non-BZD. It acts by stimulating ω_1 receptors (α_1 subunit of $GABA_A$), which are also known as BZD1 receptor. Non-BZDs do not affect REM sleep; hence, there is no REM rebound. These do not produce tolerance, addiction, and dependence. Zaleplon has an even shorter half-life. Therefore, it is preferred if the patient has midnight awakenings.

Antihistaminics

Antihistaminics are used for the treatment of anxiety and insomnia and are nonaddicting. These have some anticholinergic drugs effects. Drugs like diphenhydramine are popular and are used at doses of 25 to 100 mg at night for sleep or 10 to 25 mg for anxiety as per need basis. Similarly, hydroxyzine is another alternative. The drug is given at doses of 25 to 100 mg sleep time. Hydroxyzine is used at doses of 10 to 25 mg one to three times daily.

Gamma Hydroxybutyrate

This is an outdated drug but is now sold in the clubs as drug—"G" or "liquid ecstasy," etc. This is bought via the illicit market and then distributed in aqueous solution. It produces relaxation, disinhibition, and euphoria. The drug has rapid onset, short half-life (20 min). Dependence and withdrawal occur. It has a narrow therapeutic window; hence, side effects can occur. Dizziness,

nausea, vomiting, respiratory depression, and coma can occur. The drug has additive effects with ethanol and other sedative hypnotics.

Beta-Blockers

Beta-blockers address physiologic component of anxiety like tachycardia, palpitations, tremor, sweating, etc. The main advantage is that they produce no CNS depression. They are nonaddicting and produce no drowsiness like BZDs. However, they should not be used in asthma, diabetes, and congestive heart failure (CHF). Monitoring of blood pressure and pulse rate should be done while being on regular treatment. The drug is quite useful for performance anxiety. Propranolol is given at a dose of 10 mg on as per needed basis.

Melatonin

This is a pineal hormone and is important in regulating sleep–wakefulness cycle. It gets disrupted during transcontinental journeys or frequent change of work shifts. It is thus the drug choice for jet lag.

Ramelteon acts as melatonin receptor agonist at receptors of melatonin, which are believed to contribute to sleep-promoting properties. These receptors when acted upon by endogenous melatonin are thought to be involved in the maintenance of circadian rhythm, underlying the normal sleep–wakefulness cycle.

Ramelteon activates MT1 and MT2 receptors and is effective in initial insomnia. Lack of sedation, addiction, and dependence are important features of this drug.

Ramelteon is a melatonin receptor agonist and is used for initial insomnia. The drug stimulates MT1 and MT2 receptors and is used commonly among the elderly or those young people having difficulty in initiating sleep. The drug is rapidly absorbed and is metabolized to long-acting metabolite. The drug is metabolized by CYP1A2 and is thus used with caution in patients with liver disease or in combination with those drugs having potential to inhibit this isoform.

Certain endocrinal alternations, including reduced serum testosterone levels, have been seen with this drug. Usual dose is 8 mg given at bedtime. Absorption is slowed down with fatty meal. Assess the patient after 1 week, and if there is no response, then the underlying psychiatric disorder should be examined. Watch the patient for possible behavioral change, especially those with depression, as it might worsen. Drugs like rifampin, ketoconazole, and fluconazole are likely to alter the levels of ramelteon and need to be watched out for.

Way Forward[16]

There are a number of new targets involved in antianxiety responses, for example, glutamate, endocannabinoids, neuropeptide systems, ion channels, etc. Drugs like D-cycloserine, MDMA, cannabinoids, and levodopa have been explored as antianxiety.

References

1. National Institute of Clinical Excellence. Doses of benzodiazepines. Available at: http://www.evidence.nhs.uk/formulary/bnf/current/4-central-nervous-system/41-hypnotics-and-anxiolytics/412-anxiolytics/benzodiazepines/chlordiazepoxide-hydrochloride. Accessed July 28, 2016
2. Physician Desk Reference. Available at: http://www.pdr.net/drug-summary/Librax-chlordiazepoxide-hydrochloride-clidinium-bromide-1626. Accessed July 28, 2016
3. Physician Desk Reference. Available at: http://www.pdr.net/drug-summary/Rozerem-ramelteon-562. Accessed July 28, 2016
4. Bighelli I, Trespidi C, Castellazzi M, et al. Antidepressants and benzodiazepines for panic disorder in adults. Cochrane Database Syst Rev 2016;9:CD011567 [Epub ahead of print] Review
5. Conway A, Rolley J, Sutherland JR. Midazolam for sedation before procedures. Cochrane Database Syst Rev 2016; (5):CD009491
6. Steenen SA, van Wijk AJ, van der Heijden GJ, van Westrhenen R, de Lange J, de Jongh A. Propranolol for the treatment of anxiety disorders: systematic review and meta-analysis. J Psychopharmacol 2016; 30(2):128–139
7. Bandelow B, Reitt M, Röver C, Michaelis S, Görlich Y, Wedekind D. Efficacy of treatments for anxiety disorders: a meta-analysis. Int Clin Psychopharmacol 2015;30(4):183–192
8. Hansen MV, Halladin NL, Rosenberg J, Gögenur I, Møller AM. Melatonin for pre- and postoperative anxiety in adults. Cochrane Database Syst Rev 2015; (4):CD009861
9. Quante A. Acute pharmacotherapy for anxiety symptoms in patients with depression. Fortschr Neurol Psychiatr 2015; 83(3):142–148.
10. Demyttenaere K. Agomelatine in treating generalized anxiety disorder. Expert Opin Investig Drugs 2014;23(6):857–864
11. Gould RL, Coulson MC, Patel N, Highton-Williamson E, Howard RJ. Interventions for reducing benzodiazepine use in older people: meta-analysis of randomised controlled trials. Br J Psychiatry 2014;204(2):98–107
12. He XY, Cao JP, He Q, Shi XY. Dexmedetomidine for the management of awake fibreoptic intubation. Cochrane Database Syst Rev 2014; (1):CD009798 Review
13. Depping AM, Komossa K, Kissling W, Leucht S. Second-generation antipsychotics for anxiety disorders. Cochrane Database Syst Rev 2010; (12):CD008120
14. Amato L, Minozzi S, Vecchi S, Davoli M. Benzodiazepines for alcohol withdrawal. Cochrane Database Syst Rev 2010; (3): CD005063
15. Ipser JC, Stein DJ, Hawkridge S, Hoppe L. Pharmacotherapy for anxiety disorders in children and adolescents. Cochrane Database Syst Rev 2009; (3):CD005170
16. Available at: https://www.sciencedirect.com/science/article/pii/S016372581930 1512. Accessed September 19, 2020

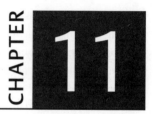

Antiepileptic Drugs

Vikas Dhikav and Kuljeet Singh Anand

Clinical Case Example

- A 5-year-old female child is brought to clinic because of episodic "blanking out," which began 1 month ago. The patient has episodes in which she abruptly stops all activities for about 10 seconds, followed by a rapid return to full consciousness. The patient's eyes are open during the episodes, and she remains motionless with occasional "fumbling" hand movements. After the episode, the patient resumes whatever activity she was previously engaged with no awareness that anything has occurred. She has 20 to 30 episodes per day and has no convulsions. Past medical, physical, and developmental histories are unremarkable. She has no history of previous or current medications; no allergies; family history is pertinent for her father having similar episodes as a child. What drug could be prescribed for this patient?

Answer: This patient has a diagnosis of absence seizures that can be confirmed by electroencephalography (EEG). Patient can be started with sodium valproate at a dose of 20 mg/kg of body weight per day; in severe cases, this may be increased but only in patients in whom plasma valproic acid levels can be monitored. Above 40 mg/kg/day, clinical biochemistry, liver function tests, and hematological parameters should be monitored.

Epilepsy[1–5]

Epilepsy is known as "recurrent convulsive disorder." Recurrent, periodic, and hypersynchronous discharges generate in the brain, leading to involuntary movements, accompanied by autonomic, sensory, and motor symptoms.

It is important to make a differentiation between epilepsy and seizures. A seizure is the clinical manifestation of an abnormal synchronization and excessive excitation of a population of cortical neurons, while epilepsy is a tendency toward recurrent seizures unprovoked by acute systemic or neurologic insults.

More than a century ago, Jackson said that seizures are "occasional, sudden, extensive, rapid, local discharges of the neurons in the brain." These synchronous discharges are strong enough to cause epileptic fits. Defective synaptic functions can contribute to epilepsies by playing their roles as well. In general, there is decrease in the inhibitory discharges and increase in stimulatory discharges, leading to imbalance of the harmony. Imbalance of glutamate and gamma-aminobutyric acid (GABA) have been demonstrated using "Kindling" model of epilepsy in amygdale and other limbic structures, and this explains partial seizures. Similarly, pilocarpine and kainic acid can produce status epileptics.

More than 50 million people worldwide have epilepsy, making it the most common neurological disorder. Roughly, around 1% people have epilepsies. It should be noted that a seizure is a transient disturbance of cerebral function due to an abnormal paroxysmal discharge in the brain.

Presently, there are about two dozen antiepileptic drugs in clinical use and the number keeps growing. Several antiepileptic drugs are under development. The most commonly used drugs in epilepsy work by sodium channel blockade (**Fig. 11.1**). A brief historical development is given in **Box 11.1**. Common choices for seizure types are given in **Table 11.1**. For simply studying antiepileptics, they are divided into generations (**Table 11.2**).

Antiepileptic Drugs[6-10]

An antiepileptic drug decreases the frequency and/or severity of seizures in people with epilepsy. In general, the inhibitory processes in the brain are augmented and the stimulatory processes are suppressed. Inhibitory processes can make the neurons more negative, while excitatory processes can make a neuron less negative. This balance is restored by antiepileptic drugs.

What Do These Drugs Do?

Antiepileptic agents treat the symptom of seizures, not the underlying epileptic condition. Several agents like ethosuximide and valproate have unique mechanisms by which they are able to reduce the transient calcium currents in the

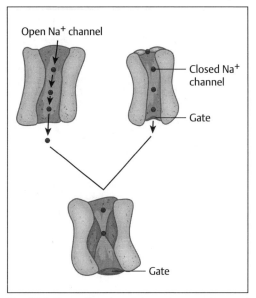

Fig. 11.1 Drugs like phenytoin, carbamazepine, and valproate act by prolonging inactivation of sodium channels.

Box 11.1: Brief history of antiepileptic drug development
• 1857—bromides.
• 1912—phenobarbital.
• 1937—phenytoin.
• 1954—primidone.
• 1960—ethosuximide.
• 1974—carbamazepine.
• 1975—clonazepam.
• 1978—valproate.
• 1993—felbamate, gabapentin.
• 1995—lamotrigine.
• 1997—topiramate, tiagabine.
• 1999—levetiracetam.
• 2000—oxcarbazepine, zonisamide.

Table 11.1 Choice of antiepileptic drugs as per the seizure types

Partial	Drugs	Generalized	Drugs
Simple	Carbamazepine	Tonic clonic	Valproate, lamotrigine, zonisamide
Complex	Carbamazepine/oxcarbazepine	Absence	Valproate/ethosuximide

Table 11.2 Generations of antiepileptic drugs

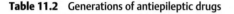

1st generation	2nd generation	3rd generation
Phenobarbitone	Vigabatrin	Talampanel
Phenytoin	Lamotrigine	Perampanel
Ethosuximide	Topiramate	Rufinamide
Valproate	Oxcarbazepine	Lacosamide
Carbamazepine	Levetiracetam	Stiripentol
Benzodiazepines	Pregabalin	
Primidone	Zonisamide	

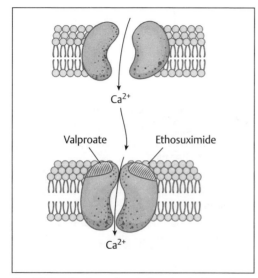

Fig. 11.2 Antiseizure drug-induced reduction of currents of T-type is the reason due to which absence seizures are controlled. However, curiously, this mechanism is shared by broad-spectrum antiepileptic drugs such as sodium valproate as well. This suppression of "spike and wave discharge" is an important mechanism by which both drugs have efficacy in this common type of epilepsy of young children.

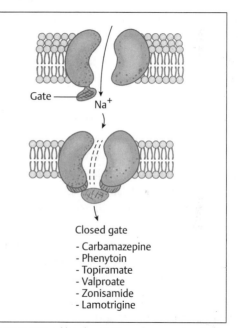

Fig. 11.3 Drugs like phenytoin, carbamazepine, topiramate, valproate, zonisamide, and lamotrigine can block repetitive activation of sodium channels. This can interfere with both origin and spread of seizure activity.

thalamic area of the brain (**Fig. 11.2**). However, the most commonly used drugs in epilepsy work by blocking sodium channels (**Fig. 11.3**). Blockade of the repetitive firing of sodium channels can prevent origin and spread of seizure activity (**Fig. 11.4**).

Antiepileptic drugs decrease the excitability of the membranes of brain neurons by acting on the receptors or ion channels or both. The older drugs act upon sodium channels or neurotransmitters like GABA (e.g., phenytoin or benzodiazepines [BZDs]). High-frequency repetitive firing of action potential mediated by sodium channels is reduced by several conventional antiepileptic drugs, for example, phenytoin, carbamazepine, etc. New drugs bind with high affinity to neuronal

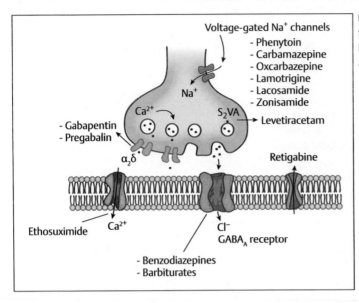

Fig. 11.4 Several drugs are able to block sodium channels and inhibit origin and spread of seizure activity.

membranes. New drugs like gabapentin act at high affinity site, which may be related to their binding sites. Decreased presynaptic release of excitatory glutamate may be related to the mechanism of action of lamotrigine. Oxcarbazepine may have a mechanism similar to that of carbamazepine and maybe reducing repetitive firing of voltage-dependent sodium channels. Vigabatrin binds irreversibly to GABA transaminase, an enzyme which degrades GABA. Increased GABA at postsynaptic receptors may be responsible for the clinical efficacy of vigabatrin in epilepsy.[19]

The goal of antiepileptic medications is to maximize quality of life by minimizing seizures and adverse drug effects.

Pathophysiology

Seizures represent paroxysmal discharge due to alteration in the electrical properties of neurons present in the cerebral cortex. There are two major mechanisms in the brain that work in opposition with each other, for example, facilitatory (glutamate) and inhibitory (GABA). Usually, a fine balance is maintained between them; a sudden imbalance between the excitatory

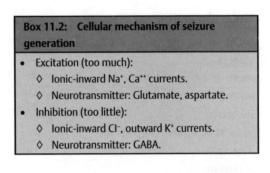

Box 11.2: Cellular mechanism of seizure generation

- Excitation (too much):
  ◊ Ionic-inward Na^+, Ca^{++} currents.
  ◊ Neurotransmitter: Glutamate, aspartate.
- Inhibition (too little):
  ◊ Ionic-inward Cl^-, outward K^+ currents.
  ◊ Neurotransmitter: GABA.

and inhibitory neurons leads to a sudden onset of seizure activity.

The neurochemical basis of the abnormal discharge is not well-understood. It may be associated with enhanced excitatory amino acid transmission, impaired inhibitory transmission, or abnormal electrical properties of the affected cells. The glutamate content in areas surrounding an epileptic focus is often raised. **Box 11.2** lists the cellular mechanisms of seizure generation. **Fig. 11.5** shows mutations in the ion channels as the cause of epilepsy.

The characteristic event in epilepsy is the seizure, which is often associated with convulsion, but may occur in many other forms. The seizure is

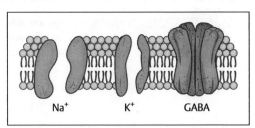

Fig. 11.5 Mutations in the ion channels like sodium, potassium, and gamma-aminobutyric acid (GABA_A) receptors have been identified. Physiologically, some such mutations have also been found in cerebellum (responsible for ataxia in some cases) and familial hemiplegic migraine.

caused by an abnormal high-frequency discharge of a group of neurons, starting locally and spreading to a varying extent to affect other parts of the brain.

Molecular Abnormalities

There are a variety of ion channel abnormalities seen in epilepsies. These include Na^+/Ca^{2+}, etc. There is an increase in channel conductance, leading to increase in excitatory discharges. Success of major antiepileptic drugs proves the point that both sodium and calcium channels play roles in epilepsies. Recently, the role of potassium channels that are known to play a role in regulating intrinsic neuronal electrical activity is coming to surface. A new drug named retigabine is being developed that interferes with functioning of voltage-gated potassium channels (Kv7).

Antiepileptic drugs work by a variety of heterogenous mechanisms: The main aim is to antagonize the action of excitatory neurotransmitters and boost the activity of inhibitory neurotransmitters.

For example, major antiepileptics like phenytoin and carbamazepine work by blocking voltage-gated sodium channels. Ethosuximide and valproate block voltage-gated calcium channels. BZDs and barbiturates stimulate GABA_A receptors and potentiate effects of an inhibitory neurotransmitter in the brain. Effect of a neurotransmitter transporter is blocked by tiagabine (GABA transporter), and metabolism of GABA is inhibited by inhibiting the metabolic enzymes called GABA transaminase (GABA-T) by vigabatrin. Synaptic proteins involved in neurotransmitter release SV2A is inhibited by levetiracetam.

Models of Epilepsies

Antiepileptic drugs have symptomatic effects. These do not have any effect on epileptogenesis. Since it is difficult to study epilepsy in humans, experimental models are used.

- **Pentylenetetrazol seizures model:** This is used to identify drugs used for absence seizures. Pentylenetetrazol is a central nervous system (CNS) stimulant with seizure-provoking properties. It has been used to study seizure phenomenon in experimental animals.

- **Maximum electroshocks seizures (MES) model:** This model is used for generalized tonic-clonic epilepsy. In this model, the graded doses of antiepileptic medications can be tested in experimental animals, for example, mice.

- **Kindling:** This is a model of temporal lobe epilepsy. First introduced in 1960s, this model can mimic the behavioral component of seizures, for example, complex partial seizures. Chemically applied or electrically induced, kindling can be used for the same.

Neurotransmitter Abnormalities

The exact cause of neurotransmitter alterations is not known in epilepsy. Increase in concentrations of ions like sodium, potassium, and calcium is known to occur inside the neurons during seizure episodes. Once this happens, alterations in neurotransmitter release occur.

Increase in glutamate and decrease in GABA transmission occurs in epilepsy. Glutamate antagonists, for example, riluzole and idrocilamide are used in treatment of amyotrophic lateral sclerosis. Some drugs like valproate increase the activity of inhibitory neurotransmitters (**Fig. 11.6**), and phenytoin and lamotrigine may reduce glutaminergic activity, leading to restoration of balance between excitatory and inhibitory neurotransmitters (**Fig. 11.7**). Common causes of epilepsies are given in **Box 11.3**.

Box 11.3: Causes of epilepsies
• Idiopathic.
• Pediatric epilepsies (e.g., congenital abnormalities/perinatal injuries).
• Metabolic disorders (alcohol withdrawal, sudden discontinuation of antiepileptic drugs, hypoglycemia, or uremia).
• Trauma.
• Space-occupying lesions.
• Vascular (e.g., cerebrovascular accidents).
• Brain infections.
• Neurodegenerative diseases.

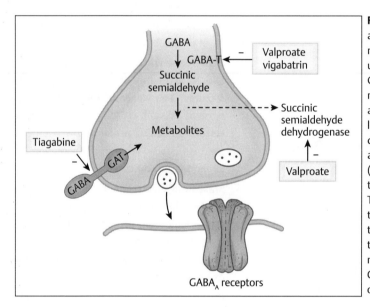

Fig. 11.6 Gamma-aminobutyric acid (GABA) binds to the GABA receptors, leading to opening up of the GABA$_A$ receptors-Cl$^-$ complex. Increase in the membrane polarization occurs as a result. Several drugs like valproate and vigabatrin decrease metabolism of GABA, and drugs like benzodiazepines (BZDs) increase the opening of this GABA$_A$-Cl$^-$ channel complex. This causes cellular inhibition in the brain. Note in the diagram, tiagabine is acting on GABA transporter but the drug does not have direct interaction with GABA receptors, which are shown on postsynaptic membranes.

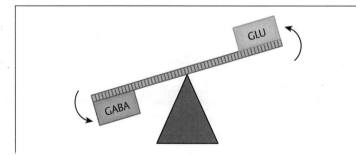
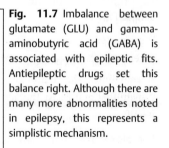

Fig. 11.7 Imbalance between glutamate (GLU) and gamma-aminobutyric acid (GABA) is associated with epileptic fits. Antiepileptic drugs set this balance right. Although there are many more abnormalities noted in epilepsy, this represents a simplistic mechanism.

Types of Epilepsies

Two common forms of generalized epilepsy are the tonic-clonic fit (grand mal) and the absence seizure (petit mal). Status epilepticus is a life-threatening condition in which seizure activity is uninterrupted.

Seizures may be partial or generalized, depending on the location and spread of the abnormal neuronal discharge. The attack may involve mainly motor, sensory, or behavioral phenomena. Unconsciousness occurs when the reticular formation is involved.

International League against Epilepsies (ILAE) classifies epilepsies in two different types: Generalized and partial; disorder in the former is diffuse, bilaterally and poorly localizable, while in the latter in hemisphere, indicating involvement of limited neuronal circuits. It is important to note that excepting a minority of cases that can be treated surgically, treatment of epilepsies rely heavily on antiepileptic drugs.

Partial seizures are of two types: Simple and complex.

Partial Seizures

The discharge begins locally and often remains localized, producing relatively simple symptoms without loss of consciousness. The lesion is located in one hemisphere.

Simple Partial

Focal motor symptoms (e.g., jerking) spread to different parts of body. Different types of sensory and mental manifestations can also occur. There is no impairment of consciousness in this form of seizure.

Complex Partial

Identical symptoms plus impaired consciousness can occur. Patients will find themselves unable to obey commands and carry out willful movements. Automatic behaviors can occur.

Generalized Seizures

These types of seizures involve the whole brain, including the reticular system, thus producing abnormal electrical activity throughout both hemispheres. Immediate loss of consciousness occurs. Seizures can be convulsive or nonconvulsive.

Generalized seizures are of many types.

Absence Seizures

These types of seizures are generally seen in young children (5–12 years) and may cease by teenage years end. However, some children may have some other generalized seizures later. Therefore, they are typical 3 Hz/seconds discharge in EEG (**Figs. 11.8** and **11.9**).

Affected children may constantly stare or may have transient impairment of consciousness, accompanied by changes in tone. More marked changes in muscle tone may signify "atypical

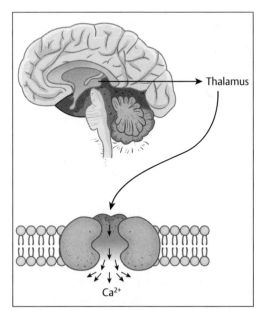

Fig. 11.8 Characteristic discharges (3 Hz/s) are recorded in electroencephalogram both in cerebral cortex and thalamus. This "spike and wave" is produced by inflow of calcium currents. These currents are also called as T-currents.

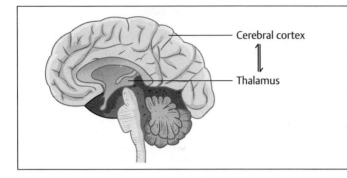

Fig. 11.9 Firing of cerebral cortex and the thalamus in a reciprocal manner can cause generalized seizures of absence type. This oscillation between thalamus and cerebral cortex can cause "trans like state" that is seen in patients with absence seizures.

Cerebral cortex

Thalamus

absence" seizures. Multiple seizure types may coexist, accompanied by developmental delay or mental retardation.

Myoclonic Jerks

Single or multiple contractions of isolated muscle groups occur in myoclonic jerks. These may be so subtle at times as to escape the attention of even a keen clinician. Sudden muscle contractions occur. These occur at all ages and may even be part of syndromes, for example, West syndrome.

Generalized Tonic-Clonic

There are two phases: Tonic phase in which there is sudden increase in muscle tone in which patient can fall on ground and lose consciousness with respiratory arrest. This phase is soon followed by a phase with repetitive jerks, leading later to development of flaccid coma. Repetitive episodes of both phases can lead to status epilepticus. Importantly, there can be mood changes, lethargy, or myoclonic jerks in some patients before frank seizures can occur (known as aura).

Causes of Seizures

It is important to know that seizure etiology can be identified only in about one-third of the patients. In the rest of them, seizures can be idiopathic, and their etiology is unknown. All focal or adult-onset seizures should be investigated with brain imaging (e.g., MRI) as there is a good chance of having an anatomical abnormality, leading to seizures. Presence of spikes of sharp waves in EEG or patterned discharge suggests epilepsies.

Individual Antiepileptic Drugs

The current drug therapy is effective in 70 to 80% of patients. Reducing electrical excitability of cell membranes, possibly through inhibition of sodium channels, is an important therapeutic goal exhibited at molecular level (**Fig. 11.10**). Drugs like ethosuximide and valproate reduce the entry of calcium in brain neurons (**Fig. 11.11**). Enhancing GABA-mediated synaptic inhibition is the main mechanism of several antiepileptic drugs. This may be achieved by an enhanced pre- or postsynaptic action of GABA, by inhibiting GABA-transaminase, or by drugs with direct GABA-agonist properties. Individual antiepileptic drugs and their clinical details are given in **Boxes 11.4** and **11.5**.

A few drugs appear to act by a third mechanism, namely, inhibition of T-type calcium channels. Newer drugs act by another mechanism, which is yet to be elucidated. Drugs that block excitatory amino acid receptors are effective in animal models but not yet developed for clinical use.

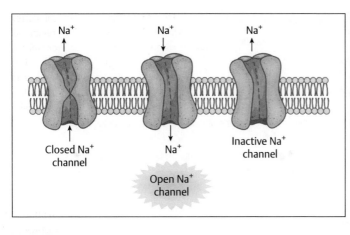

Fig. 11.10 Voltage-gated sodium channels are responsible for initiating the action potential in the brain neurons. Hence, the sodium channel blockers are used in various forms of epilepsies. As stated earlier, mutations in sodium channels are responsible for genetic syndromes associated with epilepsies.

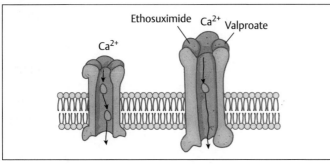

Fig. 11.11 Ethosuximide and valproate reduce the entry of calcium in the thalamic neurons, making them useful for absence seizures.

Phenytoin

It was discovered by Merit and Putnam in the year 1932. It was a result of a planned search to find a replacement for phenobarbitone.

Phenytoin acts by inhibiting depolarization shift. That means it blocks both initiation and propagation of seizure activity. At a molecular level, it does so by:

- Blocking voltage dependence Na^+ channel.
- Blocking voltage dependence Ca^{2+} channel.
- Inhibiting calcium-induced secretory processes, including release of hormones and neurotransmitters.
- Inhibiting posttetanic potentiation.

At normal or low doses, the actions are exhibited mostly at sodium channels, while at high doses, calcium channels are affected. Side effects such as lethargy and drowsiness are perhaps due to involvement of calcium channels. Release of neurotransmitters too is affected at high dose.

Pharmacokinetics

Given orally, it is well absorbed and 90% protein bound. Because phenytoin is a weak acid, its intestinal absorption is variable and plasma concentration can vary widely. Monitoring is therefore needed. It is metabolized by the microsomal system and is excreted first in the bile and then in the urine. Majority of metabolism is done by CYP2C9 and CYP2C19.

Phenytoin is available in two formulations: Immediate release (IR) and extended release (ER). The former is commonly used in multiple doses, and the latter is used when once daily doses are needed. Phenytoin equivalent can be calculated

159

Box 11.4: Summary of mechanism of actions of major antiepileptics[7-10]

- Phenytoin, carbamazepine, eslicarbazepine, oxcarbazepine:
  ◊ Block voltage-dependent sodium channels at high-firing frequencies.
- Barbiturates (e.g., phenobarbitone):
  ◊ Prolong GABA-mediated chloride channel openings.
- BZDs:
  ◊ Increase frequency of GABA-mediated chloride channel openings (cellular hyperpolarization).
- Felbamate:
  ◊ May block voltage-dependent sodium channels at high-firing frequencies.
  ◊ May modulate NMDA receptor via strychnine-insensitive glycine receptor.
- Gabapentin:
  ◊ Increases neuronal GABA concentration.
  ◊ Enhances GABA-mediated inhibition.
- Lamotrigine:
  ◊ Blocks voltage-dependent sodium channels at high-firing frequencies.
  ◊ May interfere with pathologic glutamate release.
- Ethosuximide:
  ◊ Blocks low voltage or "transient" (T-type) calcium channels in thalamic neurons.
- Valproate:
  ◊ May enhance GABA transmission in specific circuits.
  ◊ Blocks voltage-dependent sodium channels.
- Vigabatrin:
  ◊ Irreversibly inhibits GABA-transaminase (GABA-T).
- Topiramate:
  ◊ Blocks voltage-dependent sodium channels at high-firing frequencies.
  ◊ Increases frequency at which GABA opens Cl⁻ channels (different site than BZDs).
  ◊ Antagonizes glutamate action at AMPA/kainate receptor subtype.
  ◊ Inhibition of carbonic anhydrase.
- Tiagabine:
  ◊ Interferes with GABA reuptake; potentiates hippocampal inhibition.
- Levetiracetam:
  ◊ Synaptic vesicle protein 2A binding and modulation.
- Oxcarbazepine:
  ◊ Blocks voltage-dependent sodium channels at high-firing frequencies.
  ◊ Exerts effect on K⁺ channels.
- Zonisamide:
  ◊ Blocks voltage-dependent sodium channels and T-type calcium channels.
- Pregabalin/gabapentin:
  ◊ Increases neuronal GABA.
  ◊ Increase in glutamic acid decarboxylase.
  ◊ Decrease in neuronal high-voltage calcium currents by binding of alpha-2 delta subunit of the voltage-gated calcium channel.
- Lacosamide:
  ◊ Blocks slow inactivated state of sodium channels.
  ◊ Carbonic anhydrase inhibitor:
    □ Acetazolamide.

Box 11.5: Common side effects of phenytoin
• Gingival hyperplasia, hirsutism, increased collagen proliferation.
• Gastrointestinal irritation.
• Ataxia and diplopia.
• Blood dyscrasias.

by considering different formulations. It is important to note that phenytoin formulations differ in bioavailability; hence, patients should be given the same drugs from a single manufacturer. A therapeutically equivalent product should be selected if products were to be switched.

The drug is hence displaced by drugs like phenylbutazone and sulfonamides. This can increase plasma levels of phenytoin. It is an enzyme inducer and can decrease plasma levels of several drugs such as oral contraceptives, causing their failure. Its half-life is 15 to 30 hours and follows zero-order kinetics. Importantly, different formulations can have different bioavailability; therefore, patients should be encouraged to have same formulations throughout the course of their disease.

Side Effects

The most common side effect is gum hyperplasia which is seen in about 30% of the patients. Studies indicate that the enlargement of gums is related to fall in serum folic acid and the duration of drug therapy.[18] Diplopia, ataxia, and nystagmus are initial dose-dependent side effects and reflect impairment of cerebellar functions. Hypotension and cardiac depression can occur upon intravenous (IV) injection.

Hirsutism occurs due to androgenic properties of drug; therefore, the drug is avoided in young women (**Box 11.5**). Hepatitis is a rare side effect.

Hypocalcemia is a manifestation of decrease in calcium absorption from the gut wall. It could also occur due to accelerated metabolism of vitamin D.

It could contribute to refractoriness. In many patients, osteomalacia can occur. Hyperglycemia occurs due to decrease in insulin release from the pancreas. Megaloblastic anemia occurs as a result of folic acid deficiency. Inhibition of folic acid absorption also contributes toward teratogenicity.

Pseudolymphoma occurs in small number of patients and is accompanied by paracortical hyperplasia. Sometimes, enlargement of lymph nodes can be painful too. The condition is reversible upon drug discontinuation.

Leakage of the drug from circulation can cause "red glove syndrome." Fos (phenytoin) is a phosphorylated ester of phenytoin and is free from this side effect. Moreover, it could be given by intramuscular (IM) route. Its safety is also better than that of phenytoin. Fosphenytoin is a phosphate ester prodrug of phenytoin, which has been developed to overcome complications associated with parenteral phenytoin administration in the treatment of acute symptomatic seizures, short-term prophylaxis, repetitive or prolonged seizures, and status epilepticus.[7]

Allergy to phenytoin may be a part of systemic reaction, and the drug will then have to be stopped. Valproate or carbamazepine can be used as alternatives. Nystagmus, ataxia, slurred speech, nausea, vomiting, or coma may suggest gross overdose. It produces a range of long-term side effects. Peripheral neuropathy, cerebellar atrophy, Hodgkin lymphoma, osteomalacia, hyperglycemia, megaloblastic anemia, and hypocalcemia are some of the possible long-term side effects. Merritt and Putnam described its use in 1938.

Use

It is used in generalized and partial epilepsies. It is also effective in posttraumatic seizures. There is no evidence that newer drugs like levetiracetam are better than phenytoin.[14] The drug is contraindicated in absence seizures like pheno-barbitone and carbamazepine. Also, the studies have not found outcome difference in phenytoin versus valproate in generalized and partial seizures.[15] The drug can be IV administered or orally administered.

Drug Interactions

Drug interactions may occur when there is an addition of a new medication or when inducer/inhibitor is present. Addition of inducer/inhibitor to existing medication regimen or removal of an inducer/inhibitor from chronic medication regimen could result in drug interactions[8]:

- Given with isoniazid and cimetidine, the plasma levels of phenytoin could rise due to inhibition of its metabolism. Phenobarbitone can induce metabolism of phenytoin.
- Drugs like phenylbutazone and sulfonamides can displace it from protein-binding sites.
- Phenytoin can interfere with thyroid function test as it has the affinity for binding to thyroid hormone-binding globulin.
- Sodium valproate increases plasma levels of lorazepam and lamotrigine by inhibiting the enzyme UDP glucuronosyltransferase (UGT).
- Valproate can increase plasma concentrations of phenytoin and phenobarbital by inhibiting CYP2C19.
- Topiramate and oxcarbazepine by blocking the enzyme CYP2C19.
- Increase plasma concentrations of phenytoin.
- Carbamazepine metabolism is inhibited by ketoconazole, fluconazole, erythromycin, and diltiazem (mediated by CYP3A4, CYP2C8, CYP1A2).

Dosage and Administration

Oral Administration

Phenytoin capsules are approximately 90% bioavailable by the oral route. Phenytoin is 100% bioavailable by the IV route. For this reason, plasma phenytoin concentrations may increase modestly when IV phenytoin is substituted for oral phenytoin sodium therapy. Initial dose is 100 capsule orally three times a day; dosage is then adjusted to suit individual requirements. Maintenance dose for most adults will be one capsule three times a day.

Status Epilepticus

Phenytoin is given as a loading dose of 10 to 15 mg/kg IV administered slowly at a rate not exceeding 50 mg/minute (this should need approximately 20 min in an adult). The loading dose should be followed by maintenance doses of 100 mg orally or IV every 6 to 8 hours.

For children, a loading IV dose of 15 to 20 mg/kg of phenytoin will usually produce plasma concentrations of phenytoin within the therapeutic range (10–20 µg/mL). The drug should be IV injected slowly at a rate not exceeding 50 mg/minute. Continuous monitoring of the electrocardiogram and blood pressure is essential during administration. The patient should be observed for signs of respiratory depression, especially during loading dose. IV lorazepam or IM midazolam effectively controls early status epilepticus in approximately 63 to 73% of patients.[6]

Therapeutic Drug Monitoring

Determination of phenytoin plasma levels is advised when using phenytoin in the management of status epilepticus and in the subsequent establishment of maintenance dosage.

Carbamazepine

This is an iminostilbene derivative and has been used as a mood stabilizer in the past. Derivative of tricyclic antidepressants, carbamazepine is similar profile to that of phenytoin but with fewer unwanted effects. Carbamazepine is effective in most forms of epilepsy (except absence seizures) and is particularly effective in psychomotor epilepsy. It is also useful in trigeminal neuralgia and mania.

The drug has shown effectiveness in blocking kindling, a process in which repeated subthreshold stimuli can generate seizures. Conventional antiepileptics such as phenytoin and phenobarbitone are not effective in this model of epilepsy. Both carbamazepine and BZDs can block the same.

Given orally, it has good oral absorption. The drug is an autoinducer; therefore, the half-life changes over time. Hence, gradually increasing dosages are needed. Half-life is 10 to 15 hours and a toxic metabolite named 10,11 epoxide is responsible for side effects. Patients with HLA-B*15:02 genotype are at high risk of developing serious adverse cutaneous reactions to carbamazepine.[5]

Carbamazepine is a strong inducing agent; therefore, it has many drug interactions. The drug has comparatively low incidence of unwanted effects, principally sedation, ataxia, mental disturbances, and water retention.

The most common side effect is skin rashes. Carbamazepine-induced rashes appear to be more common in patients with HLA haplotype B*1502. Other side effects include neutropenia, hepatitis, and syndrome of inappropriate antidiuretic hormone (ADH) secretion.

Given with dextropropoxyphene, it can lead to increase in plasma levels of drug. Sodium valproate can reduce the metabolism of carbamazepine, leading to increase in toxicity of carbamazepine.

Use

It is the drug of choice for partial epilepsies (simple and complex) and neuralgias. It is also used in generalized epilepsies. However, it is ineffective in absence seizures. Since the drug produces epoxide, the toxic metabolite, plasma levels monitoring of drug may be needed to avoid side effects.

Carbamazepine is started in initial doses of 200 mg orally two times a day (IR and ER) or 100 mg orally four times a day (suspension for elderly). The drug dose can be increased at weekly intervals by adding up to 200 mg/day using a two-times-a-day regimen of ER or a three times a day or four-times-a-day regimen of the other formulations. The usual maintenance dose ranges between 600 and 1,200 mg/day. Dosage generally should not exceed 1,200 mg/day. IV solution can be used for patients who are not able to take oral tablets. The drug is not indicated in absence seizures.

Side Effects

Carbamazepine commonly causes morbilliform rashes which are harmless as opposed to phenytoin where the drug will have to be stopped when such rashes occur. Diplopia may be a manifestation of acute increase in plasma levels. Dizziness ataxia can occur commonly as a side effect of carbamazepine, especially during dose titration phase. Liver functions and leukocyte counts need to be monitored. Syndrome of inappropriate ADH secretion can occur (**Fig. 11.12**).

Bipolar Disorder

Carbamazepine is given for treatment of patients with acute manic or mixed episodes associated with bipolar I disorder. The drug is started at a dose of 200 mg given twice daily and is increased by increments of 200 mg/day, but the total dose should not exceed 1,600 mg daily.

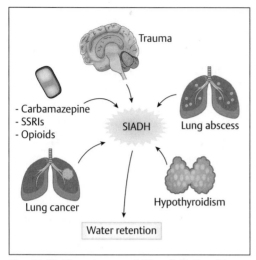

Fig. 11.12 There is a possibility of dilutional hyponatremia with carbamazepine. This is more common in elderly with oxcarbazepine. Head injury, drugs like opioids, selective serotonin reuptake inhibitors (SSRIs), and lung cancer are other causes of syndrome of inappropriate antidiuretic hormone (SIADH).

Postherpetic Neuralgia

Carbamazepine is given at doses of 100 to 200 mg daily, and the dose can be slowly increased to 1,200 mg daily.

Trigeminal Neuralgia

Trigeminal neuralgia (TN) was first reported by Fothergill; hence, it is also known as Fothergill disease. It is a major disorder of face, responsible for chronic painful state. TN affects sensory division of fifth cranial nerve and produces recurrent shock like severe pain. These pains are short-lasting but are often intense in nature. It is uncommon and has a prevalence of 4 cases per 1,00,000. The condition affects people above the age of 50 and is slightly more common in women. It has a significant impact on quality of life as even minor stimuli such as shaving, touching, and taking tea or coffee can precipitate severe pain. Etiology suggests that there is a vascular compression of trigeminal nerve, leading to focal demyelination and aberrant neural discharges.

Carbamazepine has remained the first-line drug for the last two to three decades. The drug is so effective that it has a diagnostic utility. That means patients with classical TN will respond to the drug, indicating the diagnosis. Commonly used agents in TN other than carbamazepine are given in **Box 11.6**.

Carbamazepine is started at a dose of 200 mg twice a day and can increase up to 1,200 mg a day. Attempt should be done to reduce the dose every 3 to 6 months. Oxcarbazepine is an alternative. In patients nonresponsive to both, one can use gabapentin, baclofen, lamotrigine, and pregabalin. Recently, peripheral nerve block with ropivacaine along with carbamazepine has been shown to have advantage of reduced side effects.

When drug therapy fails, minimally invasive therapy or surgery can be used. Younger patients can benefit from microvascular decompression (MVD). There is a 4% chance of cerebrospinal fluid (CSF) leak, hematoma, or infarction after MVD. Gamma knife is another treatment option which is noninvasive. Radiofrequency ablation, rhizotomy, balloon decompression, and glycerol rhizolysis are minimally invasive treatment options. Topical amethocaine has also been tried.

Sodium Valproate

This was used as a solvent for antiepileptic drugs. Antiepileptic properties were discovered accidentally.

Box 11.6: Commonly used drugs in trigeminal neuralgia
• Baclofen (10–20 mg daily).
• Lamotrigine (400 mg daily).
• Gabapentin (up to 2,400 mg/d).

The drug acts by increasing the release of GABA and decreasing degradation of GABA, which increases the seizure threshold.

Pharmacokinetically, it has good oral absorption and is a protein-bound drug like phenytoin. The drug undergoes metabolism by an oxidase enzyme and is short acting.

No dose adjustments are needed in renal failure but lower than normal doses are given in hepatic impairment. Elderly patients too need lower than normal dose.

Side Effects

The drug is well tolerated; yet few side effects are seen.

Gastrointestinal upset is most common. Tremors occur frequently. These are fine tremors; in some, however, coarse tremors also occur. Weight gain probably is a manifestation of increased appetite. It could be counteracted by caloric restriction and by encouraging mild-to-moderate exercise, for example, brisk walking. However, other forms of exercises, for example, swimming should be avoided.

Hyperammonemia, increase in liver enzymes, and hepatic failure can occur mainly in infants. Maximum incidence occurs at the age of 4 months.

Thrombocytopenia is a rare side effect of drug. Importantly, the drug does not produce any sedation. That is why it is so widely used in school-going children and working adults where sedation may be undesirable.

Drug Interactions

- Sodium valproate is not given with clonazepam. Although rare, status epilepticus can be precipitated.
- The drug can inhibit the metabolism of phenobarbitone, and this can lead to stupor or coma.

Uses

Sodium valproate could be used in the following conditions.

Epilepsy

Valproate is given at doses of 10 to 15 mg/kg/day orally initially, and then it can be increased by 5 to 10 mg/kg/day at weekly intervals; may increase dose up to 60 mg/kg/day for epilepsy. Typically, doses may vary between 250 and 1,000 mg daily. For migraine, 250 mg orally every 12 hours, adjusted on clinical response, and not to exceed 1,000 mg/day. In mania, 750 mg/day orally in divided doses; adjusted as rapidly as possible to reach desired therapeutic effect, and the dose is not to exceed 60 mg/kg/day. Despite the challenges of availability of newer drugs, valproate remains a gold standard antiepileptic drug for the treatment of children.[9]

Migraine

Valproate is given in prophylaxis of migraine when propranolol fails. The drug is not effective for acute attack of migraine like other drugs used in prophylaxis. It is started at a dose of 250 mg orally and then the dose can be increased to 1,000 mg daily.

Bipolar Mania

Valproate is given for manic episodes associated with bipolar disorders. The drug is started at divided doses (750 mg daily) and the dose is not exceeded 4,200 mg (60 mg/kg).

Ethosuximide

This is a safe antiepileptic drug which acts by inhibiting T-currents in thalamus. These are a type of calcium currents.

The drug is well-absorbed by oral route and is poorly metabolized. Elimination is renal; therefore, dose needs reduction in renal failure. It is a long-acting drug with a half-life of 50 hours.

The drug is well tolerated, and the most common side effects are hypersensitivity and gastrointestinal upset. Sodium valproate inhibits its metabolism and increases its plasma levels. It is the drug of choice for absence seizures. It is particularly favored in those with uncomplicated absence seizures. It is not effective for generalized tonic-clonic seizures. Sodium valproate is preferred in complicated absence seizures.

Absence seizures are common in childhood; therefore, it is important to recognize them clinically. Affected child may stare at object and may lose consciousness only on a very brief and temporary basis. On EEG, patients may exhibit 3 to 4 Hz/second discharge. Hyperventilation may frequently help physicians make a correct diagnosis in a school-going child.

Drug is started at dose of 7.5 mg/kg (older than 6 years) in two divided doses, and it can be increased up to 40 mg/kg, depending upon clinical and EEG response. Adverse effects include gastrointestinal upset, thrombocytopenia, and, rarely, CNS side effects.

Initial and maintenance doses of commonly used antiepileptics are given in **Table 11.3**.

Phenobarbitone

This is the most commonly used barbiturate. Others include pentobarbital, amobarbital, and thiopental. It is a GABA-mimetic drug that behaves like GABA upon binding to the GABA$_A$ receptors (**Fig. 11.13**). The drug increases presynaptic inhibition. For this reason, phenobarbitone has a linear dose response curve (DRC), and respiratory depression, coma, and death can occur in progressively higher doses. That is why it is much more toxic in overdose compared to BZDs. For the same reason, unlike benzodiazepines, which do not depress respiration to a significant degree (only reduce hypoxic derive, that too in overdose), barbiturates can impair both hypoxic and neurogenic derives of respiration.

Phenobarbitone elevates seizure threshold and reduces spread of seizure activity from a seizure focus. Sedative and hypnotic effects occur due to its action on midbrain reticular formation.

Pharmacokinetics

Phenobarbitone has slow but excellent oral absorption. Only a handful is metabolized by oxidation, and the rest of amount is eliminated unchanged. It has a long half-life due to slow redistribution from the brain. It has a quick onset of action within 30 minutes. The drug is absorbed from the stomach, being the acidic drug.

Uses

It is the drug of choice for epilepsy in pregnancy and is also used for hemolytic anemia, jaundice in newborn, and neonatal seizures. It is the most commonly used agent for hypnosedative withdrawal. It is commonly used in children as an antiepileptic.

The drug is used in dose of 30 to 120 mg daily in two or three divided doses. In children, the dose is 6 mg/kg of body weight daily in three divided doses. As an oral anticonvulsant, the dose in adult is usually between 50 and 100 mg two or three times daily. In children, the dose varies between 15 and 60 mg two or three times daily.

Side Effects

The most common side effect is sedation. Tolerance, addiction, and dependence are more marked compared to BZDs.

Aggression, hyperactivity, and rashes can occur in children. Automatic behavior is known to occur in old age. Incoordination, ataxia, and dizziness occur at high doses. Respiratory depression is likely when combined with BZDs and/or alcohol. Several issues plague barbiturates, and

Table 11.3 Initial and maintenance daily doses and important side effects of commonly used antiepileptic drugs (after Guidelines for Management of Epilepsies in India [GMIND])[5–10]

Antiepileptic drug	Initial dose	Maintenance dose	Side effects
Carbamazepine	100 mg twice daily	400–1,000 mg	Sedation, rashes, hepatitis, neutropenia
Clobazam	10 mg once daily at nighttime	10–30 mg	Sedation, ataxia, somnolence, irritability, depression, weight gain, tolerance
Lamotrigine	25 mg OD at night. Lower dose with valproate due to enzyme inhibition	100–300 mg	Sedation, ataxia, dizziness, skin rash, even Steven–Johnson syndrome
Levetiracetam	250 mg, twice daily	1,000–3,000 mg	Sedation, dizziness, cognitive slowing, psychosis, depression, suicidal ideation
Oxcarbazepine	150 mg twice daily	600–1,800 mg	Sedation, dizziness, ataxia, headache, hyponatremia, skin rash
Phenobarbitone	60–90 mg at bedtime	60–180 mg	Sedation, ataxia, depression, memory problems, skin rash, hyperactivity in children
Phenytoin	200–300 mg at bedtime	200–400 mg	Ataxia, sedation, gum hyperplasia, coarsening of facial features, hirsutism, memory problems, osteomalacia and bone loss, skin rash
Topiramate	25 mg once daily	100–400 mg	Sedation, somnolence, cognitive problems, weight loss, word-finding difficulty, renal stones, seizure worsening
Valproate	200 mg twice daily	500–2,000 mg	Anorexia, weight gain, nausea, vomiting, tremors, hair loss, polycystic ovarian syndrome, thrombocytopenia, fulminant hepatitis occurs rarely (monitor liver enzymes)
Topiramate	25 mg once daily	100–400 mg in epilepsy, 25–100 mg in migraine prophylaxis	Sedation, somnolence, cognitive problems, weight loss, word finding difficulty, renal stones, seizure worsening
Zonisamide	50 mg at bedtime	200–500 mg	Sedation, anorexia, renal stones, forgetfulness, skin rash, weight loss, distal paresthesias

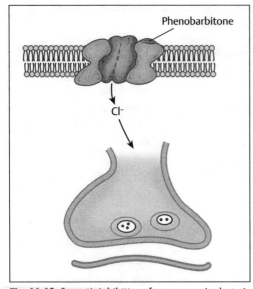

Phenobarbitone

Cl⁻

Fig. 11.13 Synaptic inhibition of gamma-aminobutyric acid (GABA) receptors by phenobarbitone is achieved at doses below needed for hypnosis. GABA$_A$ receptor-mediated increase in Cl⁻ permeability occurs.

due to availability of better agents, it is used less commonly now.

Drug interactions, several contraindications, and potential for abuse have made pheno-barbitone a less popular drug, especially as a sedative-hypnotic. It continues to be a good antiepileptic. It increases the activity of hepatic delta-aminolevulinic acid synthetase enzyme and can worsen acute intermittent porphyria. The drug suppresses ventilation in high dose and can cause respiratory depression. Supportive ventilation, diuretics, and alkalization of urine are used as treatment options.

Drug Interactions

Decrease in anticoagulant activity of warfarin occurs due to enzyme induction. Likewise, meta-bolism of glucocorticoids can be enhanced, leading to decrease in their metabolism. Absorption of phenobarbital can be reduced

by griseofulvin. Half-life of doxycycline can be shortened by phenobarbitone. Sodium valproate may inhibit metabolism of phenobarbitone; hence, the plasma levels of phenobarbitone may need to be monitored.

Contraindications

Following are the contraindications for the use of phenobarbitone:

- Acute intermittent porphyria (this induces key enzyme of porphyrin synthesis, namely, δ-aminolevulinate synthetase). This can thus increase porphyrin synthesis.
- Chronic obstructive pulmonary disorder (COPD) (bronchospasm can occur).
- Asthma (bronchospasm can occur).
- Obstructive sleep apnea (respiratory depression can occur).
- Cardiopulmonary disorders (respiratory depression can occur).

Newer Antiepileptic Drugs

Nowadays, there is an increasing trend of using newer antiepileptic drugs. The newer antiepileptics are, however, used when there are contraindications to the first-line drugs due to coexisting illnesses or when they fail or cause adverse effects or drug interactions. The first-line drugs interact with many drugs (e.g., oral contraceptives, anticoagulants, antiretrovirals or immunosuppressants, etc.). One should always consider factors such as cost and continued availability of medicines before starting newer antiepileptic drugs.

Lamotrigine

This is now a commonly used frontline anti-epileptic. The drug is similar in structure to that of other drugs inhibiting folic acid synthesis. However, on its own, it has a weak antifolate action. Of late, it has become a broad-spectrum drug and is useful in the treatment of both generalized and partial seizures.

It acts by inhibiting voltage-gated sodium channels on presynaptic neuronal membranes and thus stabilizes neurotransmission, leading to inhibition of release of glutamate. The drug also acts and blocks presynaptic calcium channel, Postsynaptic AMPA receptors have also been shown to be blocked. So, the drug comprehensively addresses neuronal excitotoxicity. Although there is a metabolic and pharmacokinetic variation, average half-life of long-acting formulation is around 24 hours when the drug is given as monotherapy.

Pharmacokinetically, oral absorption is complete, and it has a half-life of 24 hours. Carbamazepine or phenytoin may reduce its half-life by accelerating its metabolism. Lamotrigine, on the other hand, does not affect metabolism of phenytoin, carbamazepine, phenobarbitone, or valproate. Sodium valproate can block metabolism of lamotrigine, and this can elevate its levels by two times.

Dose of lamotrigine will have to be reduced; else toxicity can occur.

In 1994, lamotrigine was first approved in partial seizures. Now, it has been touted as one of the major antiepileptics and is used in generalized tonic-clonic seizures as well. A potentially life-threatening rash and renal stone may occur. The drug is relatively free from drug interactions that make it one of the easily managed drugs when multiple drugs are being used.

Lamotrigine is started at a low dose, which is gradually built, taking 6 to 8 weeks. This is one effective way of avoiding life-threatening rash (i.e., Steven–Johnson syndrome). Risk is higher in children taking combination of lamotrigine and valproate. The risk is higher in patients with a genetic particular haplotype, for example, HLA-B*15:02.[17]

Lamotrigine is started at a dose of 25 mg twice daily for 1 week and then increased to 50 mg twice daily. Maintenance dose can vary between 100 and 400 mg. Dose with valproate should be reduced to half due to enzyme inhibiting tendency of valproate. In the treatment of bipolar disorders, the drug is started in dose of 25 mg once daily and maintenance dose of 200 mg is reached in 4 to 5 weeks.

Topiramate

This is a substituted carbohydrate. The drug has remarkable structural similarities with acetazolamide and was thought to be an antidiabetic agent initially. Later, it was found to be a better antiepileptic drug. Topiramate has similar antiepileptic activities like phenytoin or carbamazepine yet has a dissimilar mechanism of action. The drug has multimodel mechanism of action, for example, it facilitates $GABA_A$ receptor-mediated inhibition, yet the drug also has major antiexcitotoxicity effects. That means it blocks AMPA and kainite receptors. Potentiation of GABA inhibition is thought to disrupt mesolimbic dopaminergic system, thus accounting for ability of this drug to have a major antialcohol-dependence property. Pharmacokinetically, it follows linear kinetics and has an average half-life of 24 hours. Protein binding is minimal. Elimination occurs via urine. Paresthesia, rashes, loss of appetite, and stones are the most common side effects. Most side effects are dose dependent and resolve upon reducing the dose. Glaucoma may worsen on this drug and is contraindicated in glaucoma patients. Due to potential of drug interactions, it is often given alone. Generally, the drug is given as 25 mg/day in evening and a weekly increment is given until target dose of 100 mg is reached.

Zonisamide

Like other drugs in this newer drug class, zonisamide too has multimodel actions. This is a benzisoxazole derivative and a weak inhibitor of carbonic anhydrase enzyme. This, however, is not the major mechanism of action of this drug. Zonisamide was approved in 1989 in Japan and 2000 in the United States. The drug blocks both voltage-dependent sodium and calcium channels. It is a sulfonamide which is used for partial seizures in adults and also has value in mixed seizure types. It is also effective as an off-label drug in mood disorders. Long half-life of this drug makes it useful as once-a-day daily dose. Absence of clinically significant drug interactions makes it useful for treatment of those who are taking multiple drugs. Side effects include rashes. It is believed to have some antioxidant, neuroprotective, and anti-Parkinson's activities. It has been suggested to be an alternative to topiramate in migraine prophylaxis in patients who are not able to tolerate topiramate. The drug is started at a dose of 100 mg once daily, and after 2 weeks, the dose can be increased to 200 mg either as a single or in divided doses.

Felbamate

Felbamate has often been touted as the drug of last resort in refractory patients with partial epilepsies. The main usefulness of this drug being its utility in a rare pediatric syndrome with multiple seizure types named Lennox–Gastaut syndrome. Aplastic anemia and hepatic failure limit its usefulness. It is an inhibitor of microsomal enzymes and prolonged use can lead to weight loss. Initial dose is 1,200 mg and can be increased till 3,600 mg. The drug is contraindicated in hepatic impairment and the dose is reduced in renal failure.

Levetiracetam

This drug is similar in structure to that of piracetam, a nootropic molecule used to be extremely popular in the past. The drug is not effective either in phenyl tetrazole (PTZ) model or maximum electroshock seizure model but is still an effective antiepileptic drug. Levetiracetam inhibits kindling in rat models of epilepsies.

Exact mechanism of action is not known, but the drug acts by blocking the action of a presynaptic protein called as SV2A. This may act by inhibiting the release of an excitatory neurotransmitter like glutamate (**Fig. 11.14**).

Pharmacokinetically, the drug is rapidly and completely absorbed, with protein binding being poor. It is partially metabolized in liver, and its half-life is not significantly affected by other drugs.

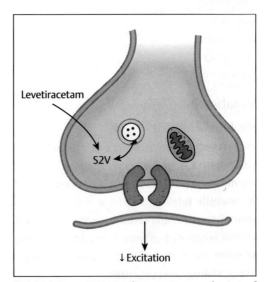

Fig. 11.14 Levetiracetam has a unique mechanism of action. The drug binds to synaptic vesicle (S2V) and decreases neuronal excitation. It seems to have no action on Na⁺/glutamate or gamma-aminobutyric acid (GABA) unlike many related drugs.

Levetiracetam is particularly effective in partial seizures, with or without secondary generalization. Usual dose is 500 mg twice daily and one can go up to 3,000 mg daily when doses are increased at a 2-week interval. Initial pediatric dose is 20 to 60 mg/kg. Change in behavior, anxiety, depression, or suicidal tendencies can occur.

Oxcarbazepine

This is a keto analogue of carbamazepine and is considered to be a less potent but safer alternative. Its mechanism of action is, however, identical to carbamazepine. The drug is completely absorbed by oral route and food does not interfere with its absorption. It gets converted by liver into carbamazepine.

Oxcarbazepine is indicated mainly for partial seizures and secondary generalized seizures. The drug is given at doses of 300 to 600 mg, and child dose is 10 mg/kg. Side effects are similar to that of carbamazepine but dilutional hyponatremia is slightly more common. Cross-allergy with carbamazepine can occur.

Vigabatrin

Vigabatrin increases GABA actions through the irreversible inhibition of an enzyme called GABA-transaminase. It is effective in partial and secondary generalized seizures. It is also effective in infantile spasm. The drug has been used throughout the world but is not approved in the United States as it has produced demyelination of white matter of spinal cord in animal models. These changes, so far, have not been seen in humans.

Pharmacokinetically, this is a water-soluble drug, and absorption is not affected by food. Drowsiness, dizziness, and weight gain can occur as side effects. Visual field constriction can also occur. The drug is started at a dose of 500 mg once daily and then can be increased to 1,500 mg. Maximum dose is 3,000 mg.

Tiagabine

Tiagabine is an adjunct antiepileptic drug used in patients above 12 years for the treatment of partial seizures. Tiagabine acts by increasing GABA activity in the brain. Hippocampal inhibition has been noted. The drug impairs the transport of GABA in neurons but does not act on GABA receptors. The drug is rapidly absorbed orally and is not a very long-acting drug. Apart from epilepsy, it is used for treatment of anxiety and panic disorders. Dizziness, weakness, confusion, and aphasia can occur as side effects. The drug is commonly used at doses of 2 to16 mg orally daily.

Pregabalin and Gabapentin

Pregabalin and gabapentin share pharmacology and therapeutic uses. Both drugs have similar mechanism of action (**Fig. 11.15**).

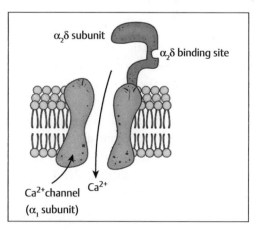

Fig. 11.15 Pregabalin reduces the synaptic release of several neurotransmitters by binding to $\alpha_2\delta$ subunit of voltage-gated Ca^{2+} channels in the brain, while gabapentin increases GABA in the brain, possibly by enhancing rate of synthesis from glutamate. Both of these drugs have no effect on $GABA_A$ or $GABA_B$ receptors.

Pregabalin is a very commonly used drug for neuropathic pain, fibromyalgia, and partial seizures as an add-on with or without secondary generalization. The drug has a GABA-ergic mechanism and binds to α-2 δ, a subtype of calcium channels. It is also effective in anxiety disorders. The drug is commonly used at doses of 75 to 300 mg daily. Sedation and weight gain can occur as side effects. It is almost free from clinically significant drug interactions.

Gabapentin is a related drug used in epilepsies, neuropathic pain, restless legs syndrome, and anxiety disorders. The drug has identical mechanism and pharmacokinetic features. Mechanism and side effect profile is also similar. Edema and sexual dysfunction has occurred in some patients. Usual adult dose for epilepsy is 300 mg orally on day 1, 300 mg orally twice a day on day 2, and 300 mg orally three times a day on day 3. Maintenance dose: 900 to 1,800 mg orally in three divided doses.

Monitoring of Antiepileptic Drugs

In general, antiepileptic serum concentrations can be used as a guide for evaluating the efficacy of medication therapy for epilepsy. This can be very useful clinically when compliance is to be ensured. Serum concentrations are also useful when optimizing antiepileptic drug therapy or teasing out drug–drug interactions. They should be used to monitor pharmacodynamic and pharmacokinetic interactions.

Serum concentrations are important when documenting positive or negative outcomes associated with antiepileptic drug therapy. Most often, individual patients define their own therapeutic levels for antiepileptic drugs. For the newly introduced antiepileptic drugs, there is no clearly defined "therapeutic range;" hence, therapeutic

Table 11.4 Plasma level guide of antiepileptic drug concentrations

Antiepileptic drugs	Serum concentration (mg/L)
Carbamazepine	4–12
Ethosuximide	40–100
Phenobarbital	10–40
Phenytoin	10–20
Valproic acid	50–100
Gabapentin	6–21
Lamotrigine	5–18
Levetiracetam	10–40
Oxcarbazepine	12–24
Topiramate	4.0–25
Zonisamide	7–40

drug monitoring is not very relevant as it is the case with older and established antiepileptics.

Commonly used antiepileptic drugs and their plasma levels are given in **Table 11.4**.

Some Add-On Antiepileptics

Clorazepate is a prodrug that gets converted into diazepam. The drug is used primarily as an antianxiety drug but is also used in treatment of partial seizures as an "add-on" agent. Clobazam, clorazepate, and clonazepam are other antiepileptic drugs of BZD types. Their mechanism is same as that of BZDs (**Fig. 11.16**).

Clonazepam is used in absence, myoclonic, and atonic seizures. However, due to better efficacy, valproate is preferred over clonazepam. Tolerance to antiepileptic effects of BZDs develops after 6 months. Therefore, these are not recommended on long-term basis. Clonazepam is started at a dose of 1.5 mg given in divided doses and maximum dose is 20 mg daily. The general rule for increment of dose is till the point where side effects appear, or seizure control is achieved.

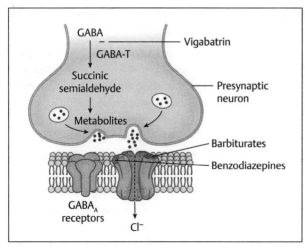

Fig. 11.16 The use of a single antiepileptic drug at the maximum tolerated dose is the standard therapy for epilepsy. However, many patients need more than one antiepileptic drug to improve seizure control. Clobazam is commonly used as an add-on therapy.

Clobazam is started at a dose of 5 mg daily, and the usual dose can be maintained at 10 to 20 mg daily. Clorazepate is given at a dose of 15 mg in divided doses, and the dose can be increased to 60 mg daily.

Drugs for Status Epilepticus

Lorazepam is the drug of choice for status epilepticus due to its better efficacy and safety. It can also be IM administered. Importantly, diazepam is avoided by this route as the absorption is poor and can lead to formation of abscess. Since lorazepam produces maximum amnesia, this has become the preferred drug for preanesthetic medication. Fosphenytoin is a prodrug of phenytoin and is safer. It can be IM administered. Due to its safety, this is preferred over phenytoin for status. It has been tried in acute TN also. Diazepam has long remained the drug of choice for status epilepticus. It is, however, the drug of choice for febrile seizures where it is given as an intrarectal gel. It is increasingly getting replaced by lorazepam. Sodium valproate is available as a parenteral solution for treatment of seizures.

A total of 10 mg of diazepam is IV administered, and the dose can be repeated once every 10 minutes. Mostly, the seizures get terminated by IV diazepam. Alternatively, lorazepam 4 mg can be IV administered. The dose is repeated every 10 minutes. Anticonvulsant effect lasts for 12 hours. Watch out for respiratory depression and hypotension. Midazolam is given at a dose of 0.2 mg/kg as a loading dose and has the same side effect profile.

Phenytoin at doses of 15 to 20 mg/kg can be IV administered. Fosphenytoin is a water-soluble analogue of phenytoin given at doses of 15 to 20 mg of phenytoin equivalent. Fosphenytoin can be IM administered also but is not as reliable as IV formulation. The drug is well tolerated but can cause paresthesia at higher rate of administration. Valproate or phenobarbitone can be given as well in refractory cases. Those who do not respond to antiepileptic drug treatment can be put under thiopentone anesthesia. A high plasma level of phenytoin (20–30 µg/dL) can be more effective than 10 to 20 µg/dL, which is usual. Sedation and ataxia are likely at high dose of phenytoin.

Antiepileptic Drug Usage in Elderly, Neonates, and Children

Pharmacokinetic and pharmacodynamic changes occur in these populations. For example, absorption has little changes. The distribution changes considerably due to decrease in lean body mass, which is very important for highly lipid-soluble drugs. There is a fall in albumin, leading to higher free fraction. Metabolism decreases due to changes in hepatic enzyme content, and blood flow becomes low. Decreased renal clearance occurs. Therefore, in neonates and elderly, lower-than-usual doses are used. In children, more frequent doses may be needed due to faster metabolism.

Antiepileptic Drugs Usage in Pregnancy[11–15]

Pharmacokinetics of antiepileptics changes in pregnancy due to increased volume of distribution. This is aided by lower serum albumin, faster drug metabolism, higher doses, but probably less than predicted by total level (measure free level). Consider more frequent dosing due to these pharmacokinetic changes. Lamotrigine is relatively well studied in pregnancy, and data on other new antiepileptics such as levetiracetam, oxcarbazepine, topiramate, zonisamide, gaba-pentin, and pregabalin are emerging. Safety issues are favorable for lamotrigine and promising for levetiracetam and oxcarbazepine.[13] There is evidence that use of valproate during pregnancy not only increases the risk of neurodevelopmental anomalies but can also cause interference with learning and memory in the child in postnatal period.[16]

Principles of Antiepileptic Use[15–20]

- In most patients with seizure of single type, satisfactory control can be achieved by use of a single drug. Treatment with two drugs may reduce seizure frequency or severity or both but the side effects could be significant. It has been seen that almost half of patients will become seizure free with one drug prescribed.

- One would have to start with low dose of an antiepileptic drug and gradually increase the dose. This will help to reduce side effects and improve compliance. This will also be useful as the tolerance to side effects will develop. Gradually, increase the dose of drugs until side effects occur or seizure control is achieved.

- If a single drug has not been able to reduce seizure frequency, add second drug without changing the first drug to a new drug. Two drugs with different mechanism of actions may be able to control seizure activity.

- Treatment with more than two drugs is not very helpful and can contribute to several side effects. This should be tried only in cases with multiple seizure types, for example, syndromic epilepsies.

- Periodic monitoring of drugs for their side effects is a must to reduce toxicity. Over 80% may have at least one adverse effect but are well-tolerated. So, management of side effects should be done. Serum levels should be determined if there is an evidence of side effects or noncompliance. It should, however, be noted that clinical response is a better guide than the serum levels per se. The most common cause of low level is poor compliance.

- Once started, antiepileptic agents need to be given for a period of at least 3 years. While stopping, the dose should be tapered. Sudden withdrawal can precipitate seizures. Dose reduction should be gradual, lasting for weeks to months. Only one drug should be withdrawn at one time.

- Some drugs are effective in particular seizure types, for example, valproate, phenytoin, carbamazepine, phenobarbi-tone, and primidone are useful in gen-eralized tonic-clonic seizures. Topiramate, zonisamide, and lamotrigine are newer broad-spectrum antiepileptic drugs useful in both partial and generalized seizures. Felbamate is particularly effective in Lennox–Gestaut syndrome. Valproate has maximum efficacy in generalized tonic-clonic seizures, more than topiramate or lamotrigine. However, its teratogenic potential in women of childbearing age should be kept in mind.

- It should be noted that majority of antiepileptic drug-induced side effects are reversible in nature and do not require hospital admission. Indian data indicate that 40% of treatment failure may be due to adverse effects. It has been recommended that patients should be started with low dose and then doses be increased gradually (start low and go slow). This is because tolerance to size effects like sedation, dizziness, etc., will develop over a period of time. These may be a cause for concern if doses are toward higher side in beginning. Even for side effects of type-B nature such as lamotrigine-induced rashes and topiramate-induced glaucoma, it may be prudent to start with low dose. Patients who are more prone to side effects such as children below 2 years are more likely to have valproate-induced hepatotoxicity. Such patients should be identified, and if possible, the drug should be avoided in this age group.

Guidelines for Epilepsy Management in India (GMIND)

- First unprovoked seizure is not treated. Treatment is started from second episode onward. Diagnosis, however, should be confirmed before starting drugs. Antiepileptic drugs do not cure the patient

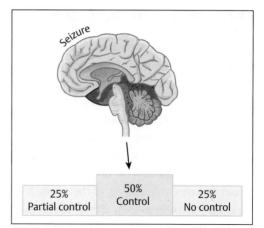

| 25% Partial control | 50% Control | 25% No control |

Fig. 11.17 In general, 75% of the patients get adequate control of seizures but about 25% remain refractory to existing antiepileptic drugs. Several therapies like limbic lobe removal and vagal nerve stimulation are tried for such patients. Several drugs are under development for such cases as well.

but are able to control the seizures in majority of patients (**Fig. 11.17**).

- If seizures continue despite using two drugs, a consultation with a neurologist should be sought.
- Failure of first medication should prompt physician to look for presence of any structural abnormality in the brain or any curable cause.
- Do not change the brand, if possible, because of potential bioavailability variations.
- It is desirable to start with conventional antiepileptic drugs as these are cheap and their side effect profiles are well known.
- Prior to initiation treatment, baselines investigations such as full blood counts, liver function tests, and kidney function test should be done.
- Routine monitoring of blood levels of antiepileptic drugs is not recommended and is indicated only based upon clinical presentations.

Choosing an Antiepileptic[10-15]

Carbamazepine and lamotrigine are good initial monotherapy options. Newer antiepileptics have proof of efficacy as monotherapy but evidence is insufficient to recommend them as first-line treatments.[10] As per the International League Against Epilepsy, the ultimate choice of an antiepileptic drug for any individual patient with newly diagnosed or untreated epilepsy should include consideration of the strength of the efficacy and effectiveness of evidence for each antiepileptic drug along with other variables such as the safety and tolerability profile, pharmacokinetic properties, formulations, and expense.[11]

Older versus Newer Antiepileptics

Little good-quality evidence from clinical trials to support the use of newer monotherapy or adjunctive therapy antiepileptics over older drugs, or to support the use of one newer antiepileptic drugs in preference to another, exists. In general, data relating to clinical effectiveness, safety, and tolerability failed to demonstrate consistent and statistically significant differences between the drugs.[12]

Recent Advances[20]

Levetiracetam was the first SV2A receptor antagonist, but behavioral side effects such as depression and suicidal thoughts limited its use. Brivaracetam is a well-tolerated alternative to this drug without behavioral side effects. Perampanel is a well-tolerated antiseizure drug with unique mechanism of action. Both of these drugs could be considered in refractory patients.

References

1. Singh G. Do no harm first-but first we need to know more: the case of adverse drug reactions with antiepileptic drugs. Available at: www.neurologyindia.com. Accessed February 18, 2011

2. Gram L. Tiagabine: a novel drug with a GABAergic mechanism of action. Epilepsia 1994;35(Suppl 5):S85–S87

3. Cheshire WP. Fosphenytoin: an intravenous option for the management of acute trigeminal neuralgia crisis. J Pain Symptom Manage 2001;21(6):506–510

4. Cheshire WP Jr. Trigeminal neuralgia. Curr Pain Headache Rep 2007;11(1):69–74

5. Franco V, Perucca E. The pharmacogenomics of epilepsy. Expert Rev Neurother 2015; 15(10):1161–1170

6. Trinka E, Höfler J, Leitinger M, Brigo F. Pharmacotherapy for status epilepticus. Drugs 2015;75(13):1499–1521

7. Eriksson K, Keränen T, Kälviäinen R. Fosphenytoin. Expert Opin Drug Metab Toxicol 2009;5(6):695–701

8. Díaz RA, Sancho J, Serratosa J. Antiepileptic drug interactions. Neurologist 2008; 14(6, Suppl 1):S55–S65

9. Guerrini R. Valproate as a mainstay of therapy for pediatric epilepsy. Paediatr Drugs 2006;8(2):113–129 Review

10. Iyer A, Marson A. Pharmacotherapy of focal epilepsy. Expert Opin Pharmacother 2014; 15(11):1543–1551

11. Glauser T, Ben-Menachem E, Bourgeois B, et al. ILAE treatment guidelines: evidence-based analysis of antiepileptic drug efficacy and effectiveness as initial monotherapy for epileptic seizures and syndromes. Epilepsia 2006;47(7):1094–1120 Review

12. Wilby J, Kainth A, Hawkins N, et al. Clinical effectiveness, tolerability and cost-effectiveness of newer drugs for epilepsy in adults: a systematic review and economic evaluation. Health Technol Assess 2005;9(15):1–157, iii–iv

13. Reimers A, Brodtkorb E. Second-generation antiepileptic drugs and pregnancy: a guide for clinicians. Expert Rev Neurother 2012;12(6):707–717

14. Yang Y, Zheng F, Xu X, Wang X. Levetiracetam versus phenytoin for seizure prophylaxis

following traumatic brain injury: a systematic review and meta-analysis. CNS Drugs 2016;30(8):677–688

15. Nolan SJ, Marson AG, Weston J, Tudur Smith C. Phenytoin versus valproate monotherapy for partial onset seizures and generalised onset tonic-clonic seizures: an individual participant data review. Cochrane Database Syst Rev 2016;4:CD001769

16. Bromley R, Weston J, Adab N, et al. Treatment for epilepsy in pregnancy: neurodevelopmental outcomes in the child. Cochrane Database Syst Rev 2014; (10): CD010236

17. Chung WH, Chang WC, Lee YS, et al; Taiwan Severe Cutaneous Adverse Reaction Consortium; Japan Pharmacogenomics Data Science Consortium. Genetic variants associated with phenytoin-related severe cutaneous adverse reactions. JAMA 2014; 312(5):525–534

18. Nayyar AS, Khan M, Vijayalakshmi KR, et al. Phenytoin, folic acid and gingival enlargement: breaking myths. Contemp Clin Dent 2014;5(1):59–66

19. Macdonald RL, Kelly KM. Antiepileptic drug mechanisms of action. Epilepsia 1995; 36(Suppl 2):S2–S12

20. Available at: https://www.tandfonline.com/doi/abs/10.1080/14656566.2019.1637420?journalCode=ieop20. Accessed September 19, 2020

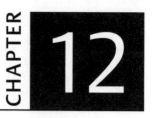

Drugs for Parkinson's Disease

Vikas Dhikav

Clinical Case Examples

Case 1

- A 58-year-old, right-handed man has a 10-year history of Parkinson's disease (PD). He is a known case of diabetes and hypertension. He has been experiencing tremor while handling utensils for 15 years. He is tired, constipated, slow, and the tremor is progressing. He has tried trihexiphenidyl which resulted in dry mouth and teeth loss. Rasagiline was tried and discontinued after 2 months. He is currently taking enalapril and metformin for hypertension and diabetes, respectively. Neurologically, his right-sided tremors are more than left. He has stooping posture and reflexes are exaggerated. How to settle this patient?

Answer: This is a patient who has not benefited from first-line drugs used for early or mild PD. He can be started with carbidopa/levodopa 25/100 mg two tablets daily. The patient should avoid taking the drugs with protein meals to ensure good bioavailability.

Case 2

- A 63-year-old male, retired bus driver, has a 10-year history of PD. He has right-sided resting tremor, rigidity, and bradykinesia. Motor symptoms initially improved with levodopa (L-dopa) 300 mg/day. Wearing-off dyskinesia and motor fluctuations occurred after a number of years of L-dopa treatment. Dopamine agonist (amantadine) and entacapone were initiated 8 years into illness, and the patient has gradual cognitive decline and recurrent visual hallucinations. He is behaviorally less motivated now, engages in excessive daytime sleepiness, is inattentive and forgetful, especially with regard to recent events and conversations, and his thought process has become slower, as he experiences trouble navigating back to his own home. He is less involved in activities at home, and he requires increased assistance in activities of daily living. What modification is required for this patient?

Answer: Patient has a diagnosis of Parkinson's disease dementia (PDD), and this needs treatment with rivastigmine either as capsules or patches.

Introduction

Parkinson's disease (PD) is a progressive neuro-degenerative disorder of the brain. It is caused by degeneration of substantia nigra in the midbrain and consequent loss of dopamine (DA) containing neurons in the nigrostriatal pathway. It was first described by James Parkinson in 1817 as a disease that presents itself with tremors, rigidity, bradykinesia, and postural hypotension. PD presents as stooping gait and afflicted patients are slow to initiate walking. They may have short-ened strides and have rapid small steps (shuffling gait). Impaired balance on turning occurs, and they may suffer falls at later stages. Tremors and rigidity are common features as well. Speech of the patient may become monotonous and tremulous, resulting in slurred speech. Cognitive impairment occurs in one-third of patients, char-acterized by loss of executive functions, including planning/decision-making/controlling emotions and frank depression. Clinical presentation of young onset PD patients could be different.[6]

Two balanced systems are important in the extrapyramidal control of motor activity at the level of the corpus striatum and substantia nigra; in the first, the neurotransmitter is acetylcholine (ACh), and in the second, DA. Tremors, rigidity, and bradykinesia and neuropsychiatric features like depression and anxiety occur due to pro-gressive degeneration of dopaminergic neurons. This results in the imbalance of ACh and DA.

Clinical Features

The symptoms of PD are connected with loss of nigrostriatal neurons and DA depletion. The symptomatic triad includes bradykinesia, rigidity, and tremor with secondary manifestations like defective posture and gait, mask-like face, and sialorrhea, along with dementia.

Generally, patients present with resting tre-mors 4 to 6 Hz/second, which is accentuated by emotional stress and land become less manifest during voluntary activity. Other manifestations include nonmotor features as depicted in **Box 12.1**.

Criteria for diagnosis of idiopathic PD requires at least two of the following points:

- Limb muscle rigidity.
- Resting tremors.
- Bradykinesia.
- Postural instability.

Drug-induced PD should be ruled out. It has been estimated that 80% of nigrostriatal neurons should be lost before symptoms of PD start appearing (**Fig. 12.1**). The goals of the treatment

Box 12.1: Other features of Parkinson's disease (nonmotor features)
• Absence of swaying arm movements.
• Mask-like faces.
• Baby steps.
• Foul-smelling breath.
• Depression.
• Intellectual decline.
• Myerson's sign (repetitive blinking upon tapping bridge of nose).

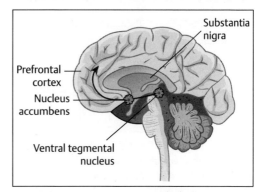

Fig. 12.1 Dopaminergic tracts in the brain.

are to treat symptoms, reduce disability, and slow down disease progression. The loss of dopaminergic neurons leads to increase in activity of ACh neurons. So, in PD, imbalance between DA and ACh occurs.

Pathophysiology

Pathophysiology of disease involves decrease in dopaminergic transmission and increase in cholinergic activity. Pathology of PD involves degeneration of DA neurons in nigrostriatal pathway. Replacing DA is a therapeutic approach to treat PD. Parkinson-like symptoms are side effects of DA receptor blockade with antipsychotic drugs. 1-methyl-4-phenyl-1,2,3,6-tetrahydropyridine (MPTP), a neurotoxin, destroys DA neurons and induces PD (**Fig. 12.2**).

Carlson in 1950s showed that L-dopa reduces symptom in patients with PD. This work won him the Nobel Prize.

PD is a common disorder of extrapyramidal system, affecting males and females equally. Mostly, the cases affect those between 45 and 65 years of age. Rarely, the disorder may have familial basis; otherwise, most cases are familial by nature.

Mutation of several genes such as parkin, synuclein, etc., have been described. MPTP has been a commonly blamed toxin for manifestations. D2 blockers could produce signs and symptoms of PD (**Box 12.2**).

Mostly, PD is diagnosed with ease. However, disorders like Huntington's (family history with dementia present), Shy–Dragger syndrome (autonomic insufficiency marked), supranuclear palsy (pseudobulbar palsy and eye involvement), Creutzfeldt–Jakob disease (dementia prominent), corticobasal degeneration (cortical dysfunction prominent), Wilson disease (hepatic and lenticular degeneration), and essential tremors (lack of family history, absence of other neurological signs) can cause diagnostic confusion.

Dopamine in Parkinson's Disease

The normally high concentration of DA in the basal ganglia of the brain is reduced in PD. The pharmacologic attempts to restore dopaminergic activity with L-dopa or with DA agonists are successful in alleviating many of the clinical features of the disorder. An alternative but complementary approach involves restoring the normal balance of cholinergic and dopaminergic influences on the basal ganglia with antimuscarinic drugs, which are cheap but not very well-tolerated treatment options.

The pathophysiologic basis for this therapy is that in idiopathic Parkinsonism, dopaminergic neurons in the substantia nigra, which normally inhibit the output of GABA-ergic cells in the corpus striatum, are lost.

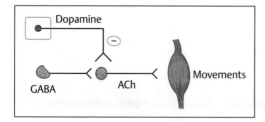

Fig. 12.2 There is a fine balance between the two motor systems regulated by acetylcholine (ACh) and dopamine (DA), which gets disturbed in patients with Parkinson's disease (PD).

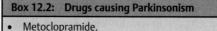

Box 12.2: Drugs causing Parkinsonism
• Metoclopramide.
• Neuroleptic drugs.
• Reserpine.

In contrast, Huntington chorea involves the loss of some cholinergic neurons and an even greater loss of the GABA-ergic cells that exit the corpus striatum. Drugs that induce Parkinsonian syndromes are DA receptor antagonists (e.g., antipsychotic agents), which lead to the destruction of the dopaminergic nigrostriatal neurons.

The cause of selective degeneration of nigrostriatal neurons in PD is not precisely known. It appears to be multifactorial. Oxidation of DA by MAO-B and aldehyde dehydrogenase generate hydroxyl-free radicals ($^{\cdot}OH$) in the presence of ferrous iron (basal ganglia are rich in iron). Normally, these radicals are quenched by glutathione and other endogenous antioxidants. Age-related (e.g., in atherosclerosis) and/or otherwise acquired defect in protective antioxidant mechanisms allows the free radicals to damage lipid membranes and DNA, resulting in neuronal degenerations. Genetic predisposition may contribute to high vulnerability of substantia nigra neurons. Environmental toxins or some infections (grippe) may accentuate these defects. Synthetic toxin N-methyl-4-phenyl tetrahydropyridine (MPTP), which occurs as a contaminant of some illicit drugs, produces nigrostriatal degenerations similar to PD. Neuroleptics and other DA blockers may cause temporary PD too.

Treatment Options for Parkinson's Disease

Several treatments are available for PD (**Fig. 12.3**) which include medical, surgical, and physical treatments. There are several goals that need to be achieved while treating a case with PD (**Box 12.3**). Many drugs are available to achieve these goals. Newer formulations of older drugs like inhaled formulation of L-dopa are under consideration.[12]

Treating Parkinson's Disease

The dopaminergic/cholinergic balance may be restored by two mechanisms:

- Enhancement of DA-ergic activity by drugs which may:
    ◊ Replenish neuronal DA by supplying L-dopa, which is its natural precursor;

Box 12.3: Goals of treating Parkinson's disease
• Symptomatic treatment (treating rigidity and bradykinesia).
• Treatment of motor complications (wearing-off phenomenon).
• Prevention of motor complications (on and off phenomenon).
• Prevention of nonmotor complications (e.g., delusions, hallucinations, constipation, etc.).

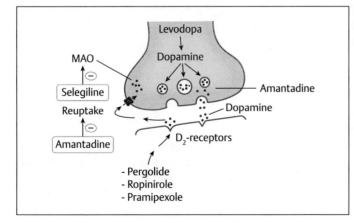

Fig. 12.3 Mechanism of commonly used anti-Parkinson drugs explained diagrammatically.

administration of DA itself is ineffective as it does not cross the blood–brain barrier (BBB).

◇ Act as DA agonists (bromocriptine, pergolide, cabergoline, etc.).

◇ Prolong the action of DA through selective inhibition of its metabolism (selegiline).

◇ Release DA from stores and inhibit reuptake (amantadine).

- **Reduction of cholinergic activity by antimuscarinic** drugs; this approach is most effective against tremor and rigidity, and less effective in the treatment of bradykinesia.

Levodopa

Loss of substantia nigra is the hallmark of PD patients. On visual inspection, this structure of basal ganglia appears pale, indicating DA depletion. This is believed to produce cardinal manifestations of PD.

This is the most effective anti-Parkinson drug which reduces mortality in PD. L-dopa was introduced by Hornequez and Cotzias in the year 1962. Since then, the drug has become the drug of choice for this disabling disease. Clinical data indicates that the drug has favorable effect on the course of the disease. Studies indicate that the drug does not have a neurodegenerative potential and does not hasten neuron loss in Parkinson's patients.

Pharmacokinetics

Given orally, the absorption is reduced by protein meal. Therefore, nonvegetarian diet should be prohibited while the patient is taking this drug. It gets metabolized in the wall of small intestine; therefore, bioavailability is low. It gets converted into DA (**Fig. 12.4**). This is shear wastage as the drug does not enter the BBB. Moreover, this contributes to the side effects. Given along with

carbidopa, the bioavailability increases and risk of nausea and vomiting becomes less.

Levodopa–Carbidopa Combination

L-dopa is a derivative of small amino acid and hence has bioavailability issues. Therefore, it is combined with carbidopa. The main function of carbidopa is to block its conversion to DA in the systemic circulation before it crosses BBB. This prevents gastrointestinal (GI) side effects. This is because the drug increases the fraction of L-dopa entering the brain. The drug is needed in doses of 75 to 200 mg daily to be able to do it. It comes as a combination of L-dopa and carbidopa (10:100, 25:100, 25:200) to block peripheral conversion. Controlled-release formulations are available with a good bioavailability. With increasing disease severity, one would have to start with L-dopa–carbidopa combination with or without entacapone, depending upon the severity. A peripheral COMT inhibitor (e.g., entacapone) is added to levodopa and carbidopa combination becomes weak or pharmacological effect wanes.

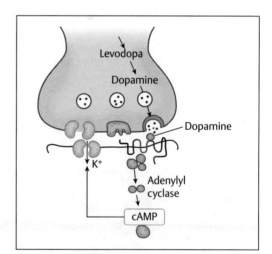

Fig. 12.4 Levodopa (L-dopa) is an isomer of dopamine (DA) that is presynaptically converted into DA. This then stimulates dopaminergic receptors to generate a G-protein–mediated response, leading to activation of adenylyl cyclase. Cyclic AMP thus generated can open K+ channels and this can cause cellular inhibition.

One can consider adding selegiline if the control becomes too difficult. Apomorphine can be used to control the "off" period in advanced patients. The drug is used subcutaneously due to its high first-pass metabolism.[3]

Advantages and Disadvantages

Advantages

L-dopa is a prodrug that is metabolized by dopa decarboxylase in the wall of the gut. The drug is therefore combined with carbidopa or benserazide. The main advantage of using the combination is lesser rise of side peripheral effects such as nausea, vomiting, postural hypotension, and cardiac arrhythmias. The main disadvantage is, however, higher risk of psychiatric side effects such as hallucinations, etc.

Another advantage of L-dopa is that it is the most potent anti-Parkinson drug which is well-tolerated and acts quickly. The drug is relatively inexpensive and is quite effective in PD.

The main clinical advantage of the drug combination is that with combination, patients can use higher dose of L-dopa (at least one-fourth reduction could be expected).

Disadvantages

Long-term side effects such as dyskinesia and on and off phenomenon could be quite bothersome. Absorption is affected by dietary proteins and hallucinations, and behavioral changes can occur.

It is, however, important to note that L-dopa–carbidopa combination does not give any benefit whatsoever in motor fluctuations. Only long-acting DA agonists such as ropinirole and pramipexole can provide such benefits.

Once absorbed, L-dopa has an extensive tissue distribution, and the drug is metabolized by several enzymes.

Risk of motor fluctuation is, however, not affected with this combination. Moreover, since more amount of L-dopa enters the brain, risk of mental side effects is increased. Importantly, carbidopa gets ionized at physiological pH; hence, it does not enter the BBB. Thus, carbidopa is a peripherally acting drug.

Treatment is generally started with low dose, that is, one tablet of sinemet containing 25 mg of carbidopa and 100 mg of L-dopa (1:4 combination) given three times a day. Fluctuations in clinical response can be reduced by using a sustained-release (SR) preparation of sinemet.

Side Effects

The most common side effect is nausea. GI issues are common with L-dopa therapy. Constipation, defined as fewer than three bowel movements per week, is the most widely recognized GI symptom of PD. This may come even before motor symptoms. Anticholinergics, amantadine, etc., can also accentuate this. Eating balanced diet, fruits, and vegetables; engaging in exercises; and consuming lots of fluids can help these patients. Giving the drug with meals can minimize the side effects. Long-term side effects can be disabling and can be seen in 50% of cases after 5 years of treatment. Nausea, vomiting, postural hypotension, arrhythmias, and hallucinations are manifestations of DA excess (**Box 12.5**). Many delayed side effects also occur.

Arrhythmias and hallucinations are rare. Long-term side effects include dyskinesias, which are types of motor fluctuations. "On and off" phenomenon is a severe form of dyskinesia. Choreoathetoid movements are common in patients who are on long-term treatment with L-dopa.

Box 12.5: Chronology of side effects of levodopa
• Early side effects: Nausea, vomiting, postural hypotension.
• Late: Dyskinesia and mental symptoms.
• Later: "On and off" phenomenon.

For initial 1 to 3 years, L-dopa has appropriate therapeutic response. After that, the "honeymoon phase" is over and response becomes erratic. This is accompanied by involuntary movements such as athetosis and dystonia. It has been estimated that each year, 5 to 10% of patients will develop dyskinesia. Although they can be pharmacologically managed, in refractory cases, pallidotomy may relieve them.

This may be associated with motor fluctuations such as "on and off" phenomenon or "end of dose." The drug effect could also wear with time. Infusions of DA or long-acting DA agonists can be used in these patients. The National Institute of Clinical Excellence recommends use of L-dopa as an early therapy in Parkinson's patients. Dyskinesias are troublesome side effects of L-dopa which occur due to increase in thalamocortical activity and replacement of DA in palatal neurons.

"End of dose" has been related to loss of DA storage capacity of brain neurons. More frequent DA administration or SR formulations can be used. DA agonists may be needed if L-dopa becomes unhelpful.

Amantadine is the most effective "response smoothening" agent and is the drug of choice for motor fluctuations. This is used in 100 mg twice daily. Dose can be increased as well if patients do not have many side effects.

End-of-dose deterioration is managed by increasing the frequency of dosing with L-dopa (e.g., to 2 or 3 hourly), but this tends to worsen the dyskinesia. The motor response then becomes more brittle, with abrupt swings between hyper- and hypomobility (the on and off phenomenon). In this case, a more effective approach is to use a COMT inhibitor, for example, entacapone, which can sometimes allay early end-of-dose deterioration without causing dyskinesia.

Some 20% of the patients with PD, notably the elderly ones, develop impairment of memory and speech with a fluctuating confusional state and hallucinations. As these symptoms are often aggravated by medication, it is preferable to gradually reduce the anti-Parkinsonian treatment.

Therapeutic Status of Levodopa

The main features that require alleviation are tremor, rigidity, and bradykinesia. Drug therapy plays the most important role in symptom relief, but it does not alter the progressive course of PD. Treatment should begin only when it is judged necessary in each individual case.

Two conflicting objectives have to be balanced: The desire for satisfactory relief of current symptoms and the avoidance of adverse reactions (ARs) as a result of long-continued treatment. There is a debate as to whether the treatment should commence with L-dopa or a synthetic DA agonist.

L-dopa provides the biggest improvement in motor activity, but its use is associated with the development of dyskinesia (involuntary movement of the face and limbs) after 5 to 10 years and sometimes sooner.

Drug Interactions

- The drug is not recommended with monoamine oxidase (MAO) inhibitors due to the fear of increase in levels of dopaminergic transmission. A hypertensive crisis may occur.
- Drugs that increase motility of intestine, for example, cisapride can increase absorption of L-dopa and drugs like atropine which decrease GI motility which, in turn, can reduce absorption.
- Antipsychotic drugs, for example, D2 blockers reduce the therapeutic activity; hence, they should not be given. Clozapine is the drug of choice for psychotic behavior

in Parkinsonian patients. Quetiapine is an alternative drug.

- Antiemetics like metoclopramide which are also D2 blockers should not be given for nausea and vomiting in PD. Instead, domperidone, which despite being a D2 blocker, can be used, as the drug does not enter BBB. Hence, it does not affect the therapeutic action of L-dopa.

Dose

Starting dose of L-dopa is 200 to 300 mg/day and is given with carbidopa. Maximum dose is 800 mg/day. Dose of carbidopa required to reduce risk of peripheral side effect is 75 mg (L-dopa–carbidopa: 300:75; 1:4). The most widely used formulation of L dopa and carbidopa is 100.25 tablet. Other strengths are however available.

Contraindications

The drug is avoided in patients with psychotic disorders, peptic ulcer, malignant melanoma, and those with acute narrow-angle glaucoma. The drug should not be given with MAO-A inhibitors as hypertensive crises may occur.

Unsuspecting patients with these contra-indications may make the situation worse; psychosis is relevant in dementia patients with behavioral and psychological symptoms. Glaucoma and peptic ulcer are general contra-dictions but may lend patients in ophthalmic and gastroenterological departments.

Dopaminergic Agonists

DA agonists have a much less powerful motor effect but are less likely to produce dyskinesias. The treatment usually begins with L-dopa in low doses to get a good motor response, adding a DA agonist when the initial benefit begins to wane (**Box 12.6**).

A typical course is about 2 to 4 years on treatment with L-dopa or DA agonist, with the patient's disability and motor performance remaining near

normal despite progression of the underlying disease. After some 5 years, about 50% of patients exhibit problems of long-term treatment, namely, dyskinesia and end-of-dose deterioration with the "on and off" phenomenon.

After 10 years, virtually 100% of patients are affected.

These are short-acting drugs and are given either in the beginning as monotherapy or given in the following:

- Patients not able to tolerate L-dopa.
- Those experiencing fluctuations in response to L-dopa.
- Those with limited response to L-dopa.

Dopaminergic agonists could improve therapeutic response to L-dopa. Use of dopamine agonists is associated with lesser risk of response fluctuations as these drugs act directly on dopaminergic receptors. These are generally indicated in those cases which have not responded to L-dopa or have developed motor fluctuations ("on and off phenomenon").

One should find the least possible dose and titrate dose to enhance tolerance to adverse

Box 12.6: Dopaminergic agonists
• **D1 agonists:**
◊ Apomorphine.
◊ Pergolide.
◊ Piribedil.
◊ Lergotrile.
◊ Rotigotine.
• **D2 agonists:**
◊ Bromocriptine.
◊ Cabergoline.
◊ Ropinirole.
◊ Quinagolide.
• **D3 agonist:**
◊ Pramipexole.

Note: Pergolide was withdrawn from the market some years back due to its association with cardiac valvular defects.

effects of dopamine agonist. This may ensure best pharmacological response. Pramipexole and ropinirole are more potent and longer acting compared to other DA agonists and are used as monotherapies. Younger patients tend to develop more motor fluctuations compared to older patients; hence, DA agonist monotherapy is more suited to these patients. Older patients are more likely to develop hallucinations and other psychotic symptoms with dopamine agonists; hence, L-dopa-carbidopa combination may be the best initial medicine in them. Both drugs are likely to cause hallucinations.[4] Sedation appears more common when DA agonists are used with L-dopa.[5]

Apomorphine

Apomorphine is related chemically to morphine but does not bind to opioid receptors. Instead, it binds to DA receptors. The drug is used in "freezing" episodes; times when the immobility of a Parkinson's patient is maximum. It is seen in advanced patients. It is given via injection; response produced is brief. Nausea occurs in almost all patients due to strong chemoreceptor trigger zone (CTZ) stimulation. Domperidone can treat this.

Bromocriptine

This is a D2 partial agonist and is a short-acting drug. Elimination is by bile. The drug is useful for treatment of acromegaly, impotence, and drug-induced hyperprolactinemia. The drug is no longer recommended for suppression of unwanted lactation. Due to several side effects like nausea, vomiting, postural hypotension, and digital vasospasm ("ergotism"), the drug is used less frequently nowadays. It has however found a new use as an antidiabetic agent.

Usual dose of bromocriptine is 1.25 mg once a day. Dose can be increased in increments of 1.25 or 2.5 mg, and maximal tolerated dose should be maintained.

Bromocriptine is beneficial in delaying motor complications like dyskinesias, etc., if started early.[1]

Cabergoline is a safer alternative drug for this. Vitamin B6 (pyridoxine) can also be used. Side effects include nausea, vomiting, and postural hypotension. Psychiatric side effects can occur due to dopaminergic activity.

Ropinirole and pramipexole are newer D2 and D3 stimulant drugs and are used both in early and advanced PD. Pramipexole is started as 0.125 mg three times a day and most patients will require between 0.5 and 1.5 mg three times a day.

Ropinirole is given as 2 to 8 mg/day. Initial dose is 0.25 mg three times a day. Details of doses and side effects are given in **Table 12.1**.

Table 12.1 Doses and adverse effects of commonly used dopamine agonists in Parkinson's disease

Drug	Dose	Side effects
Dopamine agonists		
Pramipexole	1.5–4.5 mg/d	Headache, dizziness, drowsiness, swelling in limbs, appetite or weight changes, nightmares, amnesia
Ropinirole	0.25 mg three times daily to a maximum of 4 mg daily	Nausea, vomiting, stomach pain, loss of appetite, worsened restless legs syndrome symptoms early in the morning, diarrhea, constipation, dry mouth, sweating, headache, dizziness, drowsiness, agitation, or anxiety

These are longer acting, safer, and more potent than D1 stimulants. Ropinirole is metabolized by CYP1A2, and its metabolism is inhibited by ciprofloxacin. It is eliminated by tubular secretion, which is blocked by cimetidine, leading to increase in its plasma levels. Both of these drugs have usefulness either as monotherapy in early or as adjuvant in late stage.

Ropinirole (0.25–4 mg daily) is the drug of choice for restless leg syndrome apart from its role in PD. Pramipexole can also be used (0.125–0.5 mg once a day). Patients not responding to other measures can be put on L-dopa.

Restless legs syndrome can occur as a primary (idiopathic) disorder or can occur in various forms of neuropathies (e.g., diabetic). Several genetic loci have been identified as well. Disturbed sleep and daytime sleepiness can occur.

Pramipexole was approved more than 10 years back and is used both in early and advanced cases of PD. Both of these drugs have significant advantage in terms of their ability to control motor fluctuations.

Side effects include excessive sedation akin to narcolepsy. Importantly, in narcolepsy, modafinil is the drug of choice. The drug is an enzyme inducer; therefore, plasma levels of many drugs can fall including oral contraceptives.

Rotigotine is a new nonergoline derivative that is given in the form of a patch. The drug is not given orally because of high first-pass metabolism. A 24-hour patch is available to allow smooth drug concentrations.

Uses of Dopamine Agonists in Parkinson's Disease

- DA agonists are recommended either as initial drugs in early Parkinson's or as adjuvants in late PD.
- Dose of DA agonists should be slowly titrated until side effects appear. Another drug of other class can be used in case of side effects.
- Since ergot alkaloids may have more side effects, a nonergot alkaloid is preferable.

Amantadine

Amantadine is a serendipitously discovered drug that has been an antiviral drug used in prophylaxis of influenza A2. Over 40 years back, the drug was discovered serendipitously and is in clinical use since then. The interest in this drug has now reemerged due to its role in treating motor fluctuations (especially on and off phenomenon).

This is a dopaminergic drug with anticholinergic activity and has been used in PD for last two decades. Though, traditionally, the drug has been considered to be a dopamine transmission enhancer, recent evidence suggests that the drug acts by blocking NMDA receptors of glutamate type.

This is useful in early and mild cases. It is useful either for mild PD or as an adjunct to other drugs as a "response smoothener." It is safer than L-dopa or DA agonists, but it also has lesser efficacy.

Oral absorption of the drug is good, and it has a short half-life. It is not metabolized and is eliminated unchanged. Drug is either avoided in renal failure or dose is reduced. Recommended doses include 200 to 300 mg given twice or thrice daily. Duration of action of a single oral dose may extend up to 8 hours. Still, the drug is given in divided doses to ensure smooth plasma concentrations.

The most common side effect is ankle edema, and this is a manifestation of dilation of arterioles at the level of ankle. Livedo reticularis (diffuse mottling of skin) is another common side effect and is reversible.

It is recommended as an initial drug in early Parkinson's patients or those with motor fluctuations.

The drug is contraindicated in patients with psychiatric diseases and those with epilepsies. Being a dopaminergic drug, it can accentuate psychiatric symptoms. It reduces seizure threshold. Anxiety symptoms can also occur. It is used in 100 mg twice daily doses. CNS side effects are predominant reasons for concern in patients upon amantadine. Mostly, the side effects are mild but can be severe in elderly patients. Side effects due to its alpha blocking and anticholinergic properties can also occur. These may include hypotension, blurring of vision, and constipation. Due to imbalance between filling and ejection, the drug has caused worsening of congestive heart failure as well.

It does not have good activity upon tremors but treats bradykinesia and rigidity more effectively.

Metabolic Inhibitors

Two kinds of drugs are used as metabolic inhibitors: COMT inhibitors (tolcapone and entacapone) and MAO-B inhibitors (selegiline and rasagiline).

These include drugs like carbidopa that inhibit the gut enzyme and are known as dopa-decarboxylase. This enzyme is responsible for peripheral decarboxylation of L-dopa. However, this is not the only enzyme decarboxylating the drug. Entacapone and tolcapone are drugs that also inhibit the degradation of L-dopa and hence are useful. These are therefore given in association with L-dopa.

COMT Inhibitors

COMT inhibitors reduce metabolism of L-dopa to its metabolite O-hydroxymethyldopa and therefore lead to better availability of L-dopa in the brain. This can increase duration of action of L-dopa ("on time") by 1 hour. These drugs are best used in cases that are refractory to other treatment modalities. It has been seen that COMT inhibition is relatively more effective in providing consistent extensions of pharmacological effects of L-dopa and avoids delay to achieve maximal effect compared to SR tablets of L-dopa.

Tolcapone is more potent; however, it is more toxic. The drug has been associated with hepatic failure. Entacapone is not associated with this serious toxicity. It should be kept in mind that serial liver function testing may be required at a 15-day interval. It is contraindicated in preexisting liver function.

Entacapone is a short-acting drug that should be avoided in renal failure. Therefore, more frequent dosing may be required. Tolcapone can act both as centrally and peripherally, while entacapone does not enter the BBB. Both are well absorbed orally and are protein bound. Food does not interfere with their absorption unlike L-dopa.

Entacapone is used in combination with L-dopa and carbidopa and this combination is known as sta-levo (levo + carbi + enta). It is often used in patients with advanced PD. It is important to know that ropinirole and pramipexole can be also used in advanced Parkinson's patients.

Tolcapone is started at a dose of 100 mg twice or thrice a day given along with sinemet. To avoid side effects such as dyskinesia, hypotension, and mental side effects, dose of sinemet should be reduced by one-third. Entacapone is shorter acting and given as 200 mg with each dose of carbidopa–L-dopa combination. Brown–orange color urine can occur as a side effect of tolcapone. There is no evidence of hepatotoxicity of entacapone.

Selegiline and rasagiline are antioxidants that can scavenge free radicals (**Fig. 12.5**). These are irreversible inhibitors of MAO-B enzyme which

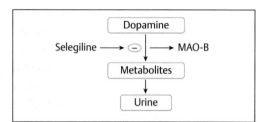

Fig. 12.5 Selegiline is an antioxidant that blocks metabolism of dopamine (DA). There has been speculation that the drug could prevent onset of Parkinson's disease (PD). MAO, monoamine oxidase.

can moderately increase duration of action of L-dopa. This may permit reduction of dose of L-dopa by half. However, the drug may increase peak effect of L-dopa and thus can worsen preexisting dyskinesia or psychiatric symptoms. Insomnia is a side effect of selegiline and occurs due to its metabolite that is structurally related to amphetamine.

It is noteworthy that one of the theories of PD states that neurodegeneration may be related to free radicals. Selegiline has been claimed to slow down this neurodegenerative response. However, objective evidence for this is not too strong.[2] It is often given to enhance action of L-dopa. However, it should be noted that L-dopa is not combined with MAO-A inhibitors. This is because they degrade DA at a fast pace and too much of DA in the brain can give rise to psychiatric symptoms.

Selegiline

Selegiline gets metabolized to amphetamines (e.g., methamphetamine), and this can cause CNS stimulation. Therefore, the drug should be given in morning to avoid insomnia. Rasagiline is not metabolized to amphetamines and is an irreversible inhibitor. There were claims in the past that the MAO-B inhibitors can potentially slow neurodegeneration. In this regard, there is renewed interest in rasagiline. However, studies done so far have shown that this effect of these drugs can be short term. The National Institute

of Clinical Excellence does not favor using these drugs for their neuroprotective role. However, MAO-B inhibitors can be used in symptomatic treatment of early Parkinson's patients. Unlike nonselective MAO inhibitors, selegiline is not associated with tyramine-mediated cheese reaction.[10]

Trihexyphenidyl

These drugs have been used historically in the treatment of PD. Indeed, these are considered to be the most widely accepted treatment options for PD patients. Deadly nightshade (Atropa belladonna) has long been tried in Parkinson's patients for excessive salivation. However, the drug is not a selective drug; hence, several side effects could emerge. Students may be familiar with the teacher of Sigmond Freud, James Charcot, who introduced anticholinergic drugs in treatment of PD. Although the drug has been in use for last 100 years, in 1945, the pathophysiological basis of its usefulness was found. Till then, it was believed that atropine helped Parkinson's patients by a peripheral mechanism! Such errors in medicine have been done earlier too!

Trihexyphenidyl is most commonly used anticholinergic drug for treatment of early PD or drug-induced PD. L-dopa is ineffective in this condition. This reduces rigidity and tremors. Importantly, although L-dopa affects all manifestations, bradykinesia is improved most commonly. The drug when given orally is rapidly absorbed. Duration of action after a single oral dose ranges from 1 to 12 hours. Finally, therefore, the drug is given twice daily. Anticholinergics can correct imbalance between striatal DA and ACh.

Anticholinergic drugs are useful in early or mild cases and are particularly useful in young patients. They are most effective for tremors/ rigidity. These can be used as monotherapy or in combination with other anti-Parkinson drugs. Most of the drugs given in **Table 12.2** have

Table 12.2 Doses of commonly used anticholinergics

Drug	Dose
Benzatropine	1–6 mg daily
Trihexyphenidyl	6–20 mg daily
Orphenadrine	60–120 mg daily
Hydroxyzine	25–50 mg daily
Promethazine	25–75 mg daily

similar efficacy or side effect profile. It should be noted that tremors or other dystonic features may improve but bradykinesia is little or not improved.

Drugs of anticholinergic class are popular but pharmacokinetics of drugs of this class, for example, benztropine, biperiden, diphenhydramine, ethopropazine, orphenadrine, procyclidine, and trihexyphenidyl is not very clear. Importantly, elderly do not tolerate these drugs as well as younger patients do. These drugs are extensively metabolized and eliminated by urine and bile.[11]

Patients need to be monitored for side effects such as acute-angle glaucoma, retention of urine, constipation, psychiatric disturbances, etc. Preferably, in these situations, the drugs are avoided. Elderly are particularly sensitive to their adverse reactions.

Drug-induced Parkinsonism is treated by anticholinergics and not by L-dopa or DA agonist because antipsychotics block D_2-receptors by which these drugs act. The piperazine phenothiazines (e.g., trifluoperazine) and butyrophenones (e.g., haloperidol) often cause Parkinsonism because they block D_2-receptors. Commonly used drugs are given in **Table 12.2.**

Contraindications
- Narrow-angle glaucoma.
- Prostatic enlargement.
- GI obstruction.

Biperiden and procyclidine are other anticholinergic drugs that could be used as a substitute of trihexyphenidyl. Patients should be watched for anticholinergic side effects such as dryness of mouth, blurring of vision, urinary retention, constipation, and confusion while these drugs are being used. Prolonged dryness of mouth can cause gingivitis and dental caries. Frequently, foul-smelling breath can be found. Anticholinergic drugs could be used in young Parkinson's patients with early disease.

Psychiatric Symptoms in Parkinson's Disease

A variety of symptoms such as confusion, anxiety, and psychosis can occur.[7] At times, disorders of impulse control can also occur. Most often, these are caused by dopaminergic drugs. It should however be kept in mind that Parkinson per se can also cause these. Depression too is an accompaniment of PD, especially in the early phase. Studies have shown that tricyclic antidepressants can delay the need for anti-Parkinson's treatment.[8] Mood in PD patients has been shown to be improved by pramipexole.[9]

Atypical antipsychotics can be used to treat psychotic symptoms and include quetiapine, risperidone, and olanzapine. It should be noted that risperidone and olanzapine can potentially worsen Parkinson's features. The drug of choice is, however, a dibenzodiazepine clozapine. It is a D4 blocker with 5-HT2 receptor blockade. Periodic count of blood cells should be done to rule out agranulocytosis that can occur. Drug should be stopped in case of low neutrophils (e.g., below 500 cells/cmm³).

Principles of Anti-Parkinsonian Treatment

- Exercise, education, and nutritional management are helpful in early cases. Always keep in mind that these patients do not get antidopaminergic drugs (e.g., D2 blockers) or metoclopramide (antiemetic drug). Loss of efficacy of L-dopa can occur and condition can worsen.
- For those with mild disease or early manifestations like tremors, anticholinergics or amantadine may be useful. Anticholinergic drugs are more likely to be effective in younger patients.
- For patients with severe functional disabilities; dopaminergic drugs are most effective. A combination of L-dopa and carbidopa are useful for such patients and is most effective in anti-Parkinson's therapy. Few physicians favor using long-acting dopamine agonists, for example, ropinirole or pramipexole for such patients as monotherapies. However, these show no response in patients who show no response to L-dopa.
- Tolcapone or selegiline can be used to increase effectiveness of L-dopa.
- "On and off" phenomenon is treated by response smootheners, for example, amantadine or tolcapone.
- Apomorphine is used for "freezing episodes." The drug has also been approved for use in patients with impotence. It acts by reducing level of prolactin.
- "Drug holiday," a relief from drug therapy for about a month, was once a popular method but is not recommended nowadays.

Drugs should not be discontinued abruptly. This can lead to neuroleptic malignant syndrome. This could be a major problem with L-dopa or DA agonists.

New Drugs/Treatments in Parkinson's Disease[13-15]

It is notable that being a neurodegenerative disease, it does not have a cure. Therefore, several new drugs are being tried such as the following:

- Dextromethorphan: This is a noncompetitive agonist of μ receptors and a synthetic opioid. The drug has a modulatory influence in dopaminergic and serotonergic transmission. The drug is being studied for symptomatic control in PD patients.
- Pimavanserin is a new antipsychotic drug that has been approved for hallucinations and delusions associated with PD psychosis.
- Istradefylline is a new class of drugs (adenosine receptor blockers), which is useful as an adjunct to L-dopa–carbidopa for treatment of on and off phenomenon.
- Safinamide is a new drug with dopaminergic and nondopaminergic effects. The drug is useful as an adjunct to L-dopa–carbidopa.
- Skin cells are being genetically reprogrammed for producing dopaminergic chemicals (personalized medicine) as the skin cells come from patient's own body.

Conclusion

Parkinson's disease is a progressive disorder of movement occurring mainly in the elderly. The chief symptoms are bradykinesia, rigidity, and tremors.

Anti-Parkinson drugs work by repleting the depleted levels of dopamine or stimulating dopamine receptors or by strengthening transmission or slowing down breakdown. Some drugs, for example, amantadine, balance the imbalance of ACh and dopamine.

References

1. van Hilten JJ, Ramaker CC, Stowe R, Ives NJ. Bromocriptine versus levodopa in early Parkinson's disease. Cochrane Database Syst Rev 2007; (4):CD002258 Review

2. Macleod AD, Counsell CE, Ives N, Stowe R. Monoamine oxidase B inhibitors for early Parkinson's disease. Cochrane Database Syst Rev 2005; (3):CD004898 Review

3. Dressler D. Apomorphine in the treatment of Parkinson's disease. Nervenarzt 2005; 76(6):681–689

4. Etminan M, Gill S, Samii A. Comparison of the risk of adverse events with pramipexole and ropinirole in patients with Parkinson's disease: a meta-analysis. Drug Saf 2003; 26(6):439–444 Review

5. Etminan M, Samii A, Takkouche B, Rochon PA. Increased risk of somnolence with the new dopamine agonists in patients with Parkinson's disease: a meta-analysis of randomised controlled trials. Drug Saf 2001;24(11):863–868

6. Dhikav V. Commentary. J Neurosci Rural Pract 2016;7(1):70–71

7. Broen MP, Narayen NE, Kuijf ML, Dissanayaka NN, Leentjens AF. Prevalence of anxiety in Parkinson's disease: a systematic review and meta-analysis. Mov Disord 2016;31(8): 1125–1133

8. Paumier KL, Siderowf AD, Auinger P, et al; Parkinson Study Group Genetics Epidemiology Working Group. Tricyclic antidepressants delay the need for dopaminergic therapy in early Parkinson's disease. Mov Disord 2012;27(7):880–887

9. Leentjens AF, Koester J, Fruh B, Shephard DT, Barone P, Houben JJ. The effect of pramipexole on mood and motivational symptoms in Parkinson's disease: a meta-analysis of placebo-controlled studies. Clin Ther 2009;31(1):89–98

10. Heinonen EH, Myllylä V. Safety of selegiline (deprenyl) in the treatment of Parkinson's disease. Drug Saf 1998;19(1):11–22 Review

11. Brocks DR. Anticholinergic drugs used in Parkinson's disease: an overlooked class of drugs from a pharmacokinetic perspective. J Pharm Sci 1999;2(2):39–46 Review

12. Lotia M, Jankovic J. New and emerging medical therapies in Parkinson's disease. Expert Opin Pharmacother 2016;17(7): 895–909

13. Available at: https://medlineplus.gov/druginfo/meds/a619053.html. Accessed September 19, 2020

14. Available at: https://journals.lww.com/ajnonline/Abstract/2017/07000/New_Drug_Approved_For_Parkinson_s_Disease.22.aspx. Accessed September 19, 2020

15. Available at: https://medicalxpress.com/news/2020-05-treatment-patient-cells-possibilities-parkinson.html. Accessed September 19, 2020

Drugs for Dementia

Vikas Dhikav

Clinical Case Example

- A man of 72 years of age is brought to you by his daughter for slow and progressive memory loss. However, he denies any problems. She reports that he was an accountant and is now unable to keep his own cheque book straight. The bank executive fails to recognize his signatures. He often forgets ways back home while going out for shopping, etc. His wife died 2 years ago, and he was diagnosed with depression at that time. In addition, he has hypertension and type II diabetes. His father was diagnosed with Alzheimer's disease at the age of 85. On physical examination, his BP is 170/90; he is oriented in time, place, and person and his minimental state examination (MMSE) score is 22/30. A few months later, his MMSE score is 18/30; on examination, it was found he has some mild cogwheel rigidity and a slightly shuffling gait but no tremors. What treatment will be appropriate?

Answer: This patient has a diagnosis of Alzheimer's disease (AD), which is the most common type of dementia. Apart from managing his diabetes and hypertension, he needs to be started with donepezil 5 mg for 4 weeks, and after this, the dose will be increased to 10 mg once daily. A regular follow-up and exercises (both physical and mental) can be recommended. The patient should be encouraged to remain social and independent.

Dementia

Dementia is characterized by a gradual loss of cognitive functioning, which can also incorporate losses of motor, emotional, and social functioning. It is a progressive disease that eventually renders people unable to care for themselves and severely interfere with activities of daily living.[1]

Dementia is a common disease of old age. Dementia to laypersons is a memory problem that interferes with day-to-day activities. There are many different causes of dementia, with Alzheimer's disease (AD) and vascular disorders being the most common types. It should however be noted that not all memory problems are dementia.[2]

Typical features of dementia are deterioration in memory, slowly and progressively with or without thinking, behavior, and impairment of activities of daily living. The disease affects older people and currently around 50 million people have dementia, with nearly 10 million new cases added every year.[3,4]

Prevention of dementia is a major aim of public health agencies and several options like cognitive activities, regular physical exercises, and drugs used for treatment of hypertension, diabetes or both are being evaluated for prevention.[4]

Impaired cognition is often accompanied by deterioration in emotional control, social behavior, and motivation. Motor problems may occur at different stages, depending on the type of dementia. For example, they occur *early* in vascular dementia and *late* in AD. Decline in activities of daily living, such as washing, eating, and toileting, are often noted. Degeneration of memory-dependent areas such as hippocampus is a feature of dementias and manifests as confusion, delirium, etc. **Fig. 13.1** describes pathophysiological details such as deposition of beta-amyloid, which is the hallmark of dementia of Alzheimer's type. **Fig. 13.2** gives details of the consequences of deposition of beta-amyloid and neurofibrillary tangles.

Dementia is a common neurodegenerative disease of old age. The disease presents as insidious onset of memory loss and then progresses to almost complete amnesia and mutism. The caregiver burden and perceived caregiver stress is significant in dementia patients.

Behavioral and psychological symptoms of dementia (BPSD) are common[5] and need special treatment. Common causes of dementias are as follows:

- Alzheimer's disease (AD).
- Vascular dementia.
- "Mixed" dementia (AD and vascular dementia).
- Dementia with Lewy bodies.
- Frontotemporal dementia.
- Parkinson's disease with dementia.
- Miscellaneous causes, for example, thyroid dementia and B12 deficiency dementia.

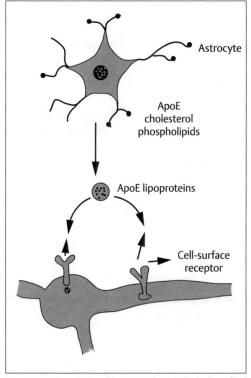

Fig. 13.1 Deposition of beta-amyloid is the hallmark of Alzheimer's disease (AD) and is often the step leading to neurodegeneration as per prevailing hypothesis.

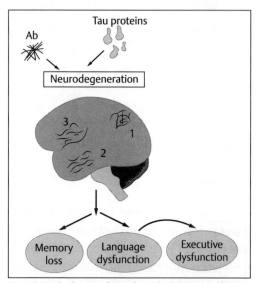

Fig. 13.2 The brains of people with Alzheimer's disease (AD) have an abundance of two abnormal structures called plaques and tangles. Plaques are made up of the beta-amyloid proteins, which are dense deposits of protein and cellular material that accumulate outside and around nerve cells. Neurofibrillary tangles are twisted fibers that build up inside the nerve cell. Both of them collectively produce degeneration of brain neurons, leading to several abnormalities in parietal area (1), temporal lobes (2), and frontal lobes (3).

194

Pathophysiology

Dementia though a heterogeneous disease involves accumulation of otherwise normal and physiological proteins in brains.

The proteins interfere with neurotransmission and cause slow death of neurons. This may lead to memory loss and other associated manifestations.

Clinical Features

Dementia has insidious onset of difficulty in episodic memory. Sementia memory is usually preserved except in case of sementic dementias. Also, depression, psychosis, aggression, and agitation may be seen.

Following is the diagnostic criteria for dementia:

- Memory impairment:
  ◊ And at least one of the following:
    □ Aphasia.
    □ Apraxia.
    □ Agnosia.
    □ Disturbances in executive functioning.

Diagnostic criteria for mild cognitive impairment are as follows:

- Memory problems.

Useful mnemonic for the diagnosis of dementia (6 As)

Memory impairment and one of the following four items:

- Apraxia.
- Aphasia.
- Agnosia.
- Abstraction and other executive functioning.

Plus

- Absence of clouding of consciousness.
- Ability to function is impaired.

- Objective memory disorder.
- Absence of other cognitive disorders or repercussions on daily life.
- Normal general cognitive function.
- Absence of dementia.

Behavioral and Psychological Symptoms of Dementias[5]

BPSD are defined by International Psychogeriatric Association (IPA) as "wide spectrum of noncognitive manifestations of dementia, including verbal and physical aggression, agitation, psychotic symptoms (hallucinations and delusions), sleep disturbances, oppositional behavior, and wandering." Some patients may become overtly violent too. Restlessness is a disturbing feature of dementia. Sleeplessness could be troublesome and could be due to disease or the side effects of drugs. It should be noted that majority of patients with dementia have BPSD.[3]

Drugs as Dementia-Causing Agents

Certain drugs can also cause dementias. Side effects to certain medications may mimic or worsen symptoms of dementia and include antihistamines, benzodiazepines, opioids, anticholinergics, tricyclic antidepressants, and antipsychotics. They should be considered in the differential diagnosis of pseudodementia, but drugs should generally be a diagnosis of exclusion when other causes have been excluded.

Drugs for Dementias[5–12]

Acetyl-cholinesterase inhibitors are intended to *preserve* functioning (i.e., delay worsening) and usually prescribed for mild-to-moderate symptoms. The drugs are effective in improving or stabilizing cognitive functioning, although the improvements can be modest.[7] A host of treatment options like antidepressants, levodopa, clozapine, etc., are used to treat dementia with Lewy bodies.[8] Likewise in patients with frontotemporal dementias, SSRIs are effective compared to anticholinesterases.[9]

Since there is no cure for irreversible dementias, we need to keep in mind the goals of dementias therapy. Dementia does not have a cure at present; the main aim of treatment is to reduce symptoms and to improve quality of life. One can use multiple medications with different modes of action together or separately across the various stages of the disease. However, drugs are one of many strategies in management of this disease.

Therapeutic goals of treating dementias are as follows:

- Cure disease.
- Prevent disease or delay onset.
- Slow progression of disease.
- Treat primary symptoms, for example, memory loss.
- Treat secondary symptoms, for example, depression and hallucinations.

The roles of drug-inhibiting cholinesterases are given in **Table 13.1**. Overall treatment options in dementia are summarized in **Table 13.2**.

Drugs used commonly for dementia are as follows:

- Drugs for BPSD:

◇ Benzodiazepines:
  □ Lorazepam.
◇ SSRIs:
  □ Escitalopram.
  □ Sertraline.
◇ Antipsychotics:
  □ Older:
    – Haloperidol.
  □ Newer:
    – Amisulpride.
    – Risperidone.
    – Quetiapine.
◇ Beta-blockers:
  □ Propranolol.

Disease modifying:

- Estrogens:
  ◇ Two trials failed to stop AD progression.
- *Ginkgo biloba:*
  ◇ Mixed results.
  ◇ Nonsteroidal anti-inflammatory drugs (NSAIDs)/prednisolone:
  ◇ No effect on symptomatic AD.
- 1,000 IU of vitamin E recommended twice daily:
  ◇ Cardiotoxicity.
  ◇ Failure to slow down conversion of mild cognitive impairment (MCI)→AD.

Table 13.1 Cholinesterase inhibiting therapy and its role in various categories of patients[10,11]

MCI*	Early stage dementia	Moderate	Severe dementia
Benefits of using cholinesterases are questionable; however, they are used commonly by physicians in anticipation of giving some potential benefits	Cognitive benefits are apparent	Cognitive benefits are apparent, activities of daily living are preserved; evidence suggests that BPSD such as agitation are reduced	Even in severe stages, the modest benefits of this class can be seen. However, adverse effects become more likely as higher doses are needed

Abbreviation: BPSD, behavioral and psychological symptoms of dementia.
*MCI, or mild cognitive impairment; now, cholinesterase inhibitors are approved for all severity categories of dementias. Although, traditionally, MCI is not a treatment category, but use of these drugs is popular for the same as well. However, the treatment should be individualized in this class.

Table 13.2 Pharmacological treatment options for AD[10,11]

MOA	Cholinesterase inhibitors			NMDA antagonist
Drug	Donepezil	Galantamine	Rivastigmine	Memantine
Indication	Mild-to-severe AD	Mild-to-moderate AD	Mild-to-severe AD	Moderate-to-severe AD
Dose	5 mg daily initially, 10 mg after 4 weeks	4 mg twice daily initially, 8 mg twice daily after 4 weeks	1.5 mg twice daily initially, later, 6 mg twice daily	5 mg twice daily initially, 10 mg twice daily after 4 weeks
			4.6 mg/cm² patch is available initially applied on exposed area of the upper back; dose is increased after 4 weeks to 9.6 mg/cm². Now a higher dosage of 13.3 mg/cm² patch is available for severe-category patients	
Side effects	Tiredness, dizziness, hallucinations, sleep alterations, abdominal cramps	Nausea, anorexia, cardiovascular side effects	GI upset, light-headedness, chest pain, muscle dystonias	Confusion, hallucinations, sleep alterations, headache, increase in blood pressure

Abbreviations: AD, Alzheimer's disease; GI, gastrointestinal; MOA, mechanism of action; NMDA, N methyl-D-aspartate.

- Antipsychotic:
  - ◊ Quetiapine, risperidone, and olanzapine:
    - □ Low dose.
    - □ Careful titration.
- Depression:
  - ◊ SSRIs:
    - □ Reduce anxiety.
    - □ Irritability.
    - □ Agitation.

Cholinesterase Inhibitors

Cholinesterase inhibitor reduces the breakdown of acetylcholine into its inactive forms, which is an important neurotransmitter in memory and cognition in the memory-dependent areas, for example, medial temporal lobes and frontal lobes. All the drugs of this class show modest improvement in cognition, function, and behavioral symptoms, but cholinesterase inhibitors are the mainstay of treatment of AD.[3] The mechanism of action (MOA) is summarized in **Fig. 13.3**. Galantamine has a dual MOA (**Fig. 13.4**).

To be able to start the patient on these drugs, one needs clear cut diagnosis of AD and an MMSE score of 10 to 24. They are not effective in mild cognitive impairment. It is generally said that we need to show an improvement on MMSE of 2 points to continue medications of this class. Side effects include gastrointestinal (nausea, vomiting, and diarrhea), cardiovascular (e.g., bradycardia, dizziness, and headache), and central (hallucinations, sleep alterations, and muscle cramps). Use carefully if gastric ulcer, heart disease, and chronic lung disease are preexisting in the patient. Overall, one-third improve, one-third stabilize, and one-third may not have any response. Cholinesterase inhibitors do not reduce progression of underlying disease.

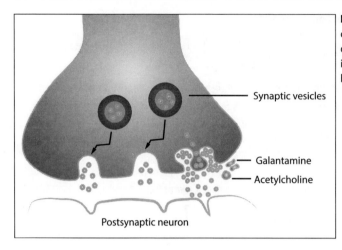

Fig. 13.3 Mechanism of action of donepezil. The drug blocks the action of acetylcholinesterase and hence increases acetylcholine activity in the brain.

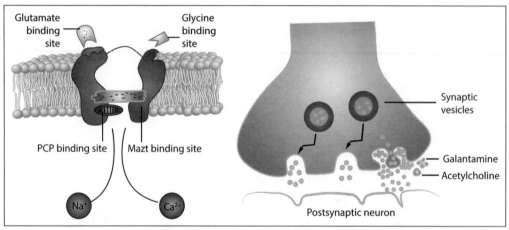

Fig. 13.4 Galantamine has dual mechanism of action and is useful in mild-to-moderate Alzheimer's disease (AD). It also has some usefulness in vascular dementia or vascular cognitive impairment. Galantamine is a reversible and competitive inhibitor of acetylcholinesterase (AchE) and is the only drug that has allosteric modulator activity of acetylcholine nicotinic receptors. PCP, phencyclidine.

Anticholinesterases are now recommended for all grades of severity of AD and Parkinson's disease dementia. Originally, they were reported to be beneficial for the treatment of moderate-to-severe AD. Improvement in cognition, behavioral disturbances, activities of daily living, and global assessment has been reported. Both donepezil and galantamine have been tried in vascular dementia.[6]

The main limitations of using donepezil is that though the symptoms of dementia go on for years,

the phase III trials of the cholinesterase inhibitors were typically of only 3 to 6 months' duration. Therefore, the limited long-term data available about the safety and efficacy in dementias pose a limitation in interpreting their long-term safety. Therefore, decision to continue them in given case should be individualized.

Table 13.3 describes major side effects of commonly used drugs in dementias. **Table 13.4** gives major differentiating pharmacological features.

Table 13.3 Common side effects of drugs used in treatment of AD

Cholinesterase inhibitors (donepezil)	NMDA-receptor antagonist (memantine)
Nausea, vomiting, diarrhea, weight loss, loss of appetite (high dose), muscle weakness, tiredness, frequent urination	Dizziness, headache, confusion, sleep alterations
Uncommon side effects include hallucinations, sleep disturbances, bad dreams, etc	Constipation can occur

Table 13.4 Major pharmacological features of anticholinesterases used in dementias[10–12]

Drug	Mechanism	Half-life	Protein biding	Metabolic enzyme isoforms
Donepezil	Reversible and noncompetitive inhibitor of acetylcholinesterase	60–80 h	>90%	CYP 2D6, CYP 3A4
Rivastigmine	Pseudoirreversible inhibitor of acetylcholinesterase and butyrylcholinesterase	2 h	40%	Acetylcholinesterase and butyrylcholinesterase (not in liver)
Galantamine	Reversible inhibitor of acetylcholinesterase and modulator of presynaptic nicotinic receptors	5–6 h	20%	CYP2D6, CYP3A4

Commonly used anticholinesterases in dementias are as follows:

- Donepezil:
  - ◊ Given once daily, dosage of 5 to 10 mg.
- Rivastigmine:
  - ◊ Given twice daily, dosages of 3 to 12 mg (orally).
  - ◊ Patch of 5 to 15 mg/cm is available to be applied transdermally.
- Galantamine:
  - ◊ Given once daily, dosages of 8 to 24 mg (can also be given twice daily).

Donepezil

Donepezil is a reversible anticholinesterase, which is specific to the brain in terms of its entry and binding ability to cholinesterase enzyme. After oral administration, the peak plasma levels are obtained after approximately 4 hours and plasma steady state after 14 to 21 days. Hence, the drug dose is doubled after 4 weeks. The drug is a long-acting one with a half-life of over 70 hours and is given once daily. The excretion is slow and occurs via the renal route and the cytochrome P450 system.

Donepezil has better tolerability compared to other drugs of this class. The drug has smoother acetylcholinesterase inhibition and achieves therapeutic concentration with longer duration of action. This avoids the fluctuations in enzyme inhibition and lessens cholinergic side effects.

Rivastigmine

Rivastigmine is a selective carbamate and is a "pseudo-irreversible" inhibitor of acetylcholinesterase and butyrylcholinesterase. The drug has a good deal of central nervous system (CNS) selectivity and achieves good concentrations in memory-dependent areas of the brain, for example, cerebral cortex and hippocampus. Rivastigmine is a short-acting drug with modest protein binding. The drug has no hepatic metabolism and is available as dermal patch (5–15 mg/cm^2) and oral capsules. Once weekly patch of rivastigmine gets developed, treatment could become simplified.[13] Odd cases with allergy to adhesive patches occur with rivastigmine. Acute muscular dystonia in elderly women can occur.[14]

Tacrine

This is the oldest cholinesterase inhibitor. The drug has been reviewed in one systematic review with five RCTs, including 1,434 patients with 1 to 39 weeks duration. The conclusion was "no difference in overall clinical improvement." Some clinically insignificant improvement in cognition has been noted. The main issue with the drug is significant risk of liver function test abnormalities. It is not used nowadays.

Metrifonate

Metrifonate is a prodrug used in schistosomiasis. The drug has a short half-life in plasma (2 h) but has long activity in the CNS due to its irreversible activity. Metrifornate has a poor protein binding and lacks brain specificity.

Side Effects of Anticholinesterases

Usually, these drugs are well-tolerated. Side effects are generally mild to moderate in intensity. Fatigue, nausea, vomiting, diarrhea, muscle cramps, sleep disturbances, hallucinations, and allergic rashes can occur due to rivastigmine. Despite the slight variations in the mode of action of the three cholinesterase inhibitors, there is no evidence of any differences between them with respect to efficacy.

Monitoring

Patients should be warned against unrealistic expectations, and one should watch for return of insight, leading to depression or anxiety. The drugs should be stopped when unacceptable side effects occur, there is lack of response to medication, disease becomes advanced, or when patients are unable to take oral medications. However, new data show that these drugs have effectiveness in advanced stages also.

Memantine

Glutamate is a transmitter in the brain that is affected by AD. Memantine blocks the pathological effects of abnormal glutamate release and allows better function of the impaired brain. It is indicated for moderate-to-severe AD. **Table 13.5** demonstrates the role of memantine in AD of varied severity.

Clinical trials show slowing in cognitive and functional decline and decrease in agitation in treated group compared to placebo.

Memantine can be used with other antidementia drugs like donepezil, galantamine, and rivastigmine. The drug has a mechanism different from the cholinesterase-inhibiting drugs (**Fig. 13.5**).

The side effects include headaches, dizziness, etc. One should not use the drug in kidney disease or seizure disorders. The drug is started with 5 mg daily and is increased to 10 mg twice daily.

Table 13.5 Role of memantine in treatment of Alzheimer's disease[10–12]

MCI*	Mild-to-moderate dementia	Moderate-to-severe dementia
Role is unknown or poorly delineated. Some physicians use this drug for patients with MCI; however, evidence does not favor the same	Effects in mild patients seem inconsistent	Benefits on cognition are apparent, and global functions seem to improve. Activities of daily living are preserved and behaviour seem to be benefited

Abbreviation: MCI, mild cognitive impairment.
*MCI is not a treatment category with memantine. However, control of risk factors that can contribute to dementia has been suggested.

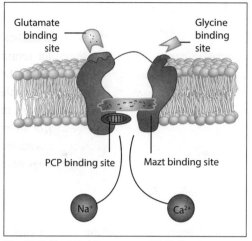

Fig. 13.5 N-methyl-D-aspartate (NMDA) receptors are glutamate-gated ion channels belonging to ionotropic receptors and have high permeability to calcium ions. A hypofunction of NMDA receptors has been associated with memory disorders and psychosis. Memantine blocks NMDA receptors. PCP, phencyclidine.

Drugs of Alternative System of Medicine

Ginkgo Biloba

Ginkgo biloba is an extract from the Ginkgo tree, which is given in doses of 120 to 240 mg daily. The drug has anti-inflammatory, anti-oxidant properties. Clinical trials show modest improvements in some measures of brain functions and memory. The drug is reasonably safe and well-tolerated, but monitoring is needed for bleeding. Clinical trials for prevention of AD using this drug are underway. Modest improvements have been shown in small and early studies in older adults with dementia.

Huperzine A

Huperzine A is a Chinese herbal medicine. The drug is a competitive and reversible cholinesterase inhibitor with both central and peripheral activity, antioxidant, and possibly has neuroprotective properties also. It is considered to be a nutraceutical given in dose of 200 to 800 μg daily.

Alzhemed

It is supposed to prevent formation and deposition of *amyloid* in the brain.

Phenserine

It is a cholinesterase inhibitor which regulates formation of amyloid in the brain. Recent clinical trials have not been encouraging about the drug.

Management of Behavioral and Psychological Symptoms of Dementia

Majority of patients with dementia develop symptoms such as agitation, aggression, depression, delusions, hallucinations, sleep disturbance, wandering, etc. Several drugs are used for the treatment of these symptoms. Antidepressants like SSRIs (e.g., citalopram, sertraline) are the mainstay. Antipsychotics such as typical antipsychotics (haloperidol) and atypical antipsychotics (risperidone, quetiapine, olanzapine) are used on and off basis and have good effect on BPSD. However, we should watch for side effects. Concerns exist with typical antipsychotics like haloperidol with regard to the significant risk of extrapyramidal side effects with prolonged use in elderly. Recent guidelines do not support the use of first-generation antipsychotics routinely for use in BPSD.[11] All antipsychotics potentially carry the risk of sedation, orthostasis, and varying amounts of anticholinergic effects. Studies show slight efficacy for behavioral problems in dementia. Moreover, they carry a black box warning (stroke) in elderly with dementias. Their prolonged use is hence not advocated. Mood stabilizers such as anticonvulsants (carbemazepine and sodium valproate) are commonly used. Major classes of drugs with examples and doses in the management of behavioral and psychological disturbances of dementias are given in **Table 13.6**. It should be noted that patients with dementia continue to use drugs of alternative system of

Table 13.6 Major classes of drugs with examples and doses in the management of BPSD[10]

Symptom/s	Class	Drug	Dose
Agitation, depression, anxiety	Antidepressant	Escitalopram is often the first drug	2.5–10 mg daily
		Sertraline is chosen for affective disturbances	25–100 mg daily
		Citalopram	5–20 mg daily
Insomnia		Trazodone	25–50 mg daily
		Mirtazapine	7.5 –30 mg daily
Aggression	Antiepileptic	Divalproex delayed release	125–1,000 mg
		Carbamazepine	100–600 mg daily

Abbreviation: BPSD, behavioral and psychological symptoms of dementia.

medicine too along with mainstream drugs, putting them at a risk of major drug interactions.[3,4,5] Anticholinesterases are effective in managing BPSD and should be the first choice.[10] These drugs are given for long term in the treatment of dementia, and weight loss could be a side effect.[12] So, nutrition could be an important issue.

Preventive Therapies

Some of the preventive therapies that are helpful in dementia are as follows:

- Antihypertensive therapy.
- Hormonal agents (estrogen).
- NSAIDs (naproxen and celecoxib).
- High-dose vitamin B, folic acid supplementation.
- Statins.
- Peroxisome receptor agonists.
- Fish oil, omega 3 fatty acids.
- Weight control, healthy diet.

Dementia Drugs under Development[1]

Beta Secretase Inhibitors

Beta secretase (BACE) inhibitor is related to the most attractive theory of dementia (beta-amyloid). However, the prior agents that have targeted this have failed. Although several agents related to this concept are in development at present.

Gamma Secretase Inhibitor

Gamma secretase inhibitors belong to various class of agents which have shown the desired biological effect. Two of them are in phase II-III trials now. Tarenflurbil, a putative gamma secretase modulator, failed to show benefit in phase III trial however. Tramiprosate failed in phase III trials as well. More work is needed on them it seems.

Antiamyloid Therapies

Antiamyloid therapies consist of a group of drugs and immunotherapies that can alter the processing of amyloid in the laboratory animal models. Drugs of this class have shown at least some ability to alter blood and spinal fluid amyloid deposition, but pathological measures of different types of amyloid in normal and/or people with AD have not been shown to be altered. Their effects on MRI, FDG PET, and other biomarkers in humans are unclear or unknown at present. Dose ranges has not been established in all cases as well. Clinical significance of encouraging proof of concept biomarkers remains unknown.

Microtubule Stabilizers

Kinase inhibitors include GSK 3, a compound that is in early development.

Unmet Needs in Dementia

Although significant progress in disease management has been made in recent years but disease modification remains a distant dream. Increasing neuroprotection against existing Aβ plaques and neurofibrillary tangles is a goal. Also, reversing existing neuronal damage remains to a probability. New and improved efficacious drugs are not only being searched for cognition but also activity of daily living and behavior. The new drugs are expected to have longer response, delay in disability/dependency, have fewer side effects, simple to administer, and have reduced number of treatment unresponsive patients, as is the case with currently available drugs.

Future Drugs in Dementia

Some of the future drugs in dementia are as follows:

- Drugs/nutraceuticals (based on epidemiologic observations).
- Neurotransmitter-based therapies.
- Glial-modulating drugs.
- Neuroprotective drugs.
- Amyloid-modulating drugs.
- Tau-modulating drugs.
- Acetylcholine-releasing drugs.
- Nicotinic agonists (alpha 7, alpha 4-beta 2 subunits).
- Serotonin: 5-HT4 partial agonists, 5-HT1A agonists/antagonists, 5-HT6 antagonists.
- Norepinephrine/dopamine: MAO-A and MAO-B inhibitors.
- GABA: GABA-B antagonists.
- Glutamate: AMPA potentiators.
- Glycine: Partial agonists.

Principles of Treating Dementias

The following principles should be kept in mind while treating dementia:

- Try nonpharmacological approaches first. Drugs are given when the behavioral approaches fail, or the condition starts interfering with activity of daily living.
- Review current medications for effectiveness, side effects, and need to continue. This is particularly true for antipsychotics drugs that are given for short-term control of BPSD.
- Identify the target symptoms like aggression, agitation, and psychotic behavior.
- Select drugs based on target symptoms and side effect profiles. Previous response to drugs could be a good guide.
- Monitor for side effects and potential drug interactions of concomitant drugs given. On an average, patients with dementias receive eight to nine drugs; hence, there is a potential for drug interactions.
- Start low, go slow, but keep going. Use in conjunction with behavioral approaches if possible. The elderly tolerate high doses poorly.
- Give medications for adequate period of time and review periodically.
- Educate patient and family about benefits and side effects. This will ensure better compliance and reduced side effects too.
- Periodically reassess medications, as repeat prescriptions are very common in old age; consider tapering or discontinuing, if needed.
- Discontinue the medications that have received black box warnings such as antipsychotics after some time. Periodically monitor side effects.

Recent Advances[15]

- **Monoclonal antibodies:** Drugs of this class, assumed to be preventing beta amyloid plaques, have long been thought to be useful. They may help clear the plaques from brain. Solanezumab is being evaluated in preclinical phase.

- **Fyn protein inhibitors:** This protein is involved in synaptic destruction in AD patients and its inhibitors are currently in development.

- **Beta-secretase inhibitors:** Verubecestat has the potential to block production of beta-amyloid.

- **Tau protein aggregation inhibitors:** Blockers of tau protein aggregations (drugs and vaccines) are under development.

- **Reducing inflammation:** Sargramostim may act by reducing inflammation in the brain.

References

1. Dementia diagnosis & Treatment. Available at: https://www.thecjc.org/(Assessed online dated 13 Dec 2020)

2. Dhikav V, Sethi M, Singhal A, Anand K. Polypharmacy and use of potentially inappropriate medications in patients with dementia and mild cognitive impairment. Asian J Pharm &. Clin Res 2014;7(2):218–220

3. Dhikav V, Sethi M, Mishra P, Singh Anand K. Behavioral and psychological symptoms among Indian patients with mild cognitive impairment. Int Psychogeriatr 2015;27(12): 2097–2098 No abstract available.

4. Dhikav V, Singh P, Anand KS. Medication adherence survey of drugs useful in prevention of dementia of Alzheimer's type among Indian patients. Int Psychogeriatr 2013;25(9):1409–1413

5. Pasqualetti G, Tognini S, Calsolaro V, Polini A, Monzani F. Potential drug-drug interactions in Alzheimer patients with behavioral symptoms. Clin Interv Aging 2015;10:1457–1466

6. Chen YD, Zhang J, Wang Y, Yuan JL, Hu WL. Efficacy of cholinesterase inhibitors in vascular dementia: an updated meta-analysis. Eur Neurol 2016;75(3-4):132–141

7. Kobayashi H, Ohnishi T, Nakagawa R, Yoshizawa K. The comparative efficacy and safety of cholinesterase inhibitors in patients with mild-to-moderate Alzheimer's disease: a Bayesian network meta-analysis. Int J Geriatr Psychiatry 2016;31(8):892–904

8. Stinton C, McKeith I, Taylor JP, et al. Pharmacological management of Lewy body dementia: a systematic review and meta-analysis. Am J Psychiatry 2015;172(8): 731–742

9. Portugal MdaG, Marinho V, Laks J. Pharmacological treatment of frontotemporal lobar degeneration: systematic review. review Br J Psychiatry 2011;33(1): 81–90 Review

10. Figiel G, Sadowsky C. A systematic review of the effectiveness of rivastigmine for the treatment of behavioral disturbances in dementia and other neurological disorders. Curr Med Res Opin 2008;24(1):157–166 Review

11. Lochhead JD, Nelson MA, Maguire GA. The treatment of behavioral disturbances and psychosis associated with dementia. Psychiatr Pol 2016;50(2):311–322

12. Soysal P, Isik AT, Stubbs B, et al. Acetylcholinesterase inhibitors are associated with weight loss in older people with dementia: a systematic review and meta-analysis. J Neurol Neurosurg Psychiatry 2016;87(12):1368–1374

13. An Update on the Safety of Current Therapies for Alzheimer's Disease: Focus on Rivastigmine. Available at: https://www.ncbi.nlm.nih.gov/pmc/articles/PMC5810854/. Accessed April 18, 2020

14. Dhikav V, Anand KS. Acute dystonic reaction with rivastigmine. Int Psychogeriatr 2013; 25(8):1385–1386

15. Mayo Clinic. What's on the Horizon. Available at: https://www.mayoclinic.org/diseases-conditions/alzheimers-disease/in-depth/alzheimers-treatments/art-20047780. Accessed April 18 2020

Pharmacotherapy of Stroke

Vikas Dhikav

Cerebrovascular Accidents

Cerebrovascular accident or stroke manifests as sudden neurological deficit. Risk factors include hypertension, valvular heart disease, diabetes, and dyslipidemias. The pattern of neurological deficits can give us an idea about the type of stroke. High-serum homocysteine levels are emerging as a significant risk factors.[1]

Acute stroke is also known as brain attack. In such a situation, every minute matters, and hence there is a popular saying, "time is brain." Stroke occurs due to sudden vascular occlusion.[1] Embolism from heart or aorta is common. Long-term disability resulting from occlusion and significant mortality are major issues in contemporary neurology. Time since the beginning of treatment which can prevent morbidity and mortality is shown in **Fig. 14.1**.

Transient ischemic attacks (TIA) is the brief episode of neurological dysfunction caused by a focal disturbance of brain or retinal ischemia, with clinical symptoms typically lasting less than 1 hour, and without evidence of infarction. TIA precedes ischemic stroke in 60% of cases. About 35% of untreated patients will develop stroke within 5 years of TIA. Stroke on the other hand is a stable and permanent damage with no expected improvement/deterioration. However, improvement occurs with the return of previously lost neurologic function over days to weeks. Sometimes it may progress and the patient continues to deteriorate following initial

onset of focal deficit. India is silently witnessing a stroke epidemic.[1]

Epidemiology[3–6]

Stroke is the second most common cause of death with 1.5 crore (15 million) people suffering from stroke every year. Almost 50 lakh people die every year due to stroke worldwide. Stroke is a major cause for loss of life, limbs, and speech in India, with the Indian Council of Medical Research estimating that in 2004, there were 9.3 lakh cases of stroke and 6.4 lakh deaths due to stroke in India, most of the people being less than 45-years old. Stroke is one of the leading causes of death and disability in India. The estimated adjusted prevalence rate of stroke ranges 84-262/100,000

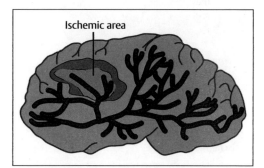

Fig. 14.1 "Time is brain" because, every minute, patients lose 200,000 neurons if left untreated. Lacunar infarcts may have pure motor or sensory deficits. Ataxia, hemiparesis, and clumsy hand syndrome may occur. The deficits may progress for 1 to 2 days before stabilizing. On computed tomography (CT) scan, the lesions may resemble "punched out" appearance. Risk of death in lacunar infarcts is less compared with nonlacunar infarcts.

in rural and 334-424/100,000 in urban areas. The incidence rate is 119-145/100,000 based on the recent population-based studies.

Stroke incidence is higher in developing countries like India compared to the West and in people who have large vessel disease due to atherosclerosis. This occurs due to hypertension, diabetes, dyslipidemia, etc.[7]

Types

Majority of the ischemic strokes are caused by embolism from the heart, aortic arch, or extracranial arteries to the brain, as stated previously, and evolution of infarct leads to progression of neurological disability as well (**Fig. 14.2**). The other type is hemorrhagic stroke. The former is of the ischemic variety.

- Lacunar infarcts: These are smaller than 5 mm and are often seen in basal ganglia, pons, internal capsule, and thalamus. Since the fibers in these areas, especially internal capsule, are so densely packed, even smaller infarcts may have widespread neurological impact. Long-standing hypertension or diabetes is most commonly associated with these types of infarction.

- Cerebral infarction: Thrombotic or embolic occlusion may occur, leading to infarction.

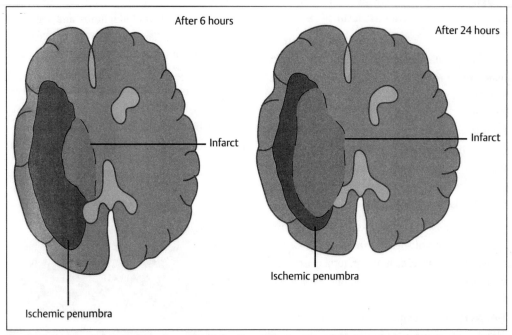

Fig. 14.2 Evolving ischemic stroke in cerebral infarction. Deterioration of the neurological deficits occurs within hours or days after initial presentation. Onset of cerebral infarct is usually abrupt, and progression occurs due to brain swelling. Sudden and brief loss of vision due to occlusion of ophthalmic artery (Amaurosis fugax—blackout) is usually encountered. Occlusion of anterior cerebral artery may cause weakness and cortical sensory loss of opposite side. Middle cerebral artery involvement can cause contralateral hemiplegia and hemisensory loss with homonymous hemianopia. Global aphasia is present if dominant hemisphere is present. Drowsiness, stupor, or coma can occur. Involvement of cortical vessels in posterior circulation causes memory defects, perseveration, and visual defects. Central branches of the circulation can cause spontaneous pain due to thalamic involvement. Cranial nerve involvements due to brainstem are common.

Atherosclerosis of cerebral arteries is a major cause. Ischemia can mediate calcium-mediated excitotoxicity insult in the neurons, leading to damage.

The World Health Organization (WHO) defines stroke as "neurological deficit, which is sudden onset, with focal rather than global dysfunction, in which after adequate investigations, symptoms are presumed to be of nontraumatic vascular origin and last for more than 24 hours." If the focal ischemic brain or retinal symptoms persist for less than 1 hour, then they are known as TIA. There is no infarction in TIA.

Middle Cerebral Artery Syndromes

Left Middle Cerebral Artery Syndrome

This is a common type of stroke, and when patients have left-sided lesion, they have right hemisensory loss, right visual field defect with aphasia (loss of language).

Right Middle Cerebral Artery Syndrome

This includes the following:

- Left hemineglect.
- Left hemiparesis.
- Left hemisensory loss.
- Left visual field defects.

Pharmacotherapy

Pharmacotherapy of stroke depends upon the stage in which the patient is seen. In acute phase, the focus is on stabilizing the patient and thrombolysing, while in the chronic phase, the goals are to prevent recurrence. In the latter phase, the lipid-lowering drugs, antiplatelets/anticoagulants, and antihypertensives are mainstay.

- Thrombolysis[7-9]:

In patients with acute ischemic stroke in whom treatment can be initiated within 3 hours of symptom onset, it is recommended that intravenous (IV) recombinant tissue plasminogen activator (rtPA) be given. tPA reverses under perfusion of brain cells by activating plasmin, allowing ischemic penumbra to recover. Plasmin is the enzyme that degrades fibrin, the protein which is the main constituent of blood clots. After 4.5 hours, the benefits of thrombolysis are doubtful. Endovascular therapy has recently been introduced as adjunctive management of acute ischemic stroke.[8]

Dissolution of clots is an important aim for the treatment of acute stroke. Streptokinase and tPA are commonly used agents. If a baseline CT scan shows absence of intracranial bleeding and there is a time window shorter than 3 hours, then IV infusion of 0.9 mg/kg of rtPA could be used. The long-term outcome for thrombolysis is favorable. A 30% benefit of having minimal or no disability was demonstrated in patients on tPA. However, the patients on tPA were more likely to be symptomatic with intracranial bleeding as a side effect.

Thrombolysis reduces the size of ischemic damage (infarct) by restoring blood flow. Neurons die over time. Prompt treatment with a thrombolytic agent (rtPA-alteplase) may promote reperfusion and improve functional outcomes. It must be given within 4.5 hours of stroke and is based upon strict inclusion criteria. It is also licensed for IV use in patients below 80 years of age. Increase in poststroke quality of life can occur if thrombolysis is done on time.

- Antihypertensives:

  Following considerations need to be borne in mind while dealing with hypertensive patients:

  ◊ Elevated blood pressure (BP) (e.g., up to 200 mm Hg systolic or 110 mm Hg diastolic) may be tolerated in the acute phase of ischemic stroke without intervention.

  ◊ BP may be lowered if this is required by cardiac conditions.

  ◊ Upper level of systolic BP in patients undergoing thrombolytic therapy is 180 mm Hg.

  ◊ Avoid and treat hypotension.

  ◊ Avoid drastic reduction in BP.

- Management of blood sugar:

  ◊ High-glucose levels in acute stroke may increase the size of the infarction and reduce functional outcome.

  ◊ Hypoglycemia can mimic acute ischemic infarction.

  ◊ Routine use of glucose potassium insulin (GKI) infusion regimes in patients with mild-to-moderate hyperglycemia did not improve outcome.

- It is a common practice to treat hyperglycemia with insulin when blood glucose exceeds 180 mg/dL.

Management of Acute Stroke[10–12]

First focus is on maintaining the airway, breathing, and circulation (ABC). After that, the cause should be investigated by conducting tests like the following: Glasgow coma scale (GCS) score should be noted; electrocardiogram and blood glucose should be obtained. An urgent CT scan should be obtained, and one should continue with ABC.

CT should be done within the time in which thrombolysis is conducted; preferably, within

4 hours. The National Institutes of Health Stroke Scale (NIHSS) score should be calculated, and there should be no hemorrhage or contraindications to thrombolysis. Consent should be obtained, and one should be aware of the age of the patient.

Alteplase-tPA is given in dose of 0.9 mg/kg (10% of total dose—bolus given over the period of 2–3 min, and 90% of total dose to be infused over 60 min). Very high BP should first be reduced (e.g., reducing BP from 180/110 to 140/90) to have best response from thrombolysis. Presence of seizures or neurological deficits or advanced age (>80 y) themselves are not contraindications to the use of thrombolytic therapy.

Do not mix tPA with any other medications. Do not use IV tubing with infusion filters. All patients must be on a cardiac monitor. When infusion is complete, saline flush with normal saline tPA must be used within 8 hours of mixing when stored at room temperature or within 24 hours if refrigerated.

Side Effects of Thrombolysis

There is a significant risk of intracerebral hemorrhage (1.7%–1 in 77 patients) which could be fatal also. Minor bleeding is common at infusion site. Anaphylaxis and angioedema can occur. Risk factors for bleeding are summarized in the Box 14.1.

Treating associated factors is important. For example, fever is associated with poorer neurological outcome after stroke. Fever increases infarct size in experimental models of stroke. It is a common practice to treat fever (and its cause) when the temperature reaches 37.5 °C in patients with stroke. Other general basic associated things are listed in Box 14.2.

The European Stroke Organization recommends intermittent monitoring of neurological status, pulse, BP, temperature, and oxygen

Box 14.1: Risk factors for bleeding after thrombolysis in patients with acute ischemic stroke

- Diabetes.
- Severe case/advanced age.
- Increased time to treatment.
- Previous aspirin use.
- History of congestive heart failure.

Box 14.2: General guidelines for stroke patients

- Head elevation up to 30°.
- Pain relief and sedation.
- Osmotic agents (glycerol, mannitol, hypertonic saline).
- Ventilatory support.
- Barbiturates, hyperventilation.
- Achieve normothermia.

saturation. This is recommended for 72 hours in patients with significant persisting neurological deficits. Also, oxygen should be administered if SpO$_2$ falls below 95%. Regular monitoring of fluid balance and electrolytes is recommended in patients with severe stroke or swallowing problems.

Risk Factor Approach[13,14]

Several pharmacologically modifiable risk factors exist in patients with stroke. These include diabetes, hypertension, dyslipidemias, obesity, hyperhomocysteinemia, etc. Aspirin, lipid-lowering drugs, and effective antihypertensive agents can reduce the risk of stroke recurrence significantly.

Secondary Prevention of Stroke[15]

Patients who had stroke or TIA are at a higher risk of developing acute stroke in the coming weeks or months. About 10% of the patients surviving acute stroke will have another stroke within the next 1 month. It has been estimated that 80% of the strokes could be prevented if the risk factors such as diabetes, dyslipidemias, and hypertension are managed.[6] The following classes of drugs are useful in preventing acute stroke in such cases:

- **Antihypertensives:**
  ◊ Angiotensin-converting enzyme inhibitors (ACEIs).
  ◊ Angiotensin receptor blockers (ARBs).
  ◊ Diuretics such as thiazides.
  ◊ Calcium channel blockers (CCBs), for example, clevidipine and amlodipine.
- **Lipid-lowering agents:**
  ◊ Statins:
    □ Rosuvastatin.
    □ Atorvastatin.
  ◊ Fibrate:
    □ Fenofibrate.
  ◊ Cholesterol absorption inhibitor:
    □ Ezetimibe.
- **Antithrombotics:**
  ◊ Antiplatelets:
    □ Aspirin.
    □ Ticlopidine.
    □ Clopidogrel.
  ◊ Anticoagulants (for atrial fibrillation):
    □ Warfarin.
- **Control diabetes:**
    □ Oral hypoglycemic.
    □ Insulins.

Goals

Primary goals of prevention of stroke are to treat hypertension and diabetes and manage lipids and clots.

Antihypertensives

Hypertension is the most significant modifiable risk factor for stroke and contributes up to 75% of all strokes. The main factor is the injury to the blood vessel walls, and the scar in the blood vessel wall is formed. This may lead to formation of plaques in the arteries, and atherosclerosis sets in. This is complicated by left ventricle dysfunction or atrial fibrillation.

Reduction of BP is a therapeutic aim following stroke. High-vascular risk patients with history of stroke, coronary artery disease, ischemic stroke, peripheral artery disease, or other risk factors such as coexisting hypertension, hyperlipidemia, smoking, or microalbuminuria need regular anti-hypertensive drugs. Several classes of drugs have been found to be useful. Beta-blockers, diuretics, and ACE inhibitors and ARBs are particularly useful.

BP management is critical to prevent stroke, and at every visit with the physician, the BP should be checked. Apart from drugs, antihypertensive drugs should be prescribed.

Target is to keep BP < 140/90 mm Hg and < 130/80 mm Hg if the patient has diabetes or chronic kidney disease. Treatment with multiple antihypertensives may be needed, and the dietary sodium consumption should be kept at its minimal levels.

Treatment with the combination of ACE inhibitors and diuretic could be used. Choice of agent will depend on the comorbidities. For example, young and stressful patients will benefit from the combination of ACE inhibitors and beta-blockers. Also, old patients will get maximum benefits from diuretics/or CCBs. Combination of ACE inhibitors and ARBs is not recommended.

ACE inhibitors are long-acting, efficacious drugs in BP control. But there are certain side effects too which should be kept in mind. Many patients may have a persistent dry cough. It can cause angioedema (in 1 out of 500 patients). Dizziness, taste disturbances, and proteinuria can also occur. Serum potassium may need to be monitored particularly in those with renal dysfunction. ACE inhibitors are to be avoided in patients with bilateral renal artery stenosis.

Lipid-Lowering Drugs

Statins are the drugs of choice for dyslipidemia. They have been shown to reduce stroke risk by 25 to 30%. Not just stroke, their roles have now been expanded to several neurological diseases like dementia, multiple sclerosis, Parkinson's disease, etc.[5] Statins decrease progression and/or induce regression of carotid artery plaque. Statins are low-density lipoprotein (LDL)-lowering agents but also have lot of nonlipid pharmacological effects such as stabilizing plaques, improving endothelial functions, anti-inflammatory, decreasing platelet aggregation, etc. Doses of commonly used statins for stroke prevention are given in **Table 14.1**.

Statins are advised for use in preventing recurrent stroke and improving neurological outcome after acute ischemic stroke. Benefits with long-term use of statins therapy have been demonstrated without any major adverse events. Current stroke prevention guidelines recommend the initiation of statins in patients with evidence of atherosclerosis and an LDL cholesterol level > 100 mg/dL without known coronary heart disease and also in patients with elevated cholesterol or comorbid coronary heart disease.

Statins are taken once a day with largest meal in evening. Several drug interactions are possible and should be kept in mind especially with antidepressants, antibiotics, and immuno-suppressants. Possible side effects include nausea, constipation, muscle pain, or weakness. Rhabdomyolysis is very rare.

Table 14.1 Doses of commonly used statins for stroke prevention

Drug	Dose
Rosuvastatin	20 mg daily
Pravastatin	40 mg daily
Simvastatin	40 mg daily
Atorvastatin	40 mg daily

Antiplatelets

Aspirin has been tested in large randomized controlled trials in acute (<48 h) stroke. Significant reduction of morbidity and mortality has been seen in recurrence of stroke. A phase III trial for the glycoprotein-IIb-IIIa antagonist abciximab was stopped prematurely because of an increased rate of bleeding.

In patients with acute ischemic stroke or TIA, early treatment (within 48 h) with aspirin therapy at a dose of 150 to 325 mg over no-aspirin therapy is recommended.

All patients with ischemic stroke or TIA should be prescribed antiplatelet therapy for secondary prevention of recurrent stroke unless there is an indication for anticoagulation. Acetylsalicylic acid 25 mg or clopidogrel may be used. Nowadays, fixed dose combinations of aspirin, clopidogrel, and rosuvastatin are available in the market.

In patients with a history of noncardioembolic ischemic stroke or TIA, it is recommended that a long-term treatment with aspirin (75–100 mg once daily)/ clopidogrel (75 mg once daily)/aspirin extended-release/dipyridamole (25/200 mg twice daily), or cilostazol (100 mg twice) should be used.

Aspirin: Aspirin irreversibly acetylates the active site of cyclooxygenase, which is required for the production of thromboxane A2, a powerful promoter of platelet aggregation. The drug is used in dose of 150 to 325 mg daily. If thrombolytic therapy is planned or given, aspirin or other antithrombotic therapy should not be initiated within 24 hours.

Anticoagulants

Warfarin: Patients with stroke and atrial fibrillation need to be treated with warfarin at a target international normalized ratio (INR) of 2.5, range 2.0 to 3.0. The drug is started in dose of 2 to 5 mg daily.

In patients with a history of ischemic stroke or TIA and atrial fibrillation, including paroxysmal atrial fibrillation, oral anticoagulants are recommended. The drug has problem of slow onset of action, drug–drug interactions, and need for regular monitoring.[2]

Heparins: Unfractionated heparin, low-molecular weight heparins (LMWH) (nadroparin, certoparin, tinzaparin, dalteparin), and heparinoids are used. LMWHs are a specific treatment for stroke.[3]

In patients with acute ischemic stroke and restricted mobility, it is suggested that prophylactic dose of subcutaneous heparin or LMWH should be given. For prophylaxis in such patients, LMWH is better compared to high-molecular weight heparins. Pharmacologic and mechanical prophylaxis should be initiated as early as possible and should be continued throughout the hospital stay or until the patient has regained mobility. Anticoagulants are given for prevention of recurrence of stroke in embolic heart disease with high risk of recurrence, in carotid stenosis, or vertebral basilar artery disease with hemodynamic impact.[4]

Anticonvulsants

Although anticonvulsants are routinely prescribed following stroke, the prophylactic administration of anticonvulsants to patients with recent stroke who have not had seizures is not recommended.

Neuroprotection

No adequately sized trial has yet shown significant effect in predefined endpoints for any neuroprotective substances. A meta-analysis has suggested a mild benefit for citicoline. Randomised controlled trials of combination treatments completed within the past 5 years have included growth factors, hypothermia, minocycline, natalizumab, fingolimod, and uric acid; the latter two drugs with alteplase produced encouraging results.[9]

Recent Advances in Stroke Management[12-15]

New risk factors, for example, antiphospholipid antibodies and homocysteine have been recognized. Role of tPA is established in stroke up to 4.5 hours from symptom onset. New protocols now suggest that tPA can also be used for mild stroke and indeed in up to 75% patients with ischemic strokes. Mechanical endovascular thrombectomy is increasingly being performed now. The same can be done till 24 hours, increasing the window of intervention. Nerinetide, a neuroprotective agent, has been reported to preserve brain cell loss in patients with acute stroke. Stem cell therapy is also an emerging treatment option in stroke. The focus is on improving stroke recovery outcomes using neuroprotective agents. Drugs to enhance motor recovery following stroke are on the horizon.

References

1. Mishra NK, Khadilkar SV. Stroke program for India. Ann Indian Acad Neurol 2010; 13(1):28–32
2. Vora A, Narasimhan C. Stroke prevention in atrial fibrillation—current standard of care and significant unmet medical need. J Assoc Physicians India 2013;61(12):904–906
3. Prasad K, Kumar A. Management of stroke: a clinical approach. J Indian Med Assoc 2009;107(6):392–394, 396–399
4. Padma V, Fisher M, Moonis M. Role of heparin and low-molecular-weight heparins in the management of acute ischemic stroke. Expert Rev Cardiovasc Ther 2006;4(3): 105–415
5. Malfitano AM, Marasco G, Proto MC, Laezza C, Gazzerro P, Bifulco M. Statins in neurological disorders: an overview and update. Pharmacol Res 2014;88:74–83
6. Prabhakaran S, Chong JY. Risk factor management for stroke prevention. Continuum (Minneap Minn) 2014;20(2 Cerebrovascular Disease):296–308
7. Banerjee TK, Das SK. Fifty years of stroke researches in India. Ann Indian Acad Neurol 2016;19(1):1–8
8. Elgendy IY, Mahmoud AN, Mansoor H, Mojadidi MK, Bavry AA. Evolution of acute ischemic stroke therapy from lysis to thrombectomy: Similar or different to acute myocardial infarction? Int J Cardiol 2016;222:441–447
9. Chamorro Á, Dirnagl U, Urra X, Planas AM. Neuroprotection in acute stroke: targeting excitotoxicity, oxidative and nitrosative stress, and inflammation. Lancet Neurol 2016;15(8):869–881
10. Explaining Stroke 101 - National Stroke Association. Available at: https://www.stroke.org/sites/default/files/resources/explaining-stroke-101.ppt. Last accessed April 3, 2021
11. Available at: https://touchneurology.com/stroke/journal-articles/latest-advances-in-the-treatment-of-acute-stroke/. Last accessed April 3, 2021
12. Available at: https://www.sciencedirect.com/science/article/abs/pii/S105230570800800099/. Last accessed April 3, 2021
13. Available at: https://www.acc.org/latest-in-cardiology/journal-scans/2020/03/03/15/26/efficacy-and-safety-of-nerinetide/. Last accessed April 3, 2021
14. Available at: https://www.pharmaceutical-technology.com/comment/stroke-research-2018/. Last accessed April 3, 2021
15. Available at: https://www.ahajournals.org/doi/full/10.1161/strokeaha.115.007433. Last accessed April 3, 2021

Deaddiction Pharmacotherapy

Vikas Dhikav

Clinical Case Example

- A 42-year-old man with a 15-year history of alcohol dependence relapsed to alcohol abuse 3 months ago. He currently reports drinking three to five drinks four to five times/week but states that when he abstains for a day or two occasionally, he does not experience alcohol withdrawal symptoms. However, his wife is upset with his drinking, and he now wants medication to help him abstain. He tried naltrexone in the past but says it "didn't help much." He takes no other medications and has no known allergies. He is not a hypertensive or diabetic patient. What of the following would you recommend: (a) Liver function tests (LFTs), (b) acamprosate 666 mg three times daily, or (c) disulfiram 250 mg/day?

Answer: Both (a) and (c) will be recommended. LFTs are needed as this patient has a long and difficult history of alcoholism. He has failed naltrexone in the past, and acamprosate is not likely to be helpful. He has felt significant consequences of his drinking and is motivated to quit; therefore, if his liver functions indicate that he does not have significant impairment, a trial of disulfiram 250 mg daily might help in this case.

What Is Addiction?

Addiction results when a substance is ingested, for example, alcohol, cocaine, nicotine, etc., and becomes pleasurable with continued use. Compulsion later on sets in, and a lot of activities such as work get postponed or left. The National Institute of Drug Abuse (NIDA) considers addiction as a "development disease, starting early in childhood."[1] Several classes of drugs are abused (**Box 15.1**). Drugs of abuse modify mental alertness and produce tolerance and dependence. Several complications like thrombophlebitis and local and systematic infections can occur (human immunodeficiency virus [HIV] and hepatitis). This is a major public health issue both in the

Box 15.1: Drugs of abuse

- Central nervous system (CNS) stimulants:
  ◊ Amphetamines.
  ◊ Cocaine.
- Narcotics:
  ◊ Heroine.
  ◊ Morphine.
  ◊ Codeine.
  ◊ Oxycodone.
  ◊ Methadone.
- CNS depressants:
  ◊ Ethanol.
  ◊ Benzodiazepines.
  ◊ Barbiturates.
- Hallucinogens:
  ◊ Lysergic acid diethylamide.
  ◊ Psilocybin.

developing and developed worlds. Nonmedical use of prescription drugs is not uncommon.[9] It is largely preventable.[7]

Mind-altering substances have been used since time immemorial.[3] There are several factors that have been linked with the abuse of drugs of this class. The following factors are important here:

- Biological—alcohol and other drugs alter the chemistry of the brain and body functioning. Continued use can cause damage or injury to vital organs.
- Psychological—altered brain chemistry affects the brain's ability to think, alters feeling states, and impacts the personality of the user.
- Sociological—behavioral interactions with family and social contacts are altered and/or misinterpreted by the abuser and those observing the behavior. Peer pressure is important here.

Routes of Drug Abuse

Drugs of abuse are abused via a variety of routes like oral, sniffing, smoking, injecting, etc. Drugs are ingested, injected, smoked, and snorted. Drugs like methadone and benzodiazepines are injected, while amphetamines, heroine, and cocaine have multiple routes. Apart from complications of drug abuse, systemic diseases like HIV, hepatitis B, and infective endocarditis are common in intravenous (IV) drug abusers.

Oral/Sublingual

When someone swallows a drug, it passes through the esophagus and stomach to the small intestine, where it is absorbed into the tiny blood vessels lining the walls. It usually takes approximately 20 to 30 minutes for pharmacological response to occur.

Snorting (Sniffing)

When drugs are taken this way, they are absorbed by the tiny blood vessels in the mucous membranes lining the nasal passages. It takes about 3 to 5 minutes for pharmacological response to occur.

Inhaling (Smoking, Huffing)

After smoking or inhaling the agents such as heroin or crack, the vaporized drug enters the lungs and is "rapidly" absorbed through tiny blood vessels lining the air sacs of the bronchi. From the lungs, the "drug laden" blood is pumped back to the heart and then directly to the body and brain, thus acting more quickly than any other methods of use. This is the most rapid method, taking just 7 to 10 seconds for pharmacological response.

Injections (IV/IM/SC)

The drug is injected with needles, either into the bloodstream, or under the skin. IV administration takes about 15 to 30 seconds, while IM takes 3 to 5 minutes for pharmacological response.

Treating Drug Abusers

Alcohol, opiates, marijuana/hashish, cocaine, and other stimulants account for almost all cases of abusers seeking and receiving treatment. Multiple drug abuse is a common abuse or dependence profile, and drug abusers have coexisting mental health problems. Thus, effective treatment programs should address polydrug abusers and include psychiatric care for those with other mental disorders. Involvement of the patient is important. No program of treatment can succeed if the drug abuser does not really want to get clean and sober. Motivation is the most important ingredient in recovery from addiction. While treating the addicts, it may be useful to remember, "addiction is a chronic brain disease, expressed as compulsive drug seeking behavior, expressed within a social context, and is prone to relapse but is treatable." Several categories of patients need treatment (**Box 15.2**). The goals of treatment should be clear (**Box 15.3**), and there are several options available (**Box 15.4**). **Table 15.1** lists the drugs of abuse for which effective pharmacological treatment is available. An attempt is being done to prevent drug abuse along with treatment, especially among young people.[8]

Box 15.2: Categories needing treatment in drug abuse
• Intoxication/overdose.
• Withdrawal/detoxification.
• Abstinence initiation/use reduction.
• Relapse prevention.
• Sequelae (psychosis, agitation, etc.).

Box 15.3: Therapeutic goals
• Promote abstinence.
• Promote functional integration in family or society.
• Encourage work.
• Treat comorbidities.

Box 15.4: Tools available for treatment
• Agonist (replacement/substitution).
• Antagonist (blockade).
• Aversive (negative reinforcement).

Alcohol Dependence

Alcohol is a potent neurotoxin which is consumed widely. Alcoholism is a serious psychiatric disorder whose signs and symptoms depend upon the amount and the frequency of alcohol consumption. Alcohol gets absorbed in stomach, small intestine, and colon. However, stomach is the most common site. Alcohol is metabolized primarily in the liver via oxidation by the enzyme alcohol dehydrogenase, and metabolism exhibits zero-order kinetics (15 mg/dL/h). In acute doses, alcohol inhibits cytochrome P450 (CYP) enzyme system, raising the levels of concomitantly administered drugs. The drug produces loss of muscular coordination and change in behavior in concentrations of 20 to 100 mg/dL and ataxia and mental impairment occur at 100 to 200 mg/dL. Coma occurs at concentrations of more than 400 mg/dL.[2]

Pharmacotherapy for Alcohol Addiction

There are two phases of alcohol dependence treatment:

- Acute alcohol withdrawal.
- Relapse prevention: Maintenance of medications to prevent relapse to alcohol use.

Several drugs like disulfiram, naltrexone (oral and injectable), and acamprosate are available for treatment. Monitoring of patients treated for an alcohol dependence should be done during

Table 15.1 List of drugs of abuse for which effective pharmacological treatment is available

Substance abuse where pharmacotherapy is effective	Substance abuse where pharmacotherapy is not available
• Opioids	• Cocaine
• Alcohol	• Methamphetamine
• Benzodiazepines	• Hallucinogens
• Tobacco (nicotine dependence)	• Cannabis
	• Solvents/inhalants

the withdrawal phase for possible emergence of depression/anxiety/suicidality, which can occur in the course of treatment.

Several drugs are used to treat alcohol dependence:

- Disulfiram.
- Naltrexone.
- Acamprosate.

Disulfiram

Disulfiram has been the first drug approved for the treatment of chronic alcohol dependence. This acts by blocking alcohol metabolism, leading to increase in blood acetaldehyde levels. This aims to motivate individuals not to drink because they gradually learn via aversive mechanisms that they will become ill if they consume alcohol. This is due to "antabuse" reaction such as flushing, weakness, nausea, tachycardia, hypotension, etc. (**Fig. 15.1**). Despite the aversive reaction, disulfiram is regarded as a safe and effective treatment for alcohol abstinence.[10]

The disulfiram–alcohol reaction usually begins within half an hour after alcohol is ingested, and the resultant effects range from moderate to severe. Treatment of alcohol/disulfiram reaction is supportive (IV fluids, oxygen, etc.). Side effects of disulfiram are metallic taste, sulfur-like odor, etc. Rare side effects include hepatotoxicity, neuropathy, and psychotic reactions. Contraindications of disulfiram include cardiac diseases, hepatic and renal diseases, esophageal varices, pregnancy, impulsivity, and psychotic disorders. Patient should avoid alcohol-containing beverages or alcohol itself. Dosage: 250 to 500 mg daily. Hepatitis is a rare side effect of disulfiram.[4]

Naltrexone

Naltrexone is an opioid antagonist. Naltrexone is known to reverse the pharmacological effects of opioids and is used in the management of alcohol and opioid dependence. Its closely related analogue is used to treat opioid-induced constipation (**Fig. 15.2**).

Oral naltrexone can be given at doses of 50 mg/day. Extended release or injectable naltrexone is also available as one injection per month. The drug can cause hepatocellular injury in very high doses (e.g., 5–10 times higher than normal).

Clinical Effects

Naltrexone is a long-acting opioid antagonist. The drug blocks action of morphine or heroin for 24 hours when taken as a single dose. This makes it reliable as an emergency drug too. However, a heroin addict first needs to be stabilized by supportive treatment. The drug "puts off" the reinforcement that the addict is receiving from heroin/morphine and generates negative reinforcement.

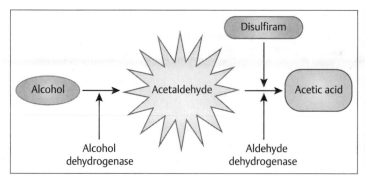

Fig. 15.1 Ethanol is converted into acetaldehyde by the enzyme alcohol dehydrogenase and is further metabolized to acetic acid (urine) by aldehyde dehydrogenase. Disulfiram inhibits aldehyde dehydrogenase; hence, every time alcohol is consumed, the patient develops high levels of acetaldehyde, leading to "acetaldehyde syndrome."

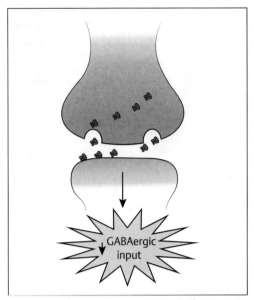

Fig. 15.2 Naltrexone is a potent opioid antagonist that increases GABA activity.

Naltrexone is contraindicated in acute hepatitis or liver failure. One should check liver function before, every month for 3 months, and then every 3 months. Be aware of concomitant opioid analgesics as naltrexone will block analgesic effect and can precipitate opioid dependence or withdrawal. Some patients may have hypersensitivity to naltrexone. Main side effects are gastrointestinal (GI) upset, leading to nausea and vomiting. Headache may occur. The drug is effective in reducing relapse and craving.

Acamprosate

Acamproste maintains alcohol abstinence and interacts with glutaminergic transmission. The drug reduces excessive glutamate transmission during alcohol withdrawal. By doing this, the drug can treat insomnia, anxiety, and restlessness, which are the common symptoms of alcohol withdrawal.

Given orally, the drug is poorly absorbed and achieves steady state in 5 days or so. It is not metabolized and is eliminated unchanged. The drug is well tolerated even in overdose. Acamprosate is given as 2 g/day. Because the drug is not metabolized in liver, it is safe in liver disease. It can be combined with naltrexone or benzodiazepines. Diarrhea is the usual side effect. Suicidal ideations have been noted.[11]

Insomnia in an Alcoholic Patient

Give the patient sleep hygiene information. Avoid the so-called "nonBenzo" sleep medications (e.g., Ambien) as these possess abuse liability, can produce intoxication syndromes, and may place patients with substance use disorders at higher risk of relapse. Consider low-dose trazodone (e.g., 25 mg) or qhs sedating antidepressant (especially if the patient has comorbid depression; e.g., Mirtazapine).

Opioid Dependence

Opioids are among the most commonly abused drugs. They have unique actions that make them useful in various acute pain syndromes. They act via G-proteins to reduce pain transmission (**Fig. 15.3**). Opioids are significantly metabolized by the CYP enzyme system and may be subject to drug–drug interactions, including codeine, hydrocodone, oxycodone, fentanyl, meperidine, methadone, buprenorphine, and tramadol. CYP2D6 metabolism is polymorphic, and hence, there are interindividual variations.[6]

Several things must be taken into account for making a diagnosis of opioid dependence. History (including previous records), confirmation from caregivers, signs of dependence (withdrawal symptoms, tracks, needle marks), and urine toxicology if needed, could be helpful. ECG can provide useful hints as opioids like methadone prolong QT interval. Naloxone challenge can be given if unsure of opioid dependence. Clinical

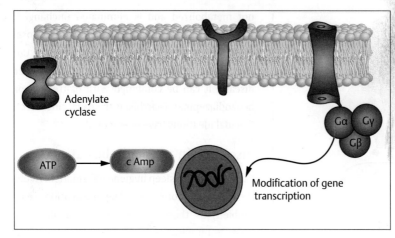

Fig. 15.3 Opioids act by G-protein–coupled receptors and may have crosstalk with ion channels also. This causes increase in permeability of inhibitory ions, leading to cellular hyperpolarization.

opiate withdrawal scale can be used to determine extent of opiate withdrawal symptoms.

Pharmacotherapy for Opioid Dependence

Several drugs are used to treat opioid dependence:

- Methadone.
- Buprenorphine.
- Naltrexone.

Methadone

Methadone, a μ-receptor agonist, is a synthetic analogue of morphine. The drug is similar to morphine in its pharmacological effects but less sedative and is used as a substitute drug in the treatment of morphine and heroin addiction. However, it is different from buprenorphine being the full agonist (**Fig. 15.4**).

Pharmacokinetics

The drug has good oral absorption, is metabolized in liver, and eliminated in urine (demethylation/cyclization). The drug is cumulative by nature and is retained in the body on long-term administration. It is a highly protein-bound drug compared to morphine. The drug achieves peak concentration in plasma 2 to 4 hours after oral administration and has a half-life of 24 hours.

The plasma steady state is achieved after 3 to 7 days. The drug can be given orally, IV, or intrarectally. There is a significant interindividual variation in metabolism of methadone.

Morphine Comparison

The drug has equal potency to that of the morphine. However, it produces less euphoria and has longer duration of action compared to morphine. Methadone can produce physical dependence similar to that of morphine. Side effects such as biliary spasm, meiosis, constipation, and respiratory depression are similar to that of morphine.

Methadone Maintenance

Any opioid addict who is an adult and has been dependent upon opioids for more than a year can be given methadone. Methadone is a long-acting μ-agonist with a duration of action of 24 to 36 hours. Dosage of 30 to 40 mg will block withdrawal, but not craving; hence, 80 to 100 mg is more effective at reducing opioid use than lower doses (e.g., 40–50 mg/d). Slow onset and longer duration of action is helpful clinically.

Methadone is started in dose of 50 mg daily, 100 mg every 2 days, and 150 mg every third day. The drug has the potential to cause

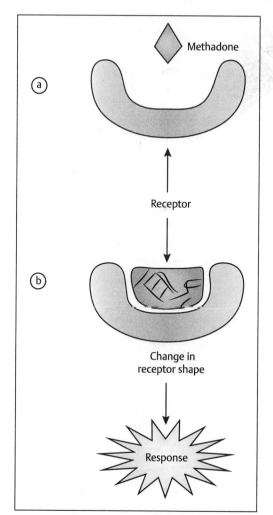

Fig. 15.4 Drug receptor complex is linked to the generation of response. A conformational change is needed for a drug to produce pharmacologically manful response, and full agonists do so with ease. However, partial agonists are unable to bring about lot of changes hence produce smaller responses.

hepatotoxicity; therefore, monitoring LFTs every 3 months is important.

Drug Interactions

Methadone is metabolized by CYP3A4 and hence can interact with many commonly used medications such as pentazocine, phenytoin, carbamazepine, rifampin, efavirenz, nevirapine,

lopinavir, etc. The drug can precipitate opiate withdrawal syndrome in opioid addicts. Increased methadone concentrations have been reported with enzyme inhibitors such as ciprofloxacin and fluvoxamine. Carbamazepine, phenobarbitone, and phenytoin are known to lower concentration of methadone due to enzyme induction.

Buprenorphine

Buprenorphine is a semisynthetic opioid, which is a mixed partial agonist of opioid μ-receptors.

Buprenorphine is used to treat opioid addiction in higher dosages to control moderate or acute pain in nonopioid-tolerant individuals. In lower-than-usual dosages, the drug can be used to control moderate chronic pain.

Buprenorphine can reach ceiling where higher doses do not result in increasing effect. The clinical advantage of this is that because it is a partial agonist, higher doses of buprenorphine can be given with fewer adverse effects (e.g., respiratory depression) than are seen with higher doses of full agonist opioids. Buprenorphine is more potent than morphine and precipitate withdrawal symptoms in opioid addicts.

The drug has high first-pass metabolism and is given by sublingual route, IV, or IM injection. When used as an analgesic, buprenorphine is usually given by injection or as a sublingual tablet. Transdermal patches are also available, where the doses are relatively low (compared with doses used in the treatment of opioid addiction). The typical analgesic dose of buprenorphine is 0.3 to 0.6 mg (IM or IV), and its analgesic effects last about 6 hours.

Both buprenorphine and methadone are used for detoxification of opioid addicts. Both are used for short- and long-term opioid substation therapy (OST). Buprenorphine has the advantage of being only a partial agonist; hence, negating the potential for life-threatening respiratory depression in cases of abuse is unlikely to occur. Moreover, the drug has a low-abuse potential of its own. Recent studies show the effectiveness of buprenorphine and methadone are almost identical, and they share adverse effect profiles as well, except more sedation with methadone. Comparative features of both methadone and buprenorphine are given in **Table 15.2**.

Sedative/Hypnotic Dependence

This type of dependence is very common in developing countries like India. It is difficult to detoxify patients with sedative/hypnotic dependence. During the withdrawal phase, seizure prophylaxis is important as a significant number may have seizures. Rebound anxiety needs to be treated as the dose is tapered. Doses of sedative-hypnotics used by the patient need to be tapered slowly on outpatient basis. The target is to reduce 10% of dose per week as too rapid tapering runs the risk of severe withdrawal leading to delirium/seizures, etc. Quick tapering may be done in the inpatients, which antiseizure medications cover. Consider valproic acid or diazepam for 30 days or more. Be aware that patients are likely to have seizure if stopped abruptly. Start valproic acid 250 mg three times daily, given for a minimum of 6 weeks. Selective serotonin reuptake inhibitors can be given if

concomitant anxiety and depression occur during withdrawal phase.

Cocaine Addiction

Cocaine is a plant-derived product that works as an indirectly acting sympathomimetic agent. This stimulates reticular activation system (**Fig. 15.5**).

The drug has a powerful reinforcement property and hence is a commonly abused drug.

Cocaine blocks dopamine, serotonin, and norepinephrine reuptake. The drug is also a weak monoamine oxidase (MAO) inhibitor.

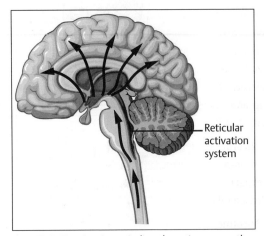

Fig. 15.5 Cocaine is an indirectly acting sympathomimetic drug that produces reinforcement and arousal. However, cocaine produces its addictive effects primarily by acting on the limbic system.

Table 15.2 Comparative profile of methadone and buprenorphine

Methadone	Buprenorphine
• Short-acting	• Long-acting
• Oral administration	• Sublingual administration
• Use limited	• Ease of use
• Tapering difficult	• Tapering easy
• Narrow safety margin	• Wider safety margin
• Respiratory depression in overdose reversed	• Respiratory depression in overdose partially reversed

Cocaine is mostly smoked. IV injection can be dangerous but produces intense euphoria among drug abusers. It is perceived as a "run of excitement." Motor and sexual activities increase and appetite decreases. Duration of action is short, and cocaine is metabolized in liver and plasma.

Apart from having euphoric property, the drug also has local anesthetic activity. It is used in ear, nose, and throat surgery. Earlier, the drug was used in eye surgeries too, where it has been replaced by lidocaine.

Nicotine Addiction

Nicotine addiction contributes to cardiovascular diseases, stroke, atherosclerosis, peptic ulcer disease, gastroesophageal reflux disease (GERD), diabetes, impotence, and cancers of lung, oral cavity, larynx, esophagus, kidney, bladder, pancreas, etc. As per one estimate, 65% of all men and 33% of all women use tobacco in some form in India.[5]

Nicotine is a major component of tobacco. Lot of gases like carbon monoxide, nitrosamines, hydrogen cyanide, and particulate matters are released when smoked.

Nicotine is a volatile liquid and is well-absorbed from the lungs. The drug is quite rapidly metabolized in liver and has a short half-life. That is why, once smoked, the smoker feels the urge to smoke again shortly thereafter.

When someone starts smoking, irritation of the airway may occur, leading to nausea and vomiting in the beginning. Soon thereafter, the psychomotor activity starts increasing and cognitive stimulation occurs. This may boost performance and confidence. On a biological level, there may be an increase in blood pressure, boosting of antidiuretic hormone activity, and increase in heart rate and GI secretions.

Nicotine soon becomes the need and psychological dependence becomes prominent. Tolerance develops quickly and at all levels like cellular and metabolic. Dopamine in nucleus accumbens increases, which provides a strong reinforcement and person becomes addicted.

Nicotine Withdrawal

Withdrawal from smoking may occur over weeks or months. Symptoms such as dizziness, tremors, increase in blood pressure, and craving occur. Anxiety, restlessness, concentration difficulty, headache, and sleep alterations also occur. GI upset and vomiting may happen as well.

Pharmacotherapy of Nicotine Addiction

Majority of smokers want to quit, but without assistance, a very small number is able to quit. Physicians can double the chances of people quitting by administering the following:

Varenicline: This is an agonist that binds and stimulates $\alpha_4\beta_2$ nicotinic acetylcholine receptors. The drug is started in dose of 0.5 mg daily for 1 to 3 days, then increased to twice daily for 1 to 4 days. Most common side effects are nausea and vivid dreams. Patients should be monitored for psychiatric symptoms. Varenicline is recommended for 12 weeks; may be repeated for 12 more.

Nicotine gums: Nicotine binds to CNS and peripheral nicotinic-cholinergic receptors. Available in 2 or 4 mg, the drug is started at weeks 1 to 6, one piece every 1 to 2 hours; then, weeks 7 to 9, one every piece 2 to 4 hours; finally, weeks 10 to 12, one every piece 4 to 8 hours. Common side effects are jaw pain and mouth soreness. Nicotine inhalers are also available. Common side effects are mouth and throat irritation and cough.

Nicotine patch: This is a transdermal patch, and the dose is decided based upon the number of

221

cigarettes smoked. For example, >25 cigarettes per day, 21 mg every 24 hours for 4 weeks; then, 14 mg for 2 weeks; finally, 7 mg for 2 weeks. Common side effects are skin irritation or sleep disturbances if worn at night.

Clonidine: Clonidine is a sympatholytic drug that stimulates α_2-adrenergic receptors (centrally acting antihypertensive) and reduces the sympathetic discharge. Nortriptyline inhibits norepinephrine and serotonin uptake and treats underlying depression.

Bupropion: This is a dopamine reuptake inhibitor and is given on the pretext that the drug treats underlying depression in smokers. The drug is given at a dose of 150 to 300 mg daily. Insomnia, nervousness, and concentration difficulties can occur as side effects.

Smoking in Pregnancy

Counseling is best choice as drugs may pose risks to the baby. Risks of premature birth or stillbirth caused by smoking may be higher than the potential risk of birth defects caused by nicotine replacement use. Bupropion and varenicline are both category C drugs (have some risks but acceptable).

Hallucinogens

Lysergic acid diethylamide (LSD), mescaline, and psilocybin are some of the many hallucinogens abused.

LSD is a synthetic chemical that can alter consciousness, increase sensory awareness, and can cause expansion of mind. Perceptual distortions are prominent.

LSD acts as agonist at 5-HT1A/1C receptors; stimulations can cause misjudgment and visual hallucinations. Cross-tolerance occurs with mescaline and psilocybin but dependence and withdrawal do not occur.

Phencyclidine is abbreviated as PCP and is commonly sold as angel dust. It has been replaced by ketamine as a general anesthetic agent. As a drug of abuse, it is taken either orally, snorted, or smoked. The drug acts as NMDA receptor blocker.

Low doses of hallucinogens can produce a sense of intoxication, and high doses can produce euphoria, hallucinations, isolation, and impaired judgment. Overdose can cause seizures, respiratory depression, cardiac arrest, and coma.

Pharmacotherapy

Treatment is generally supportive and involves maintenance of vital functions. Benzodiazepines or antipsychotics could be used.

Marijuana

Marijuana (cannabis) is heavily smoked drug in many countries. Its active component, tetrahydrocannabinol, acts via G-proteins and adenylyl cyclase. The drug exhibits pharmacological response by stimulating cannabinoid receptors (CB1).

Marijuana may be smoked or taken orally, and high doses can produce depersonalization. Increase in blood pressure, heart rate, and conjunctival injection also occur. Long-term effects are similar to cigarette smoking. Psychosis occurs and there can be an impairment of short-term memory.

Pharmacotherapy

IV fluids and benzodiazepines are given for acute treatment. Blood pressure may have to be controlled. Antipsychotics may be needed. Counseling for maladaptive behaviors will be done later.

Amphetamines

Amphetamines is a group of drugs like methylphenidate, which are not only used in the treatment of attention deficit hyperkinetic disorders but also abused.

IV injection can cause intense euphoria, increase in self-confidence, alertness, decreased sleep, hyperactivity, dangerous behavior, toxic psychosis, paranoid behaviors, and necrotizing arteritis.

Pharmacotherapy

Antipsychotics are needed. Airway, breathing, and circulation will have to be handled. Seizures and cardiac arrhythmia will need attention. Patients should be protected from physical harms.

Recent Advances in Deaddiction[12,13]

Disulfiram is the main drug in alcohol deaddiction along with naltrexone, acamprosate, nalmefene, and other drugs. Disulfiram has been proven to be effective in Indian settings as well. The Mental Healthcare Act, 2017 has recently been introduced with the objectives of providing mental health services and securing rights of persons with mental illnesses. Mental health conditions due to alcohol or drugs have been included in the definition of mental illnesses.

References

1. Addiction Pharmacotherapy. Available at: https://dgim.ucsf.edu/resources/sbirt. module4.ppt. Last accessed March 31, 2021
2. Clinical practice guidelines for treatment of alcohol dependence. Available at: www. indianjpsychiatry.org/cpg/cpg2006/cpg-mgmt_14.pdf. Last accessed March 31, 2021
3. PPT - National Institute on Drug Abuse. Available at: https://www.drugabuse.gov/ sites/default/files/addictionscience.ppt. Last accessed March 31, 2021
4. Chick J. Safety issues concerning the use of disulfiram in treating alcohol dependence. Drug Saf 1999;20(5):427–435 Review
5. Chaly PE. Tobacco control in India. Indian J Dent Res 2007;18(1):2–5
6. DePriest AZ, Puet BL, Holt AC, Roberts A, Cone EJ. Metabolism and disposition of prescription opioids: a review. Forensic Sci Rev 2015;27(2):115–145
7. Das JK, Salam RA, Arshad A, Finkelstein Y, Bhutta ZA. Interventions for adolescent substance abuse: an overview of systematic reviews. J Adolesc Health 2016;59(4S): S61–S75
8. Stockings E, Hall WD, Lynskey M, et al. Prevention, early intervention, harm reduction, and treatment of substance use in young people. Lancet Psychiatry 2016; 3(3):280–296
9. Drazdowski TK. A systematic review of the motivations for the non-medical use of prescription drugs in young adults. Drug Alcohol Depend 2016;162:3–25
10. Skinner MD, Lahmek P, Pham H, Aubin HJ. Disulfiram efficacy in the treatment of alcohol dependence: a meta-analysis. PLoS One 2014;9(2):e87366
11. Treatment improvement protocols in chapter-2; Incorporating alcohol pharma-cotherapies into medical practice. Available at: https://www.ncbi.nlm.nih.gov/books/ NBK64035/. Last accessed March 31, 2021
12. Available at: https://www.ncbi.nlm.nih.gov/ pmc/articles/PMC3056183/. Last accessed March 31, 2021
13. Available at: http://www.indianjpsychiatry. org/article.asp?issn=0019-5545;year=2019 ;volume=61;issue=10;spage=744;epage=7 49;aulast=Mohan. Last accessed March 31, 2021

Pharmacological Management of Attention-Deficit Hyperactivity Disorder

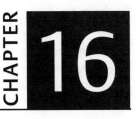

Vatsala Sharma and Vikas Dhikav

Introduction to Attention-Deficit Hyperactivity Disorder

Attention-deficit hyperactivity disorder (ADHD) places a significant impact on all domains of an individual's life, which hampers the overall functioning. In this chapter, the outline of ADHD, its pathophysiology, and treatment measures have been described.

ADHD is a neuropsychiatric condition affecting children, adolescents, and adults. It is characterized by diminished attention, hyperactivity, and increased impulsivity. The inattentive symptoms can be further divided into difficulty with selective attention, and difficulty with sustained attention and problem-solving. Problems with selective attention include making careless mistakes, paying little attention to detail, not listening, losing things, being distracted, and forgetting things. Difficulty with sustained attention comprises difficulty in finishing tasks, disorganization, and trouble sustaining mental effort.[1]

The prevalence of ADHD is more in boys compared to girls. About 60 to 85% of children diagnosed with ADHD continue to meet the diagnostic criteria in adolescence and up to 60% continue to exhibit symptoms in adulthood. However, these adults have fewer impulsive-hyperactive symptoms and mainly present with inattention.[2]

Diagnostic Criteria Changes in the Diagnostic and Statistical Manual of Mental Disorders, Fifth Edition (DSM-5)[2]

Following are the changes observed in the diagnostic criteria of ADHD as per DSM-5:

- Earlier, the symptoms had to be present by 7 years of age for making a diagnosis of ADHD. On the other hand, according to DSM-5, the "inattentive and hyperactive-impulsive symptoms" must be present by the age of 12 years.

- Earlier, two subtypes were present: Inattentive and hyperactive/impulsive type. DSM-5 has replaced it with the following three specifiers: Predominantly inattentive, predominantly hyperactive/impulsive, and combined presentation.

- According to DSM-5, a comorbid ADHD and autism spectrum diagnosis can be made.

- Rather than six, as per DSM-5, only five symptoms of either inattention or hyperactivity and impulsivity are sufficient for making the diagnosis.

Pathophysiology

Although multiple neurotransmitters are involved in the pathophysiology of ADHD, dopamine plays an important role. The prefrontal cortex of the brain has been implicated because of the high utilization of dopamine in this region. In addition to this, the prefrontal cortex has connections with other brain regions associated with attention, inhibition, decision-making, response inhibition, working memory, and vigilance.[2]

The most prominent symptom of inattention in ADHD, known as executive dysfunction, is linked to inefficient information processing in the dorsolateral prefrontal cortex (DLPFC).[1] **Table 16.1** depicts the ADHD features and the brain regions comprising the involved circuits.[1]

Locus ceruleus is made up of the noradrenergic neurons that play a role in attention. The noradrenergic system consists of the central (locus ceruleus) and peripheral components. Dysfunction of norepinephrine causes the hormone to accumulate peripherally, providing negative feedback to locus ceruleus.[2] So, the stimulants being the most effective treatment for ADHD affect both dopamine and epinephrine, supporting the neurotransmitter hypothesis.[2]

The imbalance in the dopamine and norepinephrine circuits in the prefrontal cortex causes inefficient information processing. Either too much or too little stimulation by dopamine or norepinephrine can cause ineffective processing, resulting in ADHD. For adequate functioning of

Table 16.1 Various ADHD symptoms and their corresponding brain regions

ADHD symptoms	Involved circuits
Difficulty with selective attention	DACC
Difficulty with sustained attention and problem solving	DLPFC
Hyperactivity	Prefrontal motor cortex
Impulsivity	OFC

Abbreviations: ADHD, attention-deficit hyperactivity disorder; DACC, dorsal anterior cingulate cortex; DLPFC, dorsolateral prefrontal cortex; OFC, orbitofrontal cortex.

the prefrontal cortex, the pyramidal neurons should be tuned through moderate stimulation of alpha-2A receptors by norepinephrine and D1 receptors by dopamine. The role of norepinephrine is to increase the incoming signal by promoting increased connectivity of the prefrontal network, and the role of dopamine is to decrease the noise by preventing inappropriate connections.[3]

Stress can activate norepinephrine and dopamine circuits in the prefrontal cortex, leading to an excess of phasic (bursts) firing. This causes impulsivity, inattention, and comorbidities associated with ADHD, like anxiety and substance use. So, this emphasizes on the fact that treatment of comorbid disorders is important to achieve favorable patient outcomes.[3]

Drugs for ADHD

Pharmacologic treatment is considered first-line for ADHD. Stimulants are preferred over nonstimulants due to greater efficacy and mild tolerable side effects.[4] In a study conducted to assess ADHD monotherapy, the alpha-2 agonists were found to be less efficacious as compared to psychostimulants.[5] According to a meta-analysis, both stimulants and nonstimulants were found to be effective for treating ADHD in adults, but stimulant medications showed greater efficacy for the short duration of treatment. No significant difference was observed between short- and long-acting stimulant medications.[6]

The stimulants include methylphenidate, dextroamphetamine, and dextroamphetamine–amphetamine salt combinations. Once a day, sustained release formulations are favored because of convenience and reduced rebound side effects. Nonstimulants used for ADHD include atomoxetine, alpha-adrenergic agonists (clonidine, guanfacine), and bupropion.[4] Stimulants are the first-line of treatment for children and adolescents, whereas nonstimulants like atomoxetine are prescribed as the first-line in adults with ADHD.[7]

In accordance with the pathophysiology discussed above, it is important to emphasize that to treat inattention, the release of norepinephrine and dopamine in the prefrontal cortex should be optimized. This principle is utilized for the treatment of ADHD by the stimulants and noradrenergic agents.[8]

Stimulant Medications

Methylphenidate and amphetamine are dopamine agonists but the precise mechanism of action of stimulants in ADHD is not known. Only the long-acting stimulants are FDA approved for the treatment of ADHD in adults. Here, the positive response is observed in the form of increased attention span, decreased impulsiveness, and improved mood.[4]

Dexmethylphenidate, dextroamphetamine, lisdexamfetamine, and dextroamphetamine/amphetamine salt combinations are the other stimulants. They have similar clinical benefits but the pharmacokinetic and pharmacodynamic profiles vary greatly in terms of methylphenidate.[9] Dextroamphetamine and dextroamphetamine/amphetamine salt combinations are the second drugs of choice when methylphenidate is ineffective.[4]

The stimulants may affect certain parameters like growth, vital signs, and cardiac functioning. It is advised to measure these values while starting treatment and monitoring periodically. The American Academy of Child and Adolescent Psychiatry (AACAP) practice parameters suggest the baseline record of physical examination, weight, height, pulse, and blood pressure before starting treatment with stimulants. It is also recommended that the patients on stimulants get their height, weight, and blood pressure checked on a quarterly basis and undergo a physical examination annually.[4] Due to the effect of stimulants on heart, all the stimulants are absolutely contraindicated in patients with preexisting cardiac conditions.[4] There is no universal requirement for baseline electrocardiogram (ECG), but the American Academy of Pediatrics and the American Heart Association recommend an ECG in children with a family history of heart disease or individual history of chest pain or dizziness.[9,10]

Methylphenidate

Methylphenidate is the first-line medication for ADHD. It exerts the action on both dopamine and norepinephrine transporters, increasing dopamine and norepinephrine in the prefrontal cortex.[11] Once-daily morning forms of methylphenidate are highly effective in school-going children. Some adverse effects are also noted in these children like headaches, stomach aches, nausea, and insomnia. Apart from this, the rebound effect is seen briefly when the medication wears off. It is characterized by slight hyperactivity and mild irritability.[4]

In children with motor tics, methylphenidate may cause exacerbation of the tics. In some children, tics may remain unchanged or may improve. When used over long periods, methylphenidate may cause growth suppression, if no drug holidays are given. During drug holidays on weekends or summers, the children tend to eat more and make up the growth.[4] However, based on a review article, the data regarding the effect of central nervous system (CNS) stimulants on growth were found to be variable, depending on the dose and duration of therapy.[9]

Insomnia is a major side effect of stimulants. In those patients who have responded to methylphenidate but have developed insomnia, a number of strategies can be adopted. These include the use of diphenhydramine (25–75 mg), low-dose trazodone (25–50 mg), or the addition of an alpha-adrenergic agents like guanfacine. In a few patients, insomnia disappears on its own after a few months of treatment.[4]

If adverse drug reactions occur (decreased appetite, headache), the isomeric formulation of methylphenidate and dexmethylphenidate should be considered. Even after this, if the side effects persist or if minimal benefit with stimulants is observed, nonstimulant therapy should be considered.[9]

The various available formulations of methylphenidate are as follows:

- *Immediate release*: Started for younger and smaller children (<16 kg) who are naive to stimulants. The dose is usually given twice daily about 4 hours apart (before school and at lunch time), and it can be administered up to three times daily.[4] Immediate-release preparations are available in regular and chewable forms.[8] Titration to maximum effective dose can occur quite quickly and the clinicians can titrate doses every 7 days. On titration to an appropriate dose, once-daily formulation can be considered.[4]
- *Sustained release*: Immediate-release formulation has some drawbacks. It may decrease adherence to medication due to stigma associated with multiple administrations per day, and there are adverse effects related to dosage peak. As the alternatives, sustained and extended release formulations overcome these shortcomings as well as have good efficacy and tolerability.[12]
- *Transdermal patch*: It is applied to the hip every day, typically for 9 hours. The patch should be applied in the morning, 2 hours before the desired time of effect, and removed after 9 hours. The drug's effect may continue for up to 2 to 3 hours after removing the patch. The patch may be

removed earlier than 9 hours if a shorter duration of effect is desired or if side effects develop. The patch is known to produce a rash and irritation at the application site. If irritation appears, a short course of topical corticosteroids should be used. If irritation persists, it should be changed to oral methylphenidate. Patch use should be discontinued in case leucoderma appears.[9]

The advantage of patch is that it can be used to deliver methylphenidate in children who cannot swallow the pills and can also individualize the number of hours a child is receiving medication. Apart from this, the transdermal patch has lower abuse potential and enhances adherence.[8]

Mechanism of action: Methylphenidate increases dopamine release in nucleus accumbens and dopamine along with norepinephrine in prefrontal cortex. It acts by inhibiting the reuptake through blocking the transporters, that is, dopamine active transporter (DAT) and norepinephrine transporter (NET). This causes increased synaptic availability of the neurotransmitters. The reuptake inhibition by methylphenidate is similar to that of antidepressants (selective serotonin reuptake inhibitors [SSRIs]). Unlike amphetamine, methylphenidate is not taken up into the dopamine or norepinephrine terminal by the vesicular monoamine transporter (VMAT).[8]

Amphetamine

Although amphetamine and its products are similar to methylphenidate in many ways, the amphetamine products have more potential for decreased appetite.[13] Lisdexamfetamine is the prodrug of amphetamine. It is in the combination with amino acid lysine, which gets cleaved in the stomach, releasing centrally active d-amphetamine.[8]

Mechanism of action: Amphetamine is a competitive inhibitor and acts as a pseudosubstrate.

It binds with the same site on the transporter, like of the monoamines (dopamine and norepinephrine), resulting in reuptake inhibition. At high doses, additional actions of amphetamine are observed, which makes the basis for addiction. Amphetamine is also a competitive inhibitor of VMAT. So, amphetamine is taken up in the dopamine terminal through DAT. Here, it is also transported into vesicles. At high doses, amphetamine causes displacement of dopamine from the vesicles into the terminal. This high level of dopamine on reaching a critical threshold produces two effects—massive dumping of dopamine in the synapse and reversal of DAT. The fast release of dopamine into the synapse contributes to the reinforcement, reward, euphoria, and continuing abuse.[8]

Nonstimulant Medications

Atomoxetine is a norepinephrine uptake inhibitor approved by the FDA for ADHD in children 6 years of age or older. It mediates selective inhibition of presynaptic norepinephrine transporter. It is effective for impulsivity and inattention in both children and adults. Alpha-adrenergic agonists are FDA approved for children and adolescents. The exact mechanism of action is unknown but alpha-adrenergic agonists are believed to act on the prefrontal cortex.[4]

Atomoxetine

Atomoxetine is a selective norepinephrine reuptake inhibitor (NRI) and is also called norepinephrine transporter (NET) inhibitor. It also has antidepressant action. Atomoxetine is well investigated and approved for use in children as well as adults.[8]

A black box warning was released for atomoxetine because of a potential increase in suicidal thoughts or behaviors. Therefore, the children taking this medication should be monitored for these symptoms.[4] The suicide risk is highest on starting the medication or making dose adjustments. Somnolence, dry mouth, nausea, constipation, and decreased appetite seen early in the treatment course tend to subside over time. Insomnia may also develop over time and can get worse with evening doses. Atomoxetine may cause mild tachycardia, hypertension, or orthostatic hypotension but has no impact on growth.[9]

Mechanism of action: The prefrontal cortex has a low number of DAT and dopamine is inactivated here by NET. Therefore, inhibiting NET results in an increase in dopamine as well as norepinephrine in the prefrontal cortex. Nucleus accumbens, on the other hand, has fewer NET and norepinephrine neurons; so, inhibiting NET does not increase norepinephrine or dopamine here. Therefore, atomoxetine has a selective action on prefrontal cortex, contributing to the lack of abuse potential.[8]

Ruboxetine, an antidepressant and selective NRI, has a similar mechanism of action. However, it is not approved in many countries for the treatment of ADHD.[8]

Alpha-Adrenergic Agonists

Alpha-2A receptors are widely distributed throughout the CNS and are the primary mediators of norepinephrine action. Alpha-2 adrenergic agonists used to treat ADHD are guanfacine and clonidine. These agents may put the patient at significant risk of rebound hypertension if discontinued suddenly. The extended-release versions are made available to overcome this life-threatening adverse effect. Additionally, the patients with ADHD exhibiting aggression may benefit from these medications, owing to the subtle sedative effect.[14]

The alpha-2 agonists may worsen depression and should be avoided in patients with preexisting depression. These agents can also cause hypotension and bradycardia. So, careful monitoring at fixed intervals is required.[9]

Mechanism of action: Guanfacine is more selective for alpha-2A receptors. Due to the side effects of guanfacine, only controlled release formulation is approved for ADHD treatment. Clonidine has an effect on alpha-2A, alpha-2B, and alpha-2C receptors. Apart from its action on alpha-2A receptors, the action of clonidine on other receptors is responsible for the vast side effect profile. Clonidine is approved for the use in hypertension but is not approved for ADHD. Clonidine, however, is used "off label" for ADHD in clinical practice.[8]

Compared to clonidine, guanfacine has a lower propensity for causing sedation and hypotension. At the same time, it has 25 times more potent action at the prefrontal cortex. So, guanfacine is more efficacious and has a lower side effect profile.[8]

Bupropion

Bupropion is a norepinephrine dopamine reuptake inhibitor (NDRI). In addition to DAT inhibition, it also has a weak NRI action, due to which some of the bupropion's pharmacological properties are similar to atomoxetine.[8]

Nonstandard Therapies

Modafinil, a CNS stimulant in a trial, was used to treat ADHD. Although compared to placebo (17% improved) significant improvement was noted in patients receiving modafinil (48% improved), it failed to receive FDA approval for ADHD treatment because of Stevens–Johnson skin rash that a patient had developed during the trial.[4] Venlafaxine has been used to treat ADHD with comorbid depression or anxiety. Controversies exist but no clear evidence is available to support the use of venlafaxine in the treatment of ADHD without comorbidities.[4]

Treatment of Comorbidities

The comorbid conditions and ADHD should be treated in the sequence, based on the degree of impairment. The condition causing the highest degree of impairment should be treated first. Apart from this, some medications used to treat ADHD may exacerbate the underlying comorbidity.[8] Therefore, a cautious individualized treatment plan should be adopted for each patient having ADHD with comorbidities.

ADHD, in absence of a comorbidity, is often not treated in adults. Since the comorbidity with ADHD is rare, it accounts for the reason that many of the patients with adult ADHD are not treated.[8] Adults with ADHD smoke almost equal to adults with schizophrenia. This may be due to the fact that smoking increases dopamine release, improves arousal, and appears to be effective for ADHD symptoms.[8]

Due to comorbid depression and anxiety, an SSRI is used with the stimulants. Tricyclics are not given to treat comorbid depression because of the risk of cardiac arrhythmias.[4] The stimulants used here may worsen anxiety. So, instead of stimulants, in these cases, it is advisable to administer an NRI or alpha-2A adrenergic agonist with an antidepressant.[8]

Antipsychotics are occasionally used to treat refractory severely hyperactive children and adolescents. Antipsychotics are not used generally in the treatment of ADHD due to the risk of tardive dyskinesia, withdrawal dyskinesia, weight gain, and neuroleptic malignant syndrome.[4] Another issue worth considering here is that atypical antipsychotics and CNS stimulants have opposite actions. So, the combination of these two agents is controversial. However, according to some clinician's expertise, these agents can be combined because atypical antipsychotics stimulate D1 receptors in the prefrontal cortex and block D2 receptors in the limbic areas.[8]

Therefore, it is appropriate to say that too much or too little dopamine and norepinephrine in different pathways can be difficult to manage. Treatment of ADHD symptoms (with impaired dopamine action in the cortex) with comorbidity (like tics with high-dopamine activity in the striatum) may make both deciding and implementing the treatment plan challenging for the clinician.[8]

Future Treatments for ADHD

Newer approaches for ADHD are also being targeted for cognitive symptoms of Alzheimer's disease, dementia, and schizophrenia. Several H_3 agonists are being tested to boost cognition in ADHD. Increasing acetylcholine function in the prefrontal cortex is another approach to treat cognitive symptoms associated with ADHD. Muscarinic agents are poorly tolerated; so, the emphasis is on the agents acting on cholinergic nicotinic receptors. Therefore, alpha-7–nicotinic receptor agonists are under investigation.[8]

Vortioxetine, a multifactorial antidepressant with 5-HT3 antagonist action and serotonin transporter (SERT) inhibition, also increases acetylcholine levels and is proposed as a procognitive agent for depression as well as ADHD. Varenicline, an alpha-4,beta-2–nicotinic receptor agonist, is also being tested for procognitive actions.[8]

Other agents being evaluated for their procognitive mechanisms in ADHD are as follows:

AMPAkines, 5-HT6 antagonists, and phosphodiesterase 4 (PDE_4) inhibitors.[8]

Conclusion

ADHD is characterized by inattention, impulsivity, and hyperactivity. It causes significant impairment of functioning in children, adolescents, and adults. However, adult ADHD may present with the only manifestation of inattention and is often undertreated in absence of a psychiatric comorbidity. The treatment of ADHD comprises stimulants and nonstimulants. Stimulants mainly include methylphenidate and amphetamine, whereas the nonstimulants are further divided into atomoxetine, alpha-2 adrenergic agonists, and bupropion. Some other agents like modafinil and venlafaxine are also being used. Additionally, a wide range of procognitive agents is under investigation to provide a new spectrum of treatment options for ADHD.

References

1. Stahl SM, Stahl SM. Stahl's essential psychopharmacology: neuroscientific basis and practical applications. American Psychiatric Association Publishing, USA; 2013 Apr 11:472

2. Attention deficit hyperactivity disorder. In: Benjamin JS, Virginia JS, eds. Kaplan and Sadock's Synopsis of Psychiatry: Behavioral Sciences/Clinical Psychiatry. Lippincott Williams & Wilkins; 2015:1169–1171

3. Stahl SM, Stahl SM. Stahl's essential psychopharmacology: neuroscientific basis and practical applications. American Psychiatric Association Publishing, USA; 2013 Apr 11: 475–480

4. Sadock BJ, Sadock VA. Attention deficit hyperactivity disorder. In: Benjamin JS, Virginia JS, eds. Kaplan and Sadock's Synopsis of Psychiatry: Behavioral Sciences/

Clinical Psychiatry. Lippincott Williams & Wilkins; 2015:1175–1179

5. Jain R, Segal S, Kollins SH, Khayrallah M. Clonidine extended-release tablets for pediatric patients with attention-deficit/hyperactivity disorder. J Am Acad Child Adolesc Psychiatry 2011;50(2):171–179

6. Faraone SV, Glatt SJ. A comparison of the efficacy of medications for adult attention-deficit/hyperactivity disorder using meta-analysis of effect sizes. J Clin Psychiatry 2010;71(6):754–763

7. Stahl SM, Stahl SM. Stahl's essential psychopharmacology: neuroscientific basis and practical applications. American Psychiatric Association Publishing, USA; 2013 Apr 11:484

8. Stahl SM, Stahl SM. Stahl's essential psychopharmacology: neuroscientific basis and practical applications. American Psychiatric Association Publishing, USA; 2013 Apr 11:487–501

9. Briars L, Todd T. A review of pharmacological management of attention-deficit/hyperactivity disorder. J Pediatr Pharmacol Ther 2016;21(3):192–206

10. Perrin JM, Friedman RA, Knilans TK; Black Box Working Group; Section on Cardiology and Cardiac Surgery. Cardiovascular monitoring and stimulant drugs for attention-deficit/hyperactivity disorder. Pediatrics 2008;122(2):451–453

11. Markowitz JS, Straughn AB, Patrick KS. Advances in the pharmacotherapy of attention-deficit-hyperactivity disorder: focus on methylphenidate formulations. Pharmacotherapy 2003;23(10):1281–1299

12. Cortese S, D'Acunto G, Konofal E, Masi G, Vitiello B. New formulations of methylphenidate for the treatment of attention-deficit/hyperactivity disorder: pharmacokinetics, efficacy, and tolerability. CNS Drugs 2017;31(2):149–160

13. Pelham WE, Aronoff HR, Midlam JK, et al. A comparison of ritalin and adderall: efficacy and time-course in children with attention-deficit/hyperactivity disorder. Pediatrics 1999;103(4):e43

14. Pringsheim T, Hirsch L, Gardner D, Gorman DA. The pharmacological management of oppositional behaviour, conduct problems, and aggression in children and adolescents with attention-deficit hyperactivity disorder, oppositional defiant disorder, and conduct disorder: a systematic review and meta-analysis. Part 1: psychostimulants, alpha-2 agonists, and atomoxetine. Can J Psychiatry 2015;60(2):42–51

Genetic Polymorphism in Neuropsychopharmacology

Vatsala Sharma and Vikas Dhikav

Introduction

Gene codes for enzymes provide the basis of genetic variations and the rate of metabolism by different enzymes. This principle is utilized by many specialties like neuropsychiatry for deciding the optimum treatment. Examples are emerging, which demonstrate that personalized treatment options are the way forward. The best predictor of response to psychopharmacology is either adverse drug reactions (ADRs) or past treatment response. Genetic polymorphism also depicts the severity of ADRs on an individual basis, further enhancing the requirement of personalized medicine. The importance of genetic polymorphism cannot be emphasized any further.

Pharmacokinetics is the study of the absorption, distribution, metabolization, and excretion of the drugs by the body. The cytochrome P450 (CYP) system in the liver and gut acts on the drugs, and the transformed partially active product in the blood is later excreted by kidneys. The CYP genotype variants in some patients can explain the adverse effect profile and inadequate treatment response. Pharmacodynamics, on the other hand, includes the therapeutic profile and side effects of the drugs.[1]

Types of Genetic Polymorphism

Hepatic and gut metabolizing systems are part of the CYP enzyme system, which metabolize drugs by absorption through the gut and further action in the liver. The liver detoxifies and facilitates the excretion of xenobiotics (foreign drugs or chemicals) by converting lipid-soluble compounds to water-soluble compounds with the help of enzymes. This drug metabolism occurs through phase I reactions, phase II reactions, or both. Oxidation is the most common phase I reaction catalyzed by the CYP system.[2] Enzymes in the endoplasmic reticulum of liver cells are mainly responsible for the CYP system. The enzyme complexes are also present in mitochondria, but their contribution to drug metabolism is minimal. Spectrophotometric peak depicts that the CYP system absorbs 450-nm wavelength from the spectrum of white light; hence, the name "CYP450."

There are several types of cytochrome systems, of which the following five are most important: CYP1A2, 2D6, 2C9, 2C19, and 3A4. These are classified on the basis of family, subtype, and gene product. For CYP1A2, 1 is the family, A denotes subtype (subfamily), and 2 represents gene product (isoform/individual enzyme). All the individuals do not have the same CYP enzymes; so, their enzymes are said to be polymorphic.[3] The genes that code for the enzymes of a particular cytochrome system vary from individual to another, further producing differences in each type of cytochrome system in the population. The cytochrome system is associated with two interrelated concepts—genetic polymorphisms of CYP and drug interactions. The knowledge of drug interactions is important for a clinician because these drug interactions can be life-threatening in the presence of genetic polymorphisms. With a brief note on drug interactions, the major emphasis of this chapter will be on genetic polymorphisms.

Mechanism of Genetic Polymorphism

The genes produce a phenotype that predicts variation in the metabolism of certain drugs. Individual alleles inherited from the parents pair up to produce this phenotype.[2] The genotype may comprise the following:

- *Two wild-type (functional) alleles*: Considered normal and occur in the general population. The individuals with this inheritance pattern have a normal rate of metabolization (called extensive metabolizers [EM]).
- *Two variant (defective) alleles*: Inheritance of this type has reduced or no activity (poor metabolizers [PM]).
- *One wild and other variant allele*: Produce decreased enzymatic activity (intermediate metabolizers [IM]).
- *More than two wild type alleles*: Result in greater than normal enzymatic activity (ultrarapid metabolizers [UM]).[4]

These genetic mutations cause changes in enzymes through splicing defects, amino acid substitutions, and gene deletions. Unstable enzymes are produced, contributing to altered enzyme activity.[4]

Process of Pharmacogenetic Profile Testing for Polymorphism

To elaborate on the pharmacogenetic testing in clinical practice, it is important to know the concept of single nucleotide polymorphism (SNP). Every individual has two copies of a gene, which are called alleles. Copies of a specific gene

in a population may not have identical nucleotide sequences. The single nucleotide changes, also called SNPs, are the basis for diversity. SNPs occur at every 300 to 2,000 base pairs along the genome.[5] The majority of SNPs are functionally silent but some of the SNPs lead to altered protein structure or expression, producing faulty enzymes. SNP-based "genetic profile" is a "fingerprint" for determining the susceptibility of an individual to various diseases and response to drugs.[6]

To test the pharmacogenetic profile of an individual, an oral swab is obtained for DNA samples. An assay with a technique called real-time polymerase chain reaction (PCR) is performed on the samples. SNPs are tested for each patient sample. The technique tests for the presence of specific gene variants linked with a particular symptomatic profile and response to medications.[7]

Clinical Relevance

Genetic polymorphism can lead to some unexpected treatment outcomes. Intermediate and poor metabolizers are at an increased risk of toxicity and adverse effects due to drug accumulation. These patients have hypersensitivity or low tolerance to some drugs and may require reduced doses or complete avoidance of these drugs.[2]

Due to genetic polymorphism, 5 to 10% of Caucasians have inadequate CYP2D6 action, and 20% Asians have low CYP2C19 activity, contributing to less effective means of drug metabolization and elevated blood levels. This indicates the need for a lower dose of some medications for these individuals.[8] Similarly, considering the example of antipsychotics, Asians require a lower dose compared to other races due to the lower activity level of CYP450 2D6 and higher drug levels in the blood and brain.

On the other hand, some individuals may inherit the CYP enzyme that is extremely active, contributing to a lower blood level and need for higher doses of some drugs. Therefore, genes for these CYP enzymes can condition higher or lower dose adjustments of a drug to produce an adequate response with minimal adverse effects.[8] This forms the basis of personalized medicine.

Adverse Drug Reactions

The drugs that share the common pathway of metabolism are likely to have drug–drug interactions. Alteration in the activity of CYP enzymes and certain drug–drug interactions are noteworthy in neuropsychiatry. Some are as follows (**Table 17.1**):

- CYP1A2 inhibitors like fluvoxamine and ciprofloxacin when administered with clozapine/theophylline increase the risk of seizures.
- Contrary to this, smoking acts as an inducer of CYP1A2 action, and therefore, the patients on antipsychotics may relapse when they start smoking.
- Combining powerful CYP3A4 inhibitors like ketoconazole, protease inhibitors, or erythromycin when administering 3A4 substrate pimozole can result in higher plasma pimozole levels, causing QTc prolongation and arrhythmias.

Table 17.1 Drug interactions[9]

CYP1A2	
Substrate	**Inhibitor**
- Theophylline - Duloxetine - Clozapine - Olanzapine - Zotepine - Asenapine - TCAD - Agomelatine	- Fluvoxamine Ciprofloxacin
CYP2D6	
Substrate	**Inhibitor**
- TCAD -Thioridazine - Codeine - Atomoxetine - Venlafaxine - Duloxetine -Paroxetine - Clozapine - Risperidone - Olanzapine - Aripiprazole - Iloperidone	- Paroxetine - Fluoxetine - Duloxetine - Bupropion - Quinidine - Ritonavir
CYP3A4	
Substrate	**Inhibitor**
- Pimozide - Alprazolam - Triazolam - Buspirone - HMG-CoA reductase inhibitors (statins) - Clozapine - Quetiapine - Sertindole - Aripiprazole - Zotepine - Lurasidone - Iloperidone	- Fluvoxamine - Fluoxetine - Ketoconazole - Protease inhibitors - Erythromycin - Verapamil - Diltiazem
	Inducer
-	-Carbamazepine -Rifampin

Abbreviation: TCAD, tricyclic antidepressant.

- CYP3A4 inhibitors when combined with alprazolam or triazolam can cause sedation.
- CYP3A4 inhibitors when combined with statins (except pravastatin or fluvastatin) can increase the risk of muscle damage and rhabdomyolysis.

New drug interactions mediated by CYP enzymes are being found every day. Clinicians practicing polypharmacy should be aware of the various drug interactions to prevent future mishaps.

Adverse Reactions due to Polymorphism

- Patients with CYP2D6 genetic polymorphism (PM) may have metoclopramide-induced acute dystonia.[10]
- Increased CYP2D6 activity causes increased conversion of codeine to the active metabolite, morphine. This may result in serious morphine toxicity even with small doses of codeine. It was illustrated by a case report in which the baby suffered from fatal morphine toxicity when her mother was prescribed codeine while breastfeeding. Later, it was found that the mother had an extra copy of the wild-type CYP2D6 gene. Respiratory depression can also occur after a small codeine dose in such UM.[11,12]
- Tramadol is metabolized by CYP 2D6 to O-desmethyl tramadol, which is the active product. CYP2D6 UM can develop postoperative respiratory depression while receiving tramadol intravenously (IV).[13] These UM have better pain control than EM but also have a higher frequency of nausea.[14]
- Methadone causes fatal poisonings at concentrations between 0.4 and 1.8 mg/mL. In some cases, methadone can cause death at much lower concentrations. It is associated with CYP2B6 genetic variation.[15]
- Phenytoin toxicity (mental confusion, slurred speech, memory loss, and inability

to stand) can occur in patients homozygous for the allele CYP2C9*6.[16]

Therapeutic Decision-Making through Genetic Testing

As already mentioned, genetic markers help in finding out the likelihood of treatment response and adverse effect profile. It has an additive benefit of cutting down the cost of treatment. Although after considering the patient's complete profile, these factors help the clinician in selecting the best treatment option, it cannot predict a specific drug that should be prescribed to an individual. A few examples are as follows:

- CYP2D6 converts venlafaxine to its active metabolite, desvenlafaxine. As compared to venlafaxine, desvenlafaxine has greater norepinephrine transporter (NET) inhibition. There can be two reasons for lesser conversion to the active metabolite, desvenlafaxine. If the patient is taking a CYP2D6 inhibitor with venlafaxine, there is less conversion to the active form. Also, if the patient has CYP2D6 genetic polymorphism, there will be less desvenlafaxine production, causing lower NET inhibition. Therefore, the extent of NET inhibition is unpredictable for venlafaxine, but it is relatively consistent for desvenlafaxine at a given dose. Desvenlafaxine is beneficial in this context, requiring lesser titration.[17]
- SLC 6A4 variation is the genetic variation that affects serotonin transporter (SERT) protein formation and facilitates serotonin reuptake. This variation is responsible for poor response and tolerability to selective serotonin reuptake inhibitor (SSRI)/ selective norepinephrine reuptake inhibitor (SNRI).[18]
- 5-HT2C variation affects 5-HT2C receptor synthesis and regulates dopamine and norepinephrine release. DRD2 variation

235

affects D2 receptors. It mediates positive symptoms of psychosis and movement in Parkinsonism. The therapeutic application of both of these variations is the poor tolerability and response to atypical antipsychotics.[18]

- Catechol-O-Methyltransferase (COMT) Val variation influences COMT enzyme. It regulates dopamine levels in the pre-frontal cortex and metabolizes dopamine and norepinephrine. MTHFR T variation is responsible for the regulation of L-methylfolate levels and methylation. Both of these genetic variations are responsible for reduced executive functioning.[18]

- COMT polymorphism, associated with the rapid metabolism of dopamine in the brain (UM), exacerbates the negative symptoms of schizophrenia due to low dopamine levels in the mesocortex. Amantadine, a dopamine agonist, was tried in a study which resulted in rapid short-term clinical improvement in such patients.[7]

- In patients with COMT polymorphism in schizophrenia, there is a gender variation noted. In women, COMT is required for the degradation of catechol estrogens and dopamine. The low COMT activity results in hyperdopaminergic and hypercatechol estrogens states that may be involved in the pathogenesis of a psychiatric disorder. Apart from this, estrogen has also been observed to inhibit COMT gene transcription.[19,20] So, while prescribing medications to patients with COMT polymorphism, the dose should be modified based on gender.

Other Pharmacogenomic Biomarkers

Multiple genetic determinants for detecting the development of psychiatric illness and ADRs have been studied. *CRHR1* polymorphism

haplotypes are associated with major depressive disorder, and if coupled with childhood trauma, they increase the risk of depression.[21] The dexamethasone-binding capacity of leukocytes can be used as a biomarker. It is a proxy measure for glucocorticoid receptor number, which might help screen persons likely to develop post-traumatic stress disorder (PTSD). This is based on a study involving the military personnel returning from deployment, where greater glucocorticoid receptor density was found to be predictive of the risk for PTSD symptoms.[22] The toxicity of drugs can also be predicted by variant human leukocyte antigen (HLA) class I and II alleles. It has been found that there is a strong association between HLA-B*1502 and Stevens–Johnson syndrome induced by carbamazepine.[23]

Future Directions

Even with the known impact of genotype on pharmacokinetics, there is still some controversy on whether adjustment of dosage based on genetic information can improve therapeutic efficacy and prevent adverse events to an extent of importance in clinical practice.[24] To overcome this issue, research should be encouraged to observe the long-term impact of genetic polymorphisms on treatment decisions. Further studies should also be promoted to assess the risk-benefit ratio of the clinician's dependence on the genetic profile of individuals for making therapeutic choices.

The field of pharmacogenomics in neuro-psychiatry is still at the stage of infancy but has a promising future in the form of personalized medicine. The greatest progress can be expected at the intersections of the gene-environment and genes-biomarkers categories.[25] The psychiatric disease is not due to a single gene abnormality but is due to disturbances in complex intracellular networks in the brain. To improve the diagnosis and treatment of psychiatric illness, we need to integrate the use of pharmacogenetics along with electroencephalography (EEG), magneto-encephalography (MEG), functional magnetic resonance imaging (fMRI), and diffusion tensor imaging (DTI). Drugs need to be used to target a neural network rather than its components.[26]

In addition to this, in the coming time, individuals will likely have the complete genome entered as part of the their medical record,[26] which will unfold a whole new array of diagnostic and therapeutic possibilities.

Conclusion

CYP system is complex and plays a vital role in drug metabolization and interactions. The genetic polymorphism of this CYP system can cause multiple unpredicted drug responses. The clinicians should have adequate knowledge of drugs metabolized by the common pathways to prevent this. In addition, further research across the domains of CYP systems should be promoted to expand the horizon of personalized medicine.

References

1. Stahl SM, Stahl SM. Stahl's essential psycho-pharmacology: neuroscientific basis and practical applications. American Psychiatric Association Publishing, USA; 2013:46–47

2. McDonnell AM, Dang CH. Basic review of the cytochrome p450 system. J Adv Pract Oncol 2013;4(4):263–268

3. Stahl SM, Stahl SM. Stahl's essential psycho-pharmacology: neuroscientific basis and practical applications. American Psychiatric Association Publishing, USA; 2013:47–48

4. Johansson I, Ingelman-Sundberg M. Genetic polymorphism and toxicology—with emphasis on cytochrome p450. Toxicol Sci 2011;120(1):1–13

5. Lindpaintner K. Genetics in drug discovery and development: challenge and promise of individualizing treatment in common complex diseases. Br Med Bull 1999;55(2): 471–491

6. Alwi ZB. The use of SNPs in pharmaco-genomics studies. Malays J Med Sci 2005; 12(2):4–12

7. Patel P, Sharma V, Khan T, et al. The genomics of dopamine agonists treatment of schizophrenia: a case of homozygous valine catechol-o-methyltransferase poly-morphism. J Psychol Clin Psychiatry. 2020; 11(2):66–70

8. Stahl SM, Stahl SM. Stahl's essential psycho-pharmacology: neuroscientific basis and practical applications. American Psychiatric Association Publishing, USA; 2013:47

9. Stahl SM, Stahl SM. Stahl's essential psycho-pharmacology: neuroscientific basis and practical applications. American Psychiatric Association Publishing, USA; 2013:47–51

10. van der Padt A, van Schaik RH, Sonneveld P. Acute dystonic reaction to metoclopramide in patients carrying homozygous cyto-chrome P450 2D6 genetic polymorphisms. Neth J Med 2006;64(5):160–162

11. Madadi P, Koren G, Cairns J, et al. Safety of codeine during breastfeeding: fatal mor-phine poisoning in the breastfed neonate of a mother prescribed codeine. Can Fam Physician 2007;53(1):33–35

12. Gasche Y, Daali Y, Fathi M, et al. Codeine intoxication associated with ultrarapid CYP2D6 metabolism. N Engl J Med 2004; 351(27): 2827–2831

13. Stamer UM, Stüber F, Muders T, Musshoff F. Respiratory depression with tramadol in a patient with renal impairment and CYP2D6 gene duplication. Anesth Analg 2008; 107(3):926–929

14. Kirchheiner J, Keulen JT, Bauer S, Roots I, Brockmöller J. Effects of the CYP2D6 gene duplication on the pharmacokinetics and pharmacodynamics of tramadol. J Clin Psychopharmacol 2008;28(1):78–83

15. Bunten H, Liang WJ, Pounder DJ, Seneviratne C, Osselton D. OPRM1 and CYP2B6 gene variants as risk factors in methadone-related

deaths. Clin Pharmacol Ther 2010;88(3): 383–389

16. Kidd RS, Curry TB, Gallagher S, Edeki T, Blaisdell J, Goldstein JA. Identification of a null allele of CYP2C9 in an African-American exhibiting toxicity to phenytoin. Pharmacogenetics 2001;11(9):803–808

17. Stahl SM, Stahl SM. Stahl's essential psycho-pharmacology: neuroscientific basis and practical applications. American Psychiatric Association Publishing, USA; 2013:307

18. Stahl SM, Stahl SM. Stahl's essential psycho-pharmacology: neuroscientific basis and practical applications. American Psychiatric Association Publishing, USA; 2013:362

19. Xie T, Ho SL, Ramsden D. Characterization and implications of estrogenic down-regulation of human catechol-O-methyltransferase gene transcription. Mol Pharmacol 1999; 56(1):31–38

20. Hosák L. Role of the COMT gene Val158Met polymorphism in mental disorders: a review. Eur Psychiatry 2007;22(5):276–281

21. Bradley RG, Binder EB, Epstein MP, et al. Influence of child abuse on adult depression:

moderation by the corticotropin-releasing hormone receptor gene. Arch Gen Psychiatry 2008;65(2):190–200

22. van Zuiden M, Geuze E, Willemen HL, et al. Pre-existing high glucocorticoid receptor number predicting development of post-traumatic stress symptoms after military deployment. Am J Psychiatry 2011;168(1): 89–96

23. Chung WH, Hung SI, Hong HS, et al. Medical genetics: a marker for Stevens-Johnson syndrome. Nature 2004;428(6982):486

24. Kirchheiner J, Seeringer A, Viviani R. Pharmacogenetics in psychiatry—a useful clinical tool or wishful thinking for the future? Curr Pharm Des 2010;16(2):136–144

25. Ozomaro U, Wahlestedt C, Nemeroff CB. Personalized medicine in psychiatry: problems and promises. BMC Med 2013; 11(1):132

26. Stahl SM, Stahl SM. Stahl's essential psycho-pharmacology: neuroscientific basis and practical applications. American Psychiatric Association Publishing, USA; 2013:361

Cognitive Enhancers

Vikas Dhikav and Rhythm Joshi

Introduction

Cognitive enhancers are the most commonly used drugs in cognitive neurology. A cognitive enhancer is a "drug that is aimed at enhancing individual's cognitive abilities." The increase should be done in a meaningful and sustained manner so as to add clinically meaningful increase in cognitive abilities.[1]

Learning and Memory[2]

It is important to review memory and its mechanisms before discussing the details of cognitive enhancers. Important points of consideration are as follows:

- Implicit memory is known as reflexive memory and involves memories like riding a bicycle, swimming, driving, painting, etc. The information is stored and recalled at a subconscious level and conscious effort is not needed.
- Explicit memory is memory of facts, figures, etc., which needs active recall mechanisms. These include names, date of birth, anniversary dates, dates of buying cars, house, etc.

It is important to know that once habituation and sensitization occurs, then explicit memory gets converted into implicit memory and gets recalled without any voluntary effort.[3]

Neural Substrates of Learning and Memory

- Hippocampus is the neural substrate of learning and memory. It is responsible for encoding new memories. This is a hockey-shaped structure in the brain.
- Frontal lobe is the "library" of the brain which is needed for information storage and retrieval. Strito-frontal cortex is needed for decision-making and is located deep in the frontal lobe.

Memory Storage in the Brain[4]

- **Short-term memory:**
  ◊ Lasts for few seconds to few minutes, for example, watching a picture while driving down, recalling names of people whom we met a few seconds or minutes back, etc.
- **Long-term memory:**
  ◊ This is a memory that is stored for years, for example, birthdays, schooling, marriage, etc., and can be recalled at will. It is resistant to degradation, even in advanced neurodegenerative diseases.
  ◊ Storage of memory involves mitogen-activated protein kinases, cAMP response binding elements, which eventually lead to changes in synapse structure and function. This is what

perhaps which makes this memory resistant to changes.

General Mechanisms of Action of Cognitive Enhancers[5,6]

Cognitive enhancers act by increasing blood flow to the brain and hence improve oxygen delivery. Also, increase in glucose utilization and facilitation of information exchange between cerebral cortexes results in better communication between brain parts. Increase in nerve growth factors is an additional result. Enhancement of cerebral metabolism is an overall gain, resulting in improvement in memory. **Table 18.1** gives details of mechanisms of cognitive enhancers.

Commonly Used Cognitive Enhancers in Clinical Practice[5]

Racetams

Since racetams are a major group of drugs used as cognitive enhancers, the same is being reviewed here first. These include the following:

- Piracetam.
- Aniracetam.
- Oxiracetam.
- Pramiracetam.
- Phenylpiracetam.
- Nefiracetam.
- Coluracetam.

Piracetam

Piracetam is a gamma-aminobutyric acid (GABA)-ergic drug that acts by restoring membrane fluidity. The drug has neuroprotective and anticonvulsant properties apart from being a cognitive enhancer. The drug affects neuronal plasticity. The drug is well-tolerated in treatment of cognitive disorders (e.g., dementia) and is also useful in vertigo, central myoclonus, dyslexia, and sickle cell anemia.[7]

The drug acts by increasing acetylcholine levels in the brain. Piracetam also engages in activities via NMDA and AMPA receptors. These and many more mechanisms lead to increase in membrane permeability, resulting in better neuronal functions.

Aniracetam

This is a structural analogue of piracetam and is more potent. Activation of AMPA receptors leads to better neural functions (learning and memory enhancement). The drug affects 5-HT2A, D2, and D3 receptors. The drug possesses antianxiety and antidepressant potential.

Alpha-GPC

Alpha-GPC is available in human brain and breast milk and results in higher intelligence quotients (IQs) of babies who are breastfed in comparison to being formula fed. The drug readily crosses the blood–brain barrier (BBB).

Table 18.1 Classification of cognitive enhancers

Drug	Mechanism
Piracetam	Cognitive metabolic enhancer; miscellaneous mechanisms
Neuropeptide	Various molecular mechanisms mediated by G-proteins
Cholinergic drugs	Stimulating muscarinic and nicotinic receptors
AMPAkinase	AMPA glutamate receptor activators: • Sunifiram • Unifiram
Natural nootropics	Ginkgo biloba, Panax ginseng, Bacopa monnieri, Rhodiola rosea

Citicoline

Citicoline is an intermediary in the conversion of choline to phosphatidylcholine in liver. It increases the availability of choline in the brain. Citicoline has a useful function in the brain by preserving cardiolipin and sphingomyelin. The drug decreases phospholipase stimulation. The drug is used in head trauma and stroke. It has also been used in an empirical manner in neurodegenerative diseases like Alzheimer's disease and dementia.

Ginkgo Biloba

This is one of the oldest tree species in the world and is spread across China, Japan, and Korea. People eat its leaves for nutrition or supplementation. The drug is supposed to be neuroprotective and also acts as an antioxidant.

Ginseng

Ginseng is a traditional Chinese herbal medicine which is used in cognitive dysfunction in a generic manner in some cultures. The drug is believed to act as a memory enhancer.

Bacopa Monnieri

Bacopa is a traditional Ayurvedic herbal formulation used for centuries, acting as a holistic drug.

The drug is used for Alzheimer's disease, epilepsy, and insomnia.

References

1. Nootropics. Available at: https://www.slideshare.net/ChaithanyaMalalur/cognitive-enhancers-nootropics. Accessed November 21, 2020
2. Best natural nootropics. Available at: https://exoprotein.com/blogs/nutrition/4-best-natural-nootropics. Accessed November 21, 2020
3. Learning and memory. Available at: https://www.apa.org/topics/learning. Accessed November 21, 2020
4. Learning and memory. Available at: https://www.ncbi.nlm.nih.gov/pmc/articles/PMC4248571/. Accessed November 21, 2020
5. Cognitive enhancers. Available at: https://www.webmd.com/vitamins-and-supplements/features/nootropics-smart-drugs-overview#1. Accessed November 21, 2020
6. Cognition enhancing drugs. ncbi.nlm.nih.gov/pmc/articles/PMC2690227/. Accessed November 21, 2020
7. Pharmacology of piracetam. Available at: https://.ncbi.nlm.nih.gov/16007238/. Accessed November 21, 2020

Index